The Epilepsy Prescriber's Guide to Antiepileptic Drugs

Third Edition

The Epilepsy Prescriber's Guide to Antiepileptic Drugs

Third Edition

Philip N. Patsalos
FRCPath, PhD
Professor of Clinical Pharmacology and Consultant Clinical Pharmacologist,
UCL Institute of Neurology,
The National Hospital for Neurology and Neurosurgery,
London, and the Epilepsy Society,
Chalfont St. Peter,
UK

Erik K. St. Louis
MD, MS
Associate Professor of Neurology,
Department of Neurology,
Mayo Clinic College of Medicine,
Rochester, MN, USA

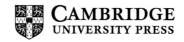

CAMBRIDGE
UNIVERSITY PRESS

University Printing House, Cambridge CB2 8BS, United Kingdom

One Liberty Plaza, 20th Floor, New York, NY 10006, USA

477 Williamstown Road, Port Melbourne, VIC 3207, Australia

314–321, 3rd Floor, Plot 3, Splendor Forum, Jasola District Centre,
New Delhi – 110025, India

79 Anson Road, #06-04/06, Singapore 079906

Cambridge University Press is part of the University of Cambridge.

It furthers the University's mission by disseminating knowledge in the pursuit of
education, learning and research at the highest international levels of excellence.

www.cambridge.org
Information on this title: www.cambridge.org/9781108453202
DOI: 10.1017/9781108669399

First edition (2010) and second edition (2014) © P. N. Patsalos and B. F. D. Bourgeois
Third edition © Philip N. Patsalos and Erik K. St. Louis

This edition published 2018

A catalogue record for this publication is available from the British Library

Library of Congress Cataloging in Publication data
Names: Patsalos, P. N. (Philip N.), author. | St. Louis, Erik K., 1965– author.
Title: The epilepsy prescriber's guide to antiepileptic drugs /
Philip N. Patsalos, Erik K. St. Louis.
Description: Third edition. | Cambridge, United Kingdom; New York, N.Y.:
Cambridge University Press, 2018. |
Includes bibliographical references and index.
Identifiers: LCCN 2018000038 | ISBN 9781108453202 (hardback)
Subjects: | MESH: Anticonvulsants | Epilepsy – drug therapy | Handbooks
Classification: LCC RM322 | NLM QV 39 | DDC 616.8/53061–dc23
LC record available at https://lccn.loc.gov/2018000038

ISBN 978-1-108-45320-2 Paperback

CONTENTS

CONTENTS

PREFACE

The purpose of the first and second edition of *The Epilepsy Prescriber's Guide to Antiepileptic Drugs* was to help those involved in the treatment of patients with epilepsy to meet the challenge of having easy access to all relevant aspects of every antiepileptic medication currently available, including the newest ones. The *Prescriber's Guide* has been very well received, and the feedback indicates that the stated goal was met at the time. Four years on from the second edition, the authors now recognize the need for a new edition in order to continue to keep up with the original goal. Up-to-date new information has been added accordingly, with no change in the easy-to-use format.

One section has been added to the book in order to cover the new drug that has become available in the meantime, brivaracetam, and another (retigabine/ezigabine) has been deleted because it has been withdrawn from the market. All sections on pharmacokinetic interactions, as well as the table at the end of the book summarizing all known pharmacokinetic interactions between antiepileptic drugs, have been extensively updated, and they represent a most comprehensive and up-to-date source of information on pharmacokinetic interactions involving antiepileptic drugs. Suggested pediatric dosage schedules have been added for several drugs. Additional adverse effects, as well as recommended precautions and monitoring, were added where applicable. The issue of bone health, as well as vitamin D monitoring and supplementation, was addressed for selected drugs, and uses in special populations have been updated where relevant. Information on teratogenicity reported in recent publications and pregnancy registries was incorporated in the sections on pregnancy. Finally, for these multiple upgrades, the relevant references were added to the list of suggested reading.

INTRODUCTION

The purpose of *The Epilepsy Prescriber's Guide to Antiepileptic Drugs* (AEDs) is to provide practical and concise information so as to allow the optimum use of AEDs in clinical practice. This quick reference guide provides a wealth of invaluable information for use by all who treat patients with epilepsy, including neurologists, neurosurgeons, general physicians, those caring for the elderly, emergency medicine doctors, medical students and trainees at all levels, general practitioners, nurses and epilepsy nurse specialists, and practice pharmacists.

All of the drugs are presented in the same design format and in alphabetical order to facilitate rapid access to information. Specifically, each drug is divided into eight sections and each section is designated by a unique color background: therapeutics, pharmacokinetics, drug interaction profile, adverse effects, dosing and use, special populations, and the overall place of the drug in the treatment of epilepsy, followed by suggested reading of key references.

Section 1: Therapeutics
This section covers the chemical name and structure; brand names in major countries; generics available; licensed indications as approved by the US Food and Drug Administration (FDA) and the European Medicines Agency or the United Kingdom Medicines and Healthcare products Regulatory Agency; non-licensed use; seizure types for which the drug is ineffective or contraindicated; mechanism of action; and efficacy profile.

Section 2: Pharmacokinetics
The second section highlights the pharmacokinetic parameters relevant to each drug's clinical therapeutics and includes absorption and distribution, metabolism, and elimination parameters.

Section 3: Drug Interaction Profile
The interaction profile of each drug is divided into three major sections which include pharmacokinetic interactions, pharmacodynamic interactions, and interaction with hormonal contraception. The pharmacokinetic interaction section is further subdivided into interactions between AEDs and interactions between AEDs and non-AED drugs. Non-interacting drugs have been omitted.

Section 4: Adverse Effects
This section explains how the drug causes adverse effects and contains a list of common, life-threatening, or dangerous adverse effects; an effect on weight is noted, and advice given on what to do about adverse effects.

Section 5: Dosing and Use
This section provides the usual dosing range; available formulations; how to dose and dosing tips; how to withdraw drug; symptoms of overdose and how to manage; what tests and therapeutic drug monitoring are needed; other warnings and precautions; and when not to use.

Section 6: Special Populations
The sixth section gives information about use of the drugs in the presence of renal and hepatic impairments, and any precautions to be taken for treating children, the elderly, and pregnant and breast-feeding women.

Section 7: The Overall Place of the Drug in the Treatment of Epilepsy
This section provides an overview, based on the authors' opinions, as to where each AED can be placed in relation to the treatment of patients with epilepsy and summarizes the primary and secondary seizure types for which it shows efficacy. Finally it highlights the potential advantages and disadvantages of each AED.

Section 8: Suggested Reading
In this section, the authors highlight the key references that were used in compiling the information contained in each drug section and readers are advised to read these if more information is needed. Readers are also encouraged to consult standard comprehensive reference books on epilepsy and AED textbooks for more in-depth information. At the back of the guide is an index by drug name. In addition, there is a list of abbreviations and a table highlighting the interactions that can occur between the different AEDs.

ACETAZOLAMIDE

A

Therapeutics

Chemical Name and Structure

Acetazolamide, N-(5-(aminosulfonyl)-1,3,4-thiadiazol-2-yl)-acetamide, is a white to faintly yellowish-white odorless crystalline powder with a molecular weight of 222.25.

Although a sulfonamide compound, it is unlike sulfonamide antibiotic compounds. It does not contain an arylamine group at the N4 position, which contributes to allergic reactions associated with sulfonamide antibiotics. The structure of acetazolamide bears some similarity to that of zonisamide. Its empirical formula is $C_4H_6N4O_3S_2$.

Brand Names

* Acetadiazol; Acetak; Albox; Apo-Acetazolamide; Azol
* Carbinib; Cetamid
* Diamox; Diamox Sequals; Diamox Sustets; Diluran; Diural; Diuramid
* Evamox
* Fonurit
* Glaupax
* Huma-Zolamide
* Ledamox; Lediamox
* Medene
* Optamide
* Renamid
* Stazol; Synomax
* Uramox
* Zolmide

Generics Available

* Yes

Licensed Indications for Epilepsy

* Adjunctive treatment of generalized tonic–clonic and partial seizures (United Kingdom Summary of Product Characteristics (UK SPC))
* Adjunctive treatment of atypical absences, atonic, and tonic seizures (UK SPC)

Licensed Indications for Non-epilepsy Conditions

* Adjunctive treatment of glaucoma (UK SPC; FDA PI)

THERAPEUTICS

1

A

ACETAZOLAMIDE

- Prevention or amelioration of symptoms associated with acute mountain sickness (FDA PI)
- Treatment of abnormal retention of fluid: congestive heart failure, drug-induced edema (UK SPC)

Non-licensed Use for Epilepsy
- Catamenial seizures
- Continuous spike and wave in slow-wave sleep
- Landau–Kleffner syndrome
- Lennox–Gastaut syndrome

Non-licensed Use for Non-epilepsy Conditions
- Idiopathic intracranial hypertension (aka benign intracranial hypertension, pseudotumor cerebri)

Ineffective (Contraindicated)
- Acetazolamide is not contraindicated for any seizure type or epilepsy; does not commonly exacerbate seizures

Mechanism of Action
- Potent inhibitor of brain carbonic anhydrase, the enzyme that reversibly catalyzes the hydration of carbon dioxide (CO_2) and the dehydration of carbonic acid
- The carbonic anhydrase inhibition results in an elevation of intracellular CO_2, a decrease of intracellular pH, and depression of neuronal activity
- Acetazolamide increases the concentration of weak acids (such as certain AEDs, e.g., phenytoin and phenobarbital) into tissue; this may account for part of the efficacy of acetazolamide as add-on therapy
- Tolerance to the effect of acetazolamide often develops, possibly as a consequence of increased carbonic anhydrase production in glial cells

Efficacy Profile
- The goals of treatment are to achieve complete seizure remission when possible, or at least improved frequency and severity of seizures, while also minimizing adverse effects and improving patient quality of life
- Onset of action may be rapid and usually within a few days
- Tolerance to the effect of acetazolamide often develops within 1–6 months
- Discontinuation of treatment may re-establish efficacy, making acetazolamide particularly appropriate for intermittent use, such as in catamenial epilepsy
- Acetazolamide is used more commonly as an add-on AED than as monotherapy
- If acetazolamide is ineffective or only partially effective, it can be replaced by or combined with another AED that is appropriate for the patient's seizure type or epilepsy syndrome

Pharmacokinetics

Absorption and Distribution

- Oral bioavailability: >90%
- Food co-ingestion: neither delays the rate of absorption nor reduces the extent of absorption
- Time to maximum concentration (Tmax): 2–4 hours
- Time to steady state: 2 days
- Pharmacokinetics: linear
- Protein binding: 90–95% (90% of the drug in the body is bound to tissue carbonic anhydrase)
- Volume of distribution: 0.3 L/kg for total concentration, 1.8 L/kg for free concentration
- Salivary concentrations: it is not known whether acetazolamide is secreted into saliva and whether such concentrations are similar to the unbound levels seen in plasma

Metabolism

- Acetazolamide is not metabolized

Elimination

- Half-life values in adults are 10–15 hours
- Renal excretion: 100% of an administered dose is excreted unchanged in urine

Drug Interaction Profile

Pharmacokinetic Drug Interactions

- Interactions between AEDs: effects on acetazolamide:
  - To date, there have been no reports of AEDs affecting the clearance of acetazolamide and affecting acetazolamide plasma levels
- Interactions between AEDs: effects by acetazolamide:
  - Acetazolamide can *increase* carbamazepine, phenobarbital, and phenytoin plasma levels
  - Acetazolamide can *decrease* the absorption of primidone
- Interactions between AEDs and non-AED drugs: effects on acetazolamide:
  - To date, there have been no reports of other non-AED drugs affecting the clearance of acetazolamide and affecting acetazolamide plasma levels
- Interactions between AEDs and non-AED drugs: effects by acetazolamide:
  - Acetazolamide can *increase* cyclosporin plasma levels
  - Acetazolamide can *decrease* lithium plasma levels

A

DRUG INTERACTION PROFILE

Pharmacodynamic Drug Interactions
- It has been suggested that the efficacy of acetazolamide in the treatment of seizures may be due in part to a pharmacodynamic interaction with other AEDs
- Acetazolamide prolongs the effects of amphetamines and quinidine
- Anorexia, tachypnea, lethargy, coma, and death have been reported in patients receiving concomitant high-dose aspirin and acetazolamide
- Acetazolamide and sodium bicarbonate in combination increase the risk of renal calculus formation

Hormonal Contraception
- Acetazolamide does not enhance the metabolism of oral contraceptives so as to decrease plasma levels of hormonal contraceptives and, therefore, does not compromise contraception control

Adverse Effects
How Drug Causes Adverse Effects
- Carbonic anhydrase inhibition by acetazolamide is likely to be the mechanism responsible for the clinical adverse effects, such as metabolic acidosis, paresthesias, and kidney stones

Common Adverse Effects
- Paresthesias, mostly tingling in the fingers and toes
- Drowsiness
- Ataxia
- Blurred vision
- Frequent urination
- Alteration of taste (parageusia), especially for carbonated beverages
- Metabolic acidosis (lowered serum bicarbonate or CO_2)
- Appetite suppression
- Gastrointestinal disturbances (nausea, vomiting, diarrhea)
- Allergic rash

Life-threatening or Dangerous Adverse Effects
- Very rarely, Stevens–Johnson syndrome, toxic epidermal necrolysis, fulminant hepatic necrosis
- Agranulocytosis, aplastic anemia, and other blood dyscrasias

Rare and not Life-threatening Adverse Effects
- Nephrolithiasis (secondary to decrease in urinary citrate)
- Blood dyscrasias
- Visual changes and transient myopia
- Tinnitus
- Depression
- Loss of libido

Weight Change
• Weight loss can occur

What to do About Adverse Effects
• Discuss common and severe adverse effects with patients or parents before starting medication, including symptoms that should be reported to the physician
• Discuss symptoms associated with kidney stones
• Some central nervous system (CNS)-related adverse effects may be lessened by slow titration, but they may persist at low doses despite slow titration
• Metabolic acidosis is usually compensated, but patients may be treated with oral bicarbonate for CO_2 values of 15–18 mEq/L or less
• Acetazolamide should generally not be administered to patients who are already receiving sulthiame, topiramate, zonisamide, or the ketogenic diet, because these treatments also predispose to metabolic acidosis and to kidney stones
• Patients should be encouraged to drink water liberally while on acetazolamide to reduce the risk of kidney stones
• Anorexia and weight loss may improve with dosage reduction

Dosing and Use
Usual Dosage Range
• Adults and children over 12 years of age: 250–1000 mg/day
• Children under 12 years of age: 10–20 mg/kg/day
• Catamenial epilepsy: 8–30 mg/kg/day

Available Formulations
• Tablet: 250 mg
• Prolonged-release capsule: 250 mg
• Parenteral solution: 500 mg powder per vial (requires reconstitution with at least 5 mL of sterile water)

How to Dose
• *For adults and children over 12 years of age:* start treatment with 250 mg/day, once or twice daily; at intervals of 3–7 days increase as needed and as tolerated by 250 mg/day; maintenance dose generally 250–1000 mg/day
• *Children under 12 years of age:* start treatment with 3–6 mg/kg/day, once or twice daily; at intervals of 3–7 days increase as needed and as tolerated by 3–6 mg/kg/day; maintenance dose generally 10–20 mg/kg/day; doses of 20–30 mg/kg/day may be necessary and are well tolerated
• *Catamenial epilepsy:* acetazolamide has been used in women with catamenial epilepsy both continuously and intermittently during the days of identified seizure exacerbation; maintenance dose generally

A

DOSING AND USE

8–30 mg/kg/day, doses up to 1000 mg/day may be necessary and are well tolerated

Dosing Tips
- Slow dose titration may delay onset of therapeutic action but enhance tolerability to sedating effects
- Some patients may do very well at relatively low doses of acetazolamide, such as 500 mg/day in adults or 10 mg/kg/day in children; the response to treatment should be assessed at these doses before increasing the dose further
- Acetazolamide may be most effective as add-on therapy and tolerance may develop later when acetazolamide is given as adjunct therapy
- When tolerance has developed, temporary withdrawal of acetazolamide usually restores the previous therapeutic effect
- In patients with catamenial epilepsy, once an effective and well-tolerated dose has been determined, this dose can be administered during the necessary number of days without gradual titration

How to Withdraw Drug
- May need to adjust dosage of concurrent medications as acetazolamide is being discontinued, because plasma levels of other drugs may change (see Pharmacokinetic Drug Interactions section)
- No data are available on potential for withdrawal seizures or symptoms upon rapid discontinuation of acetazolamide; however, rapid discontinuation after chronic use may increase the risk of seizures
- If possible, taper dose over a period of 1–3 months
- In patients receiving intermittent treatment for a few days, such as for catamenial epilepsy, gradual tapering is usually not necessary

Overdose
- To date, there have been no cases of overdose reported with acetazolamide
- Severe metabolic acidosis could develop, which can usually be corrected by the administration of bicarbonate
- The stomach should be emptied immediately by lavage or by induction of emesis
- Hemodialysis removes acetazolamide from blood and, therefore, serves as a useful procedure in cases of overdose

Tests and Therapeutic Drug Monitoring
- Serum bicarbonate (CO_2) can be measured before treatment and then periodically, but it is not routine practice to do so
- Other routine laboratory testing is not necessary
- Therapeutic drug monitoring:
  - Optimum seizure control in patients on monotherapy is most likely to occur at acetazolamide plasma concentrations of 10–14 mg/L (45–63 µmol/L)

ACETAZOLAMIDE

A

- The conversion factor from mg/L to μmol/L is 4.50 (i.e., 1 mg/L = 4.50 μmol/L)
- The reference range of acetazolamide in plasma is considered to be the same for children and adults, although no data are available to support this clinical practice
- There are no data indicating the usefulness of monitoring acetazolamide by use of saliva

Other Warnings/Precautions
- Patients should be monitored carefully for evidence of an allergic rash
- Patients should be monitored carefully for evidence of kidney stones
- In combination with carbamazepine or oxcarbazepine, there is an increased risk of hyponatremia

Do not Use
- Use with caution in patients undergoing treatments that are associated with an increase in risk of kidney stones, such as topiramate, sulthiame, zonisamide, and the ketogenic diet
- Do not use in patients with hyperchloremic acidosis
- Do not use in patients with cirrhosis because of the risk of severe hyperammonemia
- Use with caution in patients with a history of allergic rash to another medication
- A history of allergic reaction to an antibiotic sulfonamide does not appear to be an absolute contraindication for the use of acetazolamide, because there seems to be no specific cross-reactivity
- Long-term administration of acetazolamide is contraindicated in patients with chronic non-congestive angle-closure glaucoma
- Acetazolamide should not be administered to patients receiving high-dose aspirin – anorexia, tachypnea, lethargy, coma, and death have been reported to occur
- Because of its tendency to cause potassium loss, acetazolamide is contraindicated in Addison disease and adrenal insufficiency

Special Populations

Renal Impairment
- Acetazolamide is renally excreted, so the dose may need to be lowered – particularly in patients with a creatinine clearance (CrCl) of <60 mL/min; the clearance of unbound acetazolamide correlates with the CrCl
- Because acetazolamide can be removed by hemodialysis, patients receiving hemodialysis may require supplemental doses of acetazolamide

SPECIAL POPULATIONS

A

ACETAZOLAMIDE

Hepatic Impairment
- Acetazolamide is not metabolized and consequently dose adjustment will not be necessary
- Acetazolamide can increase hyperammonemia in patients with liver failure; the mechanism is probably increased renal tubular reabsorption of ammonium secondary to alkalinization of urine

Children
- Children have an increased metabolic capacity and consequently higher doses on an mg/kg/day basis are usually required to achieve the equivalent therapeutic plasma levels seen in adults
- Acetazolamide can increase hyperammonemia in children
- Age-specific higher incidence of adverse effects of acetazolamide in the pediatric age range has not been described

Elderly
- Available data on the pharmacokinetics of acetazolamide in elderly patients suggest that they have a higher unbound fraction in plasma
- The renal clearance of unbound acetazolamide is significantly lower in the elderly, and correlates with the CrCl
- Elderly patients are more susceptible to adverse effects, and therefore may not tolerate higher doses
- Because of an age-related reduction in renal and hepatic function, lower acetazolamide doses may be appropriate
- Elderly patients frequently receive concurrent drug therapies for comorbidities, and therefore may be at greater risk for pharmacokinetic and pharmacodynamic interactions; the risk of pharmacokinetic interactions with acetazolamide is low

Pregnancy
- Specialist advice should be given to women who are of childbearing potential; they should be informed about the teratogenicity of all AEDs and the importance of avoiding an unplanned pregnancy; the AED treatment regimen should be reviewed when a woman is planning to become pregnant
- Rapid discontinuation of AEDs should be avoided as this may lead to breakthrough seizures, which could have serious consequences for the woman and the unborn child
- Acetazolamide was previously classified by the US FDA as risk category C ((some animal studies show adverse effects, no controlled studies in humans); the current FDA Pregnancy and Lactation Rule has eliminated pregnancy risk category labels
- Use in women of childbearing potential requires weighing potential benefits to the mother against the risks to the fetus
- Use with other AEDs in combination may raise the risk for teratogenic effects as compared to acetazolamide monotherapy
- Taper drug if discontinuing
- Seizures may cause harm to the embryo/fetus

- Data on the pharmacokinetic changes of acetazolamide during pregnancy have not been identified

Breast Feeding
- Breast milk: in a single case report of a mother taking 1000 mg/day of acetazolamide while breast feeding, acetazolamide concentrations in breast milk were 1.3–2.1 mg/L, whereby plasma levels were 5.2–6.4 mg/L. It was calculated that the infant ingested 0.6 mg/day and the infant's plasma levels were 0.2–0.6 mg/L
- Breastfed infants: acetazolamide plasma levels in consideration of the above case are 4–9% of maternal plasma levels
- If adverse effects are observed, recommend bottle feeding

The Overall Place of Acetazolamide in the Treatment of Epilepsy

Acetazolamide is a relatively safe drug which can be used for long periods without serious adverse effects. It is used more often as a second-line add-on therapy rather than as monotherapy, especially for catamenial seizures. In some patients dramatic effects have been observed, and a worthwhile effect has been reported widely in many patients and in differing types of seizures.

Primary Seizure Types
- Absence seizures
- Partial seizures

Secondary Seizure Types
- Generalized tonic–clonic seizures
- Myoclonic seizures
- Juvenile myoclonic epilepsy
- Catamenial epilepsy

Potential Advantages
- Broad spectrum of seizure protection
- Rapid onset of action
- Associated with few and minor pharmacokinetic interactions
- Favorable adverse event profile with very rare serious adverse effects
- Does not commonly exacerbate seizures

Potential Disadvantages
- Tolerance to the effect of acetazolamide often develops within 1–6 months
- Potential teratogen

A

ACETAZOLAMIDE

Suggested Reading

Chapron DJ, Sweeney KR, Feig PU, Kramer PA. Influence of advanced age on the disposition of acetazolamide. *British Journal of Clinical Pharmacology* 1985; **19**: 363–371.

Fine AL, Wirrell EC, Wong-Kisiel LC, Nickels KC. Acetazolamide for the electrical status epilepticus in slow-wave sleep. *Epilepsia* 2015; **56**: e134–e138.

Forsythe WI, Owens JR, Toothill C. Effectiveness of acetazolamide in the treatment of carbamazepine-resistant epilepsy in children. *Developmental Medicine and Child Neurology* 1981; **23**: 761–769.

Holowach J, Thurston DL. A clinical evaluation of acetazolamide (Diamox) in the treatment of epilepsy in children. *Journal of Pediatrics* 1958; **53**: 160–171.

Katayama F, Miura H, Takanashi S. Long-term effectiveness and side effects of acetazolamide as an adjunct to other anticonvulsants in the treatment of refractory epilepsies. *Brain and Development* 2002; **24**: 150–154.

Lim LL, Foldvary N, Mascha E, Lee J. Acetazolamide in women with catamenial epilepsy. *Epilepsia* 2001; **42**: 746–749.

Oles KS, Penry K, Cole DLW, Howard G. Use of acetazolamide as an adjunct to carbamazepine in refractory partial seizures. *Epilepsia* 1989; **30**: 74–78.

Reiss WG, Oles KS. Acetazolamide in the treatment of seizures. *Annals of Pharmacotherapy* 1996; **30**: 514–519.

Resor SR, Resor LD. Chronic acetazolamide monotherapy in the treatment of juvenile myoclonic epilepsy. *Neurology* 1990; **40**: 1677–1681.

Soderman P, Hartvig P, Fagerlund C. Acetazolamide excretion into breast milk. *British Journal of Clinical Pharmacology* 1984; **17**: 599–600.

Tawil R, Moxley RT, Griggs RC. Acetazolamide-induced nephrolithiasis: implications for treatment of neuromuscular disorders. *Neurology* 1993; **43**: 1105–1106.

Vaziri ND, Saiki J, Barton CH, Rajudin M, Ness RL. Hemodialyzability of acetazolamide. *South Medical Journal* 1980; **73**: 422–423.

Watson WA, Garrelts JC, Zinn PD, Garriott JC, McLemore TL, Clementi WA. Chronic acetazolamide intoxication. *Clinical Toxicology* 1984; **22**: 549–563.

Yamamoto Y, Takahashi Y, Imai K, Mishima N, Yazawa R, Inoue K, Itoh K, Kagawa Y, Inoue Y. Risk factors for hyperammonemia in pediatric patients with epilepsy. *Epilepsia* 2013; **54**: 983–989.

ACTH

Therapeutics
Chemical Name and Structure
Adrenocorticotropic hormone (ACTH) is a peptide consisting of 39 amino acids in its natural form and 24 amino acids in its synthetic form. Its empirical formula is $C_{207}H_{308}O_{58}N_{56}S, 2AcOH,32H_2O$.

Brand Names
- Acortan
- ACTH
- Acthar, Acthelea
- Cortrosyn
- Synacthen
- Trofocortina

Generics Available
- No

Licensed Indications for Epilepsy
- ACTH is not licensed for the treatment of epileptic seizures

Licensed Indications for Non-epilepsy Conditions
- Acute exacerbations of multiple sclerosis
- Diagnostic aid in adrenocortical insufficiency
- Severe muscle weakness in myasthenia gravis

Non-licensed Use for Epilepsy
- Acquired epileptic aphasia (Landau–Kleffner syndrome)
- Infantile spasms (West syndrome)
- Lennox–Gastaut syndrome
- Myoclonic astatic epilepsy
- Ohtahara syndrome
- Rasmussen encephalitis
- Severe myoclonic epilepsy of infancy (Dravet syndrome)

Non-licensed Use for Non-epilepsy Conditions
- There are none

Ineffective (Contraindicated)
- ACTH should not be considered as a standard antiepileptic treatment and should be used only for a restricted group of severe encephalopathic epilepsies, as listed above

Mechanism of Action
- ACTH stimulates the secretion of cortisol in the adrenal gland
- Effective in patients with adrenal suppression

A

THERAPEUTICS

11

A

- Its effect on the brain and on epilepsy may be independent of steroid secretion
- ACTH suppresses the expression of corticotropin-releasing hormone, a proconvulsant neuropeptide whose expression may be enhanced in patients with infantile spasms

Efficacy Profile
- The goal is elimination of spasms and suppression of the hypsarrhythmic pattern on the electroencephalogram (EEG)
- A response is often seen within the first few days of treatment
- Relapse after full response and discontinuation of ACTH is not uncommon
- A second course of ACTH may again be effective
- In case of lack of efficacy, partial efficacy, or relapse, consider other treatments such as vigabatrin, valproic acid, topiramate, zonisamide, levetiracetam, a benzodiazepine, or vitamin B_6

Pharmacokinetics
Conventional pharmacokinetic parameters do not apply to ACTH.

Absorption and Distribution
- Because ACTH is inactivated in the gastrointestinal tract it must be administered parenterally by intramuscular (im) injection

Metabolism
- Although the precise metabolic fate of ACTH is not known, circulating ACTH is probably enzymatically cleaved at the 16–17 lysine–arginine bond by the plasma-plasminogen system

Elimination
- Half-life values are considered to be ~ 15 minutes

Drug Interaction Profile
Pharmacokinetic Drug Interactions
- Interactions between AEDs: effects on ACTH:
  - To date, there have been no reports of AEDs affecting the clearance of ACTH and affecting ACTH plasma levels
- Interactions between AEDs: effects by ACTH:
  - To date, there have been no reports of ACTH affecting the clearance of other AEDs and affecting their plasma levels
- Interactions between AEDs and non-AED drugs: effects on ACTH:
  - To date, there have been no reports of other non-AED drugs affecting the clearance of ACTH and affecting ACTH plasma levels
- Interactions between AEDs and non-AED drugs: effects by ACTH:

ACTH

– To date, there have been no reports of ACTH affecting the clearance of other non-AED drugs and affecting their plasma levels

Pharmacodynamic Drug Interactions
• To date, none have been identified

Hormonal Contraception
• The effect of ACTH on hormonal contraception is unknown, but ACTH is virtually never administered to women of childbearing age

Adverse Effects
How Drug Causes Adverse Effects
• Most adverse effects of ACTH are shared by steroids and are likely to be related to the stimulation of cortisol secretion by the adrenal gland

Common Adverse Effects
• Irritability, at times severe
• Cushingoid features
• Hypertension
• Hyperglycemia, glycosuria
• Electrolyte imbalances

Life-threatening or Dangerous Adverse Effects
• Immunosuppression and possibly impaired function of polymorpho-nuclear leukocytes
• Pneumonia, in particular *Pneumocystis pneumoniae*
• Sepsis
• Congestive heart failure

Rare and not Life-threatening Adverse Effects
• Brain atrophy
• Peptic ulcer
• Subaortic hypertrophic cardiomyopathy, usually reversible within 6 months of discontinuation
• Cataracts
• Glaucoma
• Seizure exacerbation

Weight Change
• Weight gain is common, as part of the cushingoid features

What to do About Adverse Effects
• Discuss common and severe adverse effects with parents before starting medication, including symptoms that should be reported to the physician
• Always start ACTH treatment in the hospital

A

ACTH

- ACTH is contraindicated in the presence of serious bacterial or viral infection such as tuberculosis, varicella, or cytomegalovirus
- ACTH is contraindicated in the presence of pre-existing idiopathic hypertrophic cardiomyopathy
- Prophylaxis of pneumocystis pneumonia with trimethoprim-sulfamethoxazole may be considered
- Elevated blood pressure may require treatment, initially mostly with a diuretic

Dosing and Use
Usual Dosage Range
- The optimal dosage (calculated in IU/m^2 body surface/day) and schedule have not been determined
- The highest dose is usually given at the onset, followed by a gradual tapering until discontinuation
- The initial dose used most commonly is 150 IU/m^2/day given in two divided doses, with a range between 85 and 250 IU/m^2/day; this is given for 1–2 weeks and the dose is then tapered gradually to achieve a total treatment duration of 4–6 weeks

Available Formulations
- Corticotropin (porcine pituitary extract, 39 amino acids, short-acting)

  – Gel 80 IU/mL   100 IU = 0.72 mg
  – Lyophilized powder   100 IU = 0.72 mg

- Cosyntropin/tetracosactrin (synthetic, 24 amino acids, short-acting)
  – 100 IU = 1.0 mg
- Cosyntropin/tetracosactrin (synthetic, 24 amino acids, long-acting)
  – 100 IU = 2.5 mg

How to Dose
- ACTH is administered intramuscularly as a treatment course for a limited amount of time, usually a few weeks
- A typical (but not exclusive) dosage schedule would consist of a 4-week course, with 150 IU/m^2/day given in two divided doses for 2 weeks, 30 IU/m^2/day for 3 days, 15 IU/m^2/day for 3 days, 10 IU/m^2/day for 3 days, then 10 IU/m^2 every other day for three doses; other schedules may consist of a somewhat longer tapering period

Dosing Tips
- Treatment with ACTH is usually initiated in the hospital to better facilitate:
  – Careful continuous clinical observation for early significant adverse effects and video-EEG monitoring to monitor spasm/seizure frequency and response to therapy
  – Baseline clinical and laboratory assessment of the patient
  – Teaching of im administration to parents and/or carers

How to Withdraw Drug
- There is no need to adjust dosage of concurrent medications as ACTH is being discontinued, because plasma levels of other drugs do not change (see Pharmacokinetic Drug Interactions section)
- All schedules for the administration of ACTH consist of a limited course with a predetermined withdrawal phase
- ACTH should never be stopped abruptly because it suppresses endogenous ACTH secretion
- The purpose of the tapering phase is to gradually restore normal endogenous ACTH secretion
- Monitoring of morning levels of cortisol may be useful during withdrawal

Overdose
- Doses of ACTH greater than 250 IU/m^2/day are commonly associated with serious and at times fatal complications that do not differ from those described under the Adverse Effects section

Tests and Therapeutic Drug Monitoring
- Before initiation of ACTH therapy:
  - Place a purified protein derivative skin test to rule out tuberculosis
  - Obtain chest X-ray in the presence of symptoms of respiratory illness
  - Do not administer any immunization for 10 days before and during treatment with ACTH
  - Vital signs, including blood pressure
  - Physical examination to exclude evidence of infection
  - Test urine for glucose and for evidence of urinary infection
  - Test stool for blood (guaiac)
  - Blood for complete blood count (CBC), electrolytes, blood urea nitrogen (BUN), Cr, Ca, Mg, phosphate
  - Consider baseline echocardiogram
- During ACTH therapy:
  - Blood pressure daily for 1 week, then three times weekly until ACTH discontinuation
  - Test urine for glucose twice weekly
  - Test stool for blood (guaiac)
  - Prescribe an H$_2$ antagonist, especially if stool is guaiac-positive
  - Blood for CBC, electrolytes, Cr, Ca, Mg, phosphate after 2–4 weeks
  - Consider follow-up echocardiogram after 2–4 weeks (hypertrophic cardiomyopathy)
  - Patient should be examined if fever develops

Other Warnings/Precautions
- Patients should be monitored carefully for evidence of infection
- ACTH may accentuate electrolyte loss associated with diuretic therapy

A

DOSING AND USE

THE EPILEPSY PRESCRIBER'S GUIDE TO ANTIEPILEPTIC DRUGS

- ACTH is contraindicated in the presence of pre-existing idiopathic hypertrophic cardiomyopathy

Do not Use
- ACTH is contraindicated in the presence of serious bacterial or viral infection such as tuberculosis, varicella, or cytomegalovirus

Special Populations
Renal Impairment
- There is no evidence that renal impairment requires changes in ACTH doses

Hepatic Impairment
- There is no evidence that hepatic impairment requires changes in ACTH doses

Children
- ACTH for the treatment of epilepsy is used almost exclusively in children

Elderly
- ACTH should not be used in elderly patients for the treatment of seizures

Pregnancy
- ACTH should not be used in a pregnant patient for the treatment of seizures
- ACTH was previously classified by the US FDA as risk category C (some animal studies show adverse effects, no controlled studies in humans); the current FDA Pregnancy and Lactation Rule has eliminated pregnancy risk category labels

Breast Feeding
- ACTH should not be used in a nursing mother for the treatment of seizures

The Overall Place of ACTH in the Treatment of Epilepsy
ACTH is a first-line treatment for infantile spasms (West syndrome), a condition consisting of infantile spasms, disturbed psychomotor devel-opment, and the characteristic EEG pattern of hypsarrhythmia. ACTH has an all-or-nothing effect and typically in 70–75% of children total seizure suppression occurs, but the relapse rate is relatively high. In those children who do not respond to ACTH, or who relapse after treatment, other medications should be considered, including vigabatrin (which is first-line for those with tuberous sclerosis), valproic acid, sulthiame,

ACTH

topiramate, zonisamide, levetiracetam, a benzodiazepine (especially clonazepam or nitrazepam), vitamin B_6, or dietary therapies (i.e., ketogenic, modified Atkins).

A

Primary Seizure Types
• Infantile spasms (West syndrome)

Secondary Seizure Types
• Acquired epileptic aphasia (Landau–Kleffner syndrome)
• Lennox–Gastaut syndrome
• Myoclonic astatic epilepsy
• Ohtahara syndrome
• Rasmussen encephalitis
• Severe myoclonic epilepsy of infancy (Dravet syndrome)

Potential Advantages
• ACTH has the best-documented evidence of efficacy in the treatment of infantile spasms
• A single course of 4–6 weeks of ACTH treatment can have a long-lasting or permanent anticonvulsant effect

Potential Disadvantages
• ACTH has several potentially serious or even life-threatening adverse effects

Suggested Reading

Baram TZ, Mitchell WG, Tournay A, Snead OC, Hanson RA, Horton EJ. High-dose corticotropin (ACTH) versus prednisone for infantile spasms: a prospective, randomized, blinded study. *Pediatrics* 1996; **97**: 375–379.

Bobele GB, Ward KE, Bodensteiner JB. Hypertrophic cardiomyopathy during corticotrophin therapy for infantile spasms. A clinical and echocardiographic study. *American Journal of Diseases of Children* 1993; **147**: 223–225.

Hrachovy RA, Frost JD, Kellaway P, Zion TE. Double-blind study of ACTH vs prednisolone therapy in infantile spasms. *Journal of Pediatrics* 1983; **103**: 641–645.

Kivity S, Lerman P, Ariel R, Danziger Y, Mimouni M, Shinnar S. Long-term cognitive outcomes of a cohort of children with cryptogenic infantile spasms treated with high-dose adrenocorticotropic hormone. *Epilepsia* 2004; **45**: 255–262.

Lux AL, Edwards SW, Hancock E, Johnson AL, Kennedy CR, Newton RW, O'Callaghan FJ, Verity CM, Osborne JP; United Kingdom Infantile Spasms Study. The United Kingdom Infantile Spasms Study (UKISS) comparing hormone treatment with vigabatrin on

SUGGESTED READING

A

developmental and epilepsy outcomes to age 14 months: a multi-centre randomized trial. *Lancet Neurology* 2005; **4**: 712–717.

Mackay MT, Weiss SK, Adams-Webber T, Ashwal S, Stephens D, Ballaban-Gill K, Baram TZ, Duchowny M, Hirtz D, Pellock JM, Shields WD, Shinnar S, Wyllie E, Snead OC III; American Academy of Neurology; Child Neurology Society. Practice parameter: medical treatment of infantile spasms: report of the American Academy of Neurology and the Child Neurology Society. *Neurology* 2004; **62**: 1668–1681.

Maekawa K, Ohta H, Tamai I. Transient brain shrinkage in infantile spasms after ACTH treatment. Report of two cases. *Neuropaediatrie* 1980; **11**: 80–84.

Shumiloff NA, Lam WM, Manasco KB. Adrenocorticotropic hormone for the treatment of West syndrome in children. *Annals of Pharmacotherapy* 2013; **47**: 744–754.

Tacke E, Kupferschmid C, Lang D. Hypertrophic cardiomyopathy during ACTH treatment. *Klinka Padiatrika* 1983; **195**: 124–128.

Vigevano F, Cilio MR. Vigabatrin versus ACTH as first-line treatment for infantile spasms: a randomized, prospective study. *Epilepsia* 1997; **38**: 1270–1274.

ACTH

BRIVARACETAM

B

Therapeutics

Chemical Name and Structure

Brivaracetam, (2S)-2-[(4R)-2-oxo-4-propyltetrahydro-1H-pyrrol-1-yl]
butanamide (the 4R propyl analog of levetiracetam), has a molecular
weight of 212.29 and an empirical formula of $C_{11}H_{20}N_2O_2$.

Brand Names
• Briviact

Generics Available
• No

Licensed Indications for Epilepsy
• Adjunctive treatment of partial-onset (focal) seizures, with or without
secondary generalization, in adults 16 years of age and older with epilepsy (UK SPC; FDA PI)

Licensed Indications for Non-epilepsy Conditions
• None

Non-licensed Use for Epilepsy
• None

Non-licensed Use for Non-epilepsy Conditions
• None

Ineffective (Contraindicated)
• Brivaracetam has a broad preclinical spectrum of action, but it currently lacks data or indications for use in the treatment of generalized
seizure types in the idiopathic or symptomatic generalized epilepsies
• There is no information regarding its effectiveness in adolescents less
than 16 years of age, children, or infants

B

BRIVARACETAM

Mechanism of Action
- The precise mechanism by which brivaracetam exerts its antiepileptic activity is unknown
- It binds with high and selective affinity to synaptic vesicle protein SV2A (the same target as levetiracetam), which is involved in synaptic vesicle exocytosis and may contribute to its anticonvulsant efficacy
- Brivaracetam is a partial antagonist of sodium channels, leading to blockade of voltage-dependent excitatory currents
- Brivaracetam does not appear to act via inhibition of calcium currents or α-amino-3-hydroxy-5-methyl-4-isoxazole propionic acid (AMPA) receptors, or increase in GABAergic inhibitory response

Efficacy Profile
- The goals of treatment are to achieve complete seizure remission when possible, or at least improved frequency and severity of seizures, while also minimizing adverse effects and improving patient quality of life
- Robust clinical trial evidence has demonstrated that brivaracetam possesses adjunctive efficacy in partial/focal-onset seizures in adults with refractory focal epilepsies
- Brivaracetam has no added therapeutic benefit when added to levetiracetam since these drugs each compete for the same SV2A binding site
- Brivaracetam also was suggested to have potential broad-spectrum efficacy for idiopathic generalized epilepsies
- Brivaracetam dose-dependently suppressed photoparoxysmal epileptiform activity in patients with photosensitive epilepsies
- Although its efficacy and safety have not yet been confirmed for generalized seizures in large, well-powered controlled trials, brivaracetam is not indicated for generalized epilepsies at this time
- If brivaracetam is ineffective or only partially effective, it can be replaced by or combined with another AED that is appropriate for the patient's seizure type or epilepsy syndrome

Pharmacokinetics
Absorption and Distribution
- Oral bioavailability: ~100%
- Food co-ingestion: does not affect the extent of absorption but does slow the rate of absorption
- Tmax: 0.5–1.0 hours
- Time to steady state: 2 days
- Pharmacokinetics: linear
- Protein binding: 17%
- Volume of distribution: 0.5 L/kg
- Salivary concentrations: it is unknown whether brivaracetam is secreted into saliva

Metabolism
- Brivaracetam undergoes extensive (>90%) hepatic metabolism via hydrolysis of its acetamide group, via an amidase, and secondary hydroxylation through the cytochrome P450 (CYP) 2C19 isozyme pathway
- The three major metabolites carboxylic acid, hydroxy, and hydroxyacid are not pharmacologically active
- Autoinduction is not a feature of brivaracetam metabolism

Elimination
- The elimination half-life of brivaracetam is 7–8 hours
- Renal excretion: approximately 95% of brivaracetam, including its three metabolites, is excreted in urine within 3 days, with 9% of an administered dose excreted unchanged in urine, and less than 1% excreted in feces

Drug Interaction Profile
Pharmacokinetic Drug Interactions
- Interactions between AEDs: effects on brivaracetam:
  - Carbamazepine, phenobarbital, and phenytoin can increase the clearance of brivaracetam and *decrease* brivaracetam plasma levels
- Interactions between AEDs: effects by brivaracetam:
  - Brivaracetam can increase the conversion of carbamazepine to carbamazepine-10,11 epoxide and *increase* carbamazepine-10,11 epoxide plasma levels
  - Brivaracetam can *increase* plasma levels of phenytoin
- Interactions between AEDs and non-AED drugs: effects on brivaracetam:
  - Rifampin can *decrease* brivaracetam plasma levels
- Interactions between AEDs and non-AED drugs: effects by brivaracetam:
  - To date, there have been no reports of brivaracetam affecting the clearance of other non-AED drugs and affecting their plasma levels

Pharmacodynamic Drug Interactions
- The efficacy of brivaracetam is decreased when co-administered with levetiracetam consequent to a pharmacodynamic interaction
- Brivaracetam enhances the effect of alcohol on psychomotor function, attention, and memory consequent to a pharmacodynamic interaction
- Other central nervous depressants, such as alcohol, other AEDs, and monoamine oxidase inhibitors (MAOIs) may exacerbate the depressive effect of brivaracetam

B

DRUG INTERACTION PROFILE

B

BRIVARACETAM

Hormonal Contraception
- Brivaracetam does not enhance the metabolism of oral contraceptives and therefore does not compromise contraception control
- At supratherapeutic brivaracetam doses of 200 mg twice daily (twice the recommended maximum daily dosage), oral contraceptive area under the concentration versus time curve (AUC) values were reduced by up to 27%, without impact on suppression of ovulation

Adverse Effects
How Drug Causes Adverse Effects
- Mechanism by which brivaracetam causes adverse effects has not been established
- CNS adverse effects may be due to actions on SV2A synaptic vesicle proteins

Common Adverse Effects
- Somnolence, dizziness, fatigue, and nausea/vomiting

Life-threatening or Dangerous Adverse Effects
- None known

Rare and not Life-threatening Adverse Effects
- None known

Weight Change
- Not known

What to do About Adverse Effects
- Discuss common adverse effects with patients or parents before starting medication, including symptoms that should be reported to the physician
- Risk of adverse effects is greatest in the first few months of treatment
- Slower titration may decrease incidence or severity of some adverse effects

Dosing and Use
Usual Dosage Range
- Adults: 50–200 mg/day in divided doses

Available Formulations
- Tablets: 10 mg, 25 mg, 50 mg, 75 mg, 100 mg
- Oral solution: 10 mg/mL
- Solution for intravenous (iv) injection: 50 mg/mL
- Injection: 50 mg/5 mL single-dose vial

B

How to Dose
- *For adults and adolescents over 16 years of age*: start treatment with 50 mg twice daily; at intervals of 1–2 weeks increase as needed and as tolerated to a target of 100 mg twice daily (bid) (maximal dosage 200 mg/day); maintenance dose is generally 50–200 mg/day; some patients may tolerate and respond to doses greater than 200 mg/day

Dosing Tips
- Slower titration may decrease incidence or severity of some adverse effects
- A dose for iv loading has not been determined
- iv doses can be infused undiluted, or diluted in isotonic fluids (e.g., normal saline, lactated Ringer's, 5% dextrose) over 2–15 minutes
- For intolerable sedation, most of the dose can be given at night and less during the day

How to Withdraw Drug
- There is no need to adjust dosage of most concurrent medications other than phenytoin as brivaracetam is being discontinued, because plasma levels of other drugs do not change; however, for phenytoin, consider measuring levels since phenytoin concentrations could decrease when brivaracetam is withdrawn from a polytherapy regimen containing both drugs (see Pharmacokinetic Drug Interactions section)
- Rapid discontinuation may increase the risk of seizures
- Taper dose over a period of several weeks

Overdose
- There are very limited data concerning brivaracetam overdose in humans; no fatalities have been reported; a single dose of 1400 mg was reported in one case with symptoms that included somnolence and dizziness
- Other symptoms that can be expected are vertigo, balance disorder, fatigue, nausea, diplopia, anxiety, and bradycardia
- There is no specific antidote for brivaracetam overdose
- In event of overdose, standard medical practice including securing the airway, ventilation, and monitoring of vital signs is recommended
- It is unknown whether hemodialysis removes brivaracetam from blood; since less than 10% of brivaracetam is excreted in urine, hemodialysis is not expected to enhance brivaracetam clearance

Tests and Therapeutic Drug Monitoring
- There is no need to routinely monitor any laboratory parameter during treatment with brivaracetam
- Therapeutic drug monitoring:
  - Optimum seizure control in patients on monotherapy is most likely to occur at brivaracetam plasma concentrations of 0.2–2.0 mg/L (1–9 μmol/L)

DOSING AND USE

23

- The conversion factor from mg/L to μmol/L is 4.71 (i.e., 1 mg/L = 4.71 μmol/L)
- The reference range of brivaracetam in plasma is considered to be the same for children and adults, although no data are available to support this clinical practice
- It is unknown whether brivaracetam can be monitored by use of saliva

Other Warnings / Precautions
- Patients should be monitored carefully for signs of depression or psychosis

Do not Use
- In patients with a history of allergic reaction to brivaracetam or its excipients
- Because the tablet formulation contains lactose, patients with rare hereditary problems of galactose intolerance, Lapp lactose deficiency, or glucose–galactose malabsorption should not take this formulation

Special Populations
Renal Impairment
- Dosage adjustment of brivaracetam is not required in patients with renal insufficiency
- Brivaracetam is not recommended in patients receiving hemodialysis, since it is currently unknown whether brivaracetam is removed by hemodialysis

Hepatic Impairment
- Brivaracetam is extensively metabolized in the liver and, therefore, dosage adjustment is recommended, although optimal dosing recommendations have not yet been determined
- Recommended starting dosage is 25 mg twice daily (50 mg per day)
- Recommended maximum dosage is 75 mg twice daily (150 mg per day)

Children
- There is no indication for brivaracetam yet in children or adolescents below 16 years of age, and safety and efficacy have not been established in this patient population
- One study of population pharmacokinetics in infants and children with epilepsy aged 1 month to 16 years who were receiving one to three concurrent AEDs in polytherapy has suggested that a pediatric dose adaptation of 2 mg/kg twice daily to a maximal dose of 100 mg bid for body weight >50 kg will attain steady-state concentrations comparable to adults receiving 100 mg bid dosing

Elderly
- Elderly patients are more susceptible to adverse effects (especially somnolence) and therefore often are unable to tolerate higher doses. There were insufficient numbers of elderly patients (>65 years old) in randomized trials to determine efficacy and safety of brivaracetam in this patient population; however, judicious dosing should be anticipated if the drug is used in elderly patients, similar to hepatic impairment dosing strategy (i.e., starting dosage 25 mg bid, gradually titrating to target dose of 75 mg bid, or beyond if/as tolerated by the individual patient)
- Elderly patients are often prescribed concurrent drug therapies for comorbidities and therefore may be at greater risk for pharmacokinetic and pharmacodynamic interactions; as the risk of pharmacokinetic interactions with brivaracetam is low or non-existent, brivaracetam may be advantageous for use in the elderly
- The safe profile of brivaracetam makes it a reasonable choice for adjunctive treatment of partial-onset seizures in the elderly

Pregnancy
- Specialist advice should be given to women who are of childbearing potential; they should be informed about the teratogenicity of all AEDs and the importance of avoiding an unplanned pregnancy; the AED treatment regimen should be reviewed when a woman is planning to become pregnant
- Rapid discontinuation of AEDs should be avoided as this may lead to breakthrough seizures, which could have serious consequences for the woman and the unborn child
- Brivaracetam was previously classified by the US FDA as risk category C (some animal studies show adverse effects, no controlled studies in humans); the current FDA Pregnancy and Lactation Rule has eliminated pregnancy risk category labels
- Use in women of childbearing potential requires weighing potential benefits to the mother against the risks to the fetus
- Use with other AEDs in combination could cause a higher risk for teratogenic effects than brivaracetam monotherapy
- Taper drug if discontinuing
- Seizures may cause harm to the embryo/fetus
- No data are available currently regarding brivaracetam pharmacokinetics during pregnancy; changes in brivaracetam dose may be required

Breast Feeding
- Breast milk: it is unknown whether brivaracetam is secreted in human breast milk
- Breastfed infants: it is unknown whether brivaracetam is measurable in breastfed infants of mothers receiving brivaracetam
- If drug is continued while breast feeding, infant should be monitored for possible adverse effects (irritability or sedation)

B

SPECIAL POPULATIONS

B

BRIVARACETAM

- Until breast milk secretion is known, recommend bottle feeding, or if breast feeding is chosen, recommend bottle feeding if infant adverse effects are observed

The Overall Place of Brivaracetam in the Treatment of Epilepsy

Brivaracetam is the latest AED to be licensed for clinical use (2016) and has a mechanism of action similar to that of levetiracetam. In preclinical models, brivaracetam has been shown to be more highly selective and has higher affinity for binding the brain target SV2A than levetiracetam. It is unknown whether this improved target-binding tropism may translate into superior clinical efficacy or tolerability than levetiracetam. At present, brivaracetam's efficacy is only proven for partial-onset (focal) seizures; however, this may change once trials are carried out in patients with other types of seizures or epilepsies. Because of its recent introduction, it is too early to ascertain the place of brivaracetam in the treatment of patients with epilepsy.

Primary Seizure Types
- Partial/focal seizures

Secondary Seizure Types
- None

Potential Advantages
- Has no organ toxicity (i.e., liver, kidneys, bone marrow, etc.) and has no dangerous or life-threatening adverse effects
- Simple straightforward pharmacokinetics
- Does not affect the pharmacokinetics of other drugs

Potential Disadvantages
- Limited experience and human data currently about spectrum of efficacy, although preclinical profile in animal models suggests it may be broad-spectrum
- Potential teratogen with an incomplete safety recording during pregnancy

Suggested Reading
Biton V, Berkovic SF, Abou-Khalil B, Sperling MR, Johnson ME, Lu S. Brivaracetam as adjunctive treatment for uncontrolled partial epilepsy in adults: a phase III randomized, double blind, placebo-controlled trial. *Epilepsia* 2014; **55**: 57–66.

Coppola G, Iapadre G, Operto FF, Verrotti A. New developments in the management of partial-onset epilepsy: role of brivaracetam. *Drug Design Development and Therapy* 2017; **11**: 643–657.

Klein P, Biton V, Dilley D, Barnes M, Schiemann J, Lu S. Safety and tolerability of adjunctive brivaracetam as intravenous infusion or bolus
in patients with epilepsy. *Epilepsia* 2016; **57**: 1130–1138.

Klein P, Schiemann J, Sperling MR, Whitesides J, Liang W, Stalvey T,
Brandt C, Kwan P. A randomized, double-blind, placebo-controlled,
multicenter, parallel-group study to evaluate the efficacy and safety
of adjunctive brivaracetam in adult patients with uncontrolled
partial-onset seizures. *Epilepsia* 2015; **56**: 1890–1898.

Klitgaard H, Matagne A, Nicolas JM, Gillard M, Lamberty Y, De Ryck
M, Kaminski RM, Leclercq K, Niespodziany I, Wilff C, Wood
M, Hannestad J, Kervyn S, Kenda B. Brivaracetam: rationale for
dicovery and preclinical profile of a sellective SV2A ligand for epilepsy treatment. *Epilepsia* 2016; **57**: 538–548.

Kruithof AC, Watanabe S, Peeters PA, de Kam ML, Zuiker RG,
Stevens J, van Gerven JM, Stockis A. Pharmacological interactions
between brivaracetam and ethanol in healthy males. *Journal of
Psychopharmacology* 2017; **31**: 915–926.

Kwan P, Trinka E, Van Paesschen W, Johnson ME, Lu S. Adjunctive
brivaracetam for uncontrolled focal and generalized epilepsies: results
of a phase III, double-blind, randomized, placebo-controlled,
flexible-dose trial. *Epilepsia* 2014; **55**: 38–46.

Lattanzi S, Cagnetti C, Foschi N, Provinciali L, Silvestrini M.
Brivaracetam add-on for refractory focal epilepsy: a systematic
review and meta-analysis. *Neurology* 2016; **86**: 1344–1352.

Ma J, Huang S, You C. Adjunctive brivaracetam for patients with
refractory partial seizures: a meta-analysis of randomized placebo-
controlled trials. *Epilepsy Research* 2015; **114**: 59–65.

Ryvlin P, Werhahn KJ, Blaszczyk B, Johnson ME, Lu S. Adjunctive
brivaracetam in adults with uncontrolled focal epilepsy: results from
a double-blind, randomized, placebo-controlled trial. *Epilepsia* 2014;
55: 47–56.

Schoemaker R, Wade JR, Stockis A. Brivaracetam population pharmacokinetics in children with epilepsy aged 1 month to 16 years.
European Journal of Clinical Pharmacology 2017; **73**: 727–733.

Stockis A, Sargentini-Maier ML, Brodie MJ. Pharmacokinetic interaction between brivaracetam on carbamazepine in adult patients
with epilepsy, with and without valproate co-administration.
Epilepsy Research 2016; **128**: 163–168.

Toledo M, Whitesides J, Schiemann J, Johnson ME, Eckhardt K,
McDonough B, Borghs S, Kwan P. Safety, tolerability, and seizure
control during long-term treatment with adjunctive brivaracetam
for partial-onset seizures. *Epilepsia* 2016; **57**: 1139–1151.

C

CARBAMAZEPINE

Therapeutics

Chemical Name and Structure
Carbamazepine, 5H-dibenz[b,f]azepine-5-carboxamide, is a white or yellowish-white crystalline powder, with a molecular weight of 236.27 and an empirical formula of $C_{15}H_{12}N_2O$.

Brand Names
- Actebral; Actebral Retard; Actinerval; Amizepin; Apo-Carbamazepine; Azepal
- Bamgetol; Basitrol; Brucarcer
- Carba; Carbagen SR; Carbatrol; Camapine; Carazepin; Carbabeta; Carbadac; Carbalex; Carbamazepin-B; Carbapsy; Carbatol; Carbatol CR; Carbazene; Carbazep; Carbazina; Carmapine; Carmaz; Carmian; Carmine; Carnevix; Carpin; Carzepin; Carzepine; Clostedal
- Degranol
- Elpenor; Epazin; Epikor; Epileptol; Epileptol CR; Epitol; Eposal Retard; Equetro; Espalepsin
- Finlepsin
- Gericarb SR
- Hermolepsin
- Karbamazepin
- Lepsitol
- Neugeron; Neurolep; Neurotol; Neurotop; Neurotop Retard
- Panitol
- Sepibest; Sirtal; Stazepine
- Taver; Tegol; Tegral; Tegretal; Tegretol; Tegretol CR; Tegretol Retard; Temporol; Teril-CR; Timonil; Timonil Retard; Trepina
- Vulsivan
- Zeptol CR

Generics Available
- Yes

Licensed Indications for Epilepsy
- Partial (focal) and secondary generalized seizures (UK SPC; FDA PI)
- Primary generalized tonic–clonic seizures (UK SPC; FDA PI)

Licensed Indications for Non-epilepsy Conditions
• Trigeminal neuralgia (UK SPC; FDA PI)
• Bipolar disorder unresponsive to lithium (UK SPC)

Non-licensed Use for Epilepsy
• Autosomal dominant nocturnal frontal lobe epilepsy

Non-licensed Use for Non-epilepsy Conditions
• Neuropathic pain
• Painful tonic flexor spasms in multiple sclerosis

Ineffective (Contraindicated)
• Juvenile myoclonic epilepsy
• Juvenile absence epilepsy
• Epileptic encephalopathies (e.g., Lennox–Gastaut syndrome)
• Neonatal and febrile seizures
• Exaggerates myoclonic jerks, absences, and atonic seizures

Mechanism of Action
• Acts as a use-dependent blocker of voltage-sensitive sodium channels
• Inhibits L-type calcium channels
• Inhibits release of glutamate
• Has a moderate anticholinergic action which is responsible for some of its adverse effects

Efficacy Profile
• The goals of treatment are to achieve complete seizure remission when possible, or at least improved frequency and severity of seizures, while also minimizing adverse effects and improving patient quality of life
• Continue treatment until all symptoms are gone or until improvement is stable, then continue treating indefinitely as long as improvement persists
• Continue treatment to avoid recurrence of seizures until seizure freedom persists for 2–5 years; if no known etiology, then consider withdrawal
• If carbamazepine is ineffective or only partially effective, it can be replaced by or combined with another AED that is appropriate for the patient's seizure type or epilepsy syndrome

Pharmacokinetics
Absorption and Distribution
• Oral bioavailability: 75–85%
• Food co-ingestion: neither delays the rate of absorption nor reduces the extent of absorption

C

CARBAMAZEPINE

- Tmax: 2–9 hours (immediate-release tablets); 1–7 hours (chewable tablets); 0.5–4 hours (liquid suspensions). Extended-release formulations have prolonged Tmax values
- Time to steady state: 2–4 days (adults); 2–3 days (children)
- Pharmacokinetics: non-linear due to autoinduction
- Protein binding: 75%
- Volume of distribution: 0.8–2.0 L/kg
- Salivary concentrations: carbamazepine is secreted into saliva and concentrations are similar to the unbound levels seen in plasma

Metabolism
- Metabolized in the liver, primarily by CYP3A4, with some contribution by CYP2C8, to carbamazepine-10,11-epoxide, which is pharmacologically active
- Carbamazepine-10,11-epoxide is in turn metabolized, by means of epoxide hydrolase, to an inactive *trans* carbamazepine diol
- Carbamazepine undergoes autoinduction so that clearance can increase threefold within several weeks of starting therapy and this often requires an upward dosage adjustment

Elimination
- Following a single dose, half-life values in adults and children are 18–55 hours and 3–32 hours, respectively
- During maintenance carbamazepine monotherapy half-life values in adults and children are 8–20 hours and 10–13 hours, respectively
- In the elderly carbamazepine half-life values are 30–50 hours
- Half-life of carbamazepine-10,11-epoxide is ~34 hours
- Renal excretion: <2% of an administered dose is excreted unchanged in urine

Drug Interaction Profile
Pharmacokinetic Drug Interactions
- Interactions between AEDs: effects on carbamazepine:
  - Acetazolamide, via an unknown mechanism, can *increase* carbamazepine plasma levels
  - Brivaracetam, felbamate, methsuximide, oxcarbazepine, perampanel, phenobarbital, phenytoin, primidone, and rufinamide can increase the clearance of carbamazepine and *decrease* carbamazepine plasma levels
  - Clobazam and stiripentol can decrease the clearance of carbamazepine and *increase* carbamazepine plasma levels
  - Brivaracetam, clobazam, felbamate, oxcarbazepine, phenobarbital, primidone valproic acid, and zonisamide can inhibit the metabolism of epoxide hydrolase and *increase* carbamazepine-10,11-epoxide plasma levels

- Interactions between AEDs: effects by carbamazepine:
  - Carbamazepine can *decrease* plasma levels of clobazam, clonazepam, eslicarbazepine, ethosuximide, felbamate, lamotrigine, levetiracetam, oxcarbazepine, perampanel, phenytoin, primidone, rufinamide, stiripentol, sulthiame, tiagabine, topiramate, valproic acid, and zonisamide
- Interactions between AEDs and non-AED drugs: effects on carbamazepine:
  - Cimetidine, ciprofloxacin, clarithromycin, danazol, diltiazem, erythromycin, fluconazole, fluoxetine, flurithromycin, fluvoxamine, gemfibrozil, grapefruit juice, haloperidol, indinavir, influenza virus, isoniazid, isotretinoin, josamycin, ketoconazole, Kinnow juice, lopinavir, metronidazole, miconazole, nefazodone, nelfinavir, nicotinamide, piperine, ponsinomycin, propoxyphene, resveratrol, risperidone, ritonavir, ticlopidine, trazodone, troleandomycin, verapamil, and viloxazine can *increase* carbamazepine plasma levels
  - Armodafinil, Atkins diet (modified), cisplatin, colestipol, efavirenz, Free and Easy Wanderer Plus, probenecid, rifampicin, St. John's wort, and theophylline can *decrease* carbamazepine plasma levels
  - Loxapine and quetiapine can *increase* carbamazepine-epoxide plasma levels
- Interactions between AEDs and non-AED drugs: effects by carbamazepine:
  - Carbamazepine can *increase* plasma levels of clomipramine, lithium, and oxiracetam
  - Carbamazepine can *decrease* plasma levels of acetaminophen, albendazole, alprazolam, 9-aminocamptothecin, amitriptyline, aripiprazole, armodafinil, atracurium, bromperidol, bupropion, 1-(2-chloroethyl)-3-cyclohexyl-1-nitrosourea (CCNU), chlorpromazine, cisatracurium, citalopram, clozapine, codeine, cortisol, cyclophosphamide, cyclosporin, desipramine, dexamethasone, dexmedetomidine, doxacurium, doxepin, doxycycline, efavirenz, erythromycin, felodipine, fentanyl, fexofenadine, fluphenazine, glufosfamide, haloperidol, imatinib, imipramine, indinavir, itraconazole, ivabradine, ketoconazole, lapatinib, lidocaine, mebendazole, methadone, methotrexate, methylprednisolone, mianserin, mirtazapine, moclobemide, nefazodone, nevirapine, nilvadipine, nimodipine, nortriptyline, olanzapine, omeprazole, paclitaxel, paliperidone, pancuronium, phenprocoumon, pipecuronium, pomalidomide, praziquantel, prednisolone, procarbazine, quetiapine, rapacuronium, risperidone, rocuronium, sertraline, simvastatin, tacrolimus, temozolamide, temsirolimus, teniposide, theophylline, thiotepa, trazodone, valnoctamide, vecuronium, vincristine, voriconazole, warfarin, ziprasidone, and zolpidem

Pharmacodynamic Drug Interactions
- Co-medication with lamotrigine: neurotoxicity may present as headache, nausea, diplopia, and ataxia – this occurs in the absence of any

change in lamotrigine, carbamazepine, or carbamazepine-epoxide plasma levels
- Co-medication with levetiracetam: neurotoxicity may present as nystagmus, diplopia, ataxia, nausea, and vomiting – this occurs in the absence of any change in levetiracetam, carbamazepine, or carbamazepine-epoxide plasma levels
- Co-medication with eslicarbazepine acetate: neurotoxicity may present as diplopia, abnormal coordination, and dizziness – this occurs in the absence of any change in eslicarbazepine, carbamazepine, or carbamazepine-epoxide plasma levels
- Co-medication with lacosamide: neurotoxicity may occur in the absence of any change in lacosamide, carbamazepine, or carbamazepine-epoxide plasma levels
- Co-medication with perampanel: neurotoxicity may present as increased sedation – this occurs in the absence of any change in perampanel, carbamazepine, or carbamazepine-epoxide plasma levels

Hormonal Contraception
- Carbamazepine enhances the metabolism of oral contraceptives so as to decrease plasma levels of hormonal contraceptives and to reduce their effectiveness, leading to breakthrough bleeding and contraceptive failure; medium- or high-dose oral contraceptive preparations are indicated in patients taking carbamazepine, in addition to recommendations for additional barrier contraceptives and folic acid 1,000 mg daily in all women of childbearing potential

Adverse Effects
How Drug Causes Adverse Effects
- CNS adverse effects theoretically due to excessive actions at voltage-sensitive sodium channels
- Major pharmacologically active metabolites (carbamazepine-10,11-epoxide) may be the cause of many adverse effects
- Mild anticholinergic effects may contribute to sedation and blurred vision

Common Adverse Effects
- Sedation, dizziness, confusion, unsteadiness, headache
- Nausea, vomiting, diarrhea
- Blurred vision
- Benign leukopenia (transient; in up to 10%)
- Hyponatremia, neutropenia
- Rash

Life-threatening or Dangerous Adverse Effects
- Rare aplastic anemia, agranulocytosis (unusual bleeding or bruising, mouth sores, infections, fever, sore throat)

- Rare severe dermatologic reactions (Stevens–Johnson syndrome), which have been shown to be strongly associated with the human leukocyte antigen (HLA)-B*1502 allele in Southeast Asian populations; the presence of the HLA-A*3101 allele was found to be associated with a fivefold increase in hypersensitivity reactions in subjects of Northern European ancestry
- Rare cardiac problems (e.g., bradycardia, arrhythmia, atrioventricular block)
- Rare induction of psychosis or mania
- Syndrome of inappropriate antidiuretic hormone secretion (SIADH) with hyponatremia
- Increased frequency of generalized convulsions (in patients with atypical absence seizures)
- Vitamin K-deficient hemorrhagic disease in newborns of mothers treated with carbamazepine; can be prevented by administration of vitamin K to the mother before delivery

Rare and not Life-threatening Adverse Effects
- Aseptic meningitis accompanied by myoclonus and peripheral eosinophilia
- Anaphylactic reaction
- Angioneurotic edema
- Osteomalacia/osteoporosis
- Taste disturbances
- Arthralgia, muscle pain, muscle spasm

Weight Change
- Not usual; weight gain could be related to water retention; however, increased appetite and increased weight without edema can also occur

What to do About Adverse Effects
- Discuss common and severe adverse effects with patients or parents before starting medication, including symptoms that should be reported to the physician
- Risk of serious adverse effects is greatest in the first few months of treatment
- CNS-related adverse effects are usually dose-dependent, are reversible, and are prevented by slow and upward titration following initiation of treatment
- Common adverse effects such as sedation often abate after a few months
- Take with food or split dose to avoid gastrointestinal effects
- Switch to extended-release carbamazepine because dosage frequency as well as sedation, diplopia, confusion, and ataxia may be reduced
- Extended-release carbamazepine can be sprinkled on soft food

C

ADVERSE EFFECTS

C

Dosing and Use

Usual Dosage Range
- Adults and children over 12 years of age: 800–1200 mg/day
- Children 6–12 years of age: 600–1000 mg/day
- Children under 6 years of age: 30–40 mg/kg/day

Available Formulations
- Tablets: 100 mg, 200 mg, 400 mg
- Chewable tablets: 100 mg, 200 mg
- Liquid (oral suspension): 300 mL, 450 mL (100 mg/5 mL)
- Suppositories: 125 mg, 250 mg
- Extended-release tablets: 100 mg, 200 mg, 400 mg
- Extended-release capsules: 200 mg, 300 mg

How to Dose
- When initiating carbamazepine treatment start with a low dose and titrate slowly so as to minimize adverse effects
  - *For adults and children over 12 years of age:* start treatment with 200 mg twice daily (tablet) or 1 teaspoon (100 mg) four times a day (suspension); each week increase by up to 200 mg/day in divided doses (two doses for extended-release formulation, three–four doses for other tablets); maintenance dose generally 800–1200 mg/day for adults; some patients may require up to 1600 mg/day
  - *Children 6–12 years old:* start treatment with 100 mg/day twice daily or 0.5 teaspoon (50 mg) four times a day (suspension) and increase at weekly intervals in increments of 100 mg/day in divided doses (two doses for extended-release formulation, three–four doses for all other formulations); maximum dose generally 1000 mg/day; maintenance dose generally 600–1000 mg/day
  - *Children under 6 years:* start treatment with 5–10 mg/kg/day in two or three divided doses for tablet formulations (four doses for suspension) and increase at weekly intervals in increments of 5–10 mg/kg/day; maintenance dose of 30 mg/kg/day or more is often required and dosage requirement increases twofold in children co-prescribed enzyme-inducing AEDs

Dosing Tips
- Higher peak plasma levels occur with the suspension formulation than with the same dose of the tablet formulation, so suspension should generally be started at a lower dose and titrated slowly
- Take carbamazepine with food to avoid gastrointestinal effects
- Slow dose titration may delay onset of therapeutic action but enhance tolerability to sedating effects
- Should titrate slowly in the presence of other sedating agents, such as other AEDs to best tolerate additive sedative adverse effects
- Can sometimes minimize the impact of carbamazepine upon the bone marrow by dosing slowly and monitoring closely when initiating treatment; initial trend to leukopenia/neutropenia may reverse

C

with continued conservative dosing over time and allow subsequent dosage increases with careful monitoring

• Carbamazepine often requires a dosage adjustment upward with time as the drug induces its own metabolism, thus lowering its own plasma levels over the first several weeks to months of treatment

• Do not break or chew carbamazepine extended-release tablets as this will alter the controlled-release properties

• Generally higher doses of the extended-release formulations are possible (because of the reduction in diurnal changes in plasma carbamazepine blood levels), resulting in better seizure control and reduced intermittent diurnal adverse effects

How to Withdraw Drug

• May need to adjust dosage of concurrent medications as carbamazepine is being discontinued, because plasma levels of other drugs may change (see Pharmacokinetic Drug Interactions section)

• Rapid discontinuation may increase the risk of seizures

Overdose

• Can be fatal (lowest known fatal dose in adults is 3.2 g, in adolescents is 4 g, and in children is 1.6 g): symptoms include nausea, vomiting, involuntary movements, urinary retention, trouble breathing, sedation, coma

• The stomach should be emptied immediately by lavage or by induction of emesis

• Hemodialysis removes carbamazepine from blood and, therefore, serves as a useful procedure in cases of overdose

Tests and Therapeutic Drug Monitoring

• Before starting: blood count, liver tests, serum sodium

• Because severe dermatologic reactions (Stevens–Johnson syndrome) have been shown to be strongly associated with the HLA-B*1502 allele in Southeast Asian populations, testing for this allele must be carried out before starting carbmazepine in patients of Han Chinese, Thai, and other Southeastern Asian origin

• During treatment: blood count at 3 months, then every 6 months throughout treatment

• During treatment: consider monitoring sodium levels because of possibility of hyponatremia, as well as liver, kidney, and thyroid function tests as needed

• Because carbamazepine can alter vitamin D metabolism and affect bone mass, 25-hydroxyvitamin D levels should be monitored in all patients, and vitamin D supplementation should be prescribed as needed

• Therapeutic drug monitoring:
  – Optimum seizure control in patients on monotherapy is most likely to occur at carbamazepine plasma concentrations of 4–12 mg/L (17–51 μmol/L)

- The conversion factor from mg/L to μmol/L is 4.23 (i.e., 1 mg/L = 4.23 μmol/L)
- Because children metabolize carbamazepine more rapidly, resulting in carbamazepine-10,11-epoxide levels approaching those of carbamazepine, carbamazepine-10,11-epoxide makes a greater contribution to the pharmacological effects (both beneficial and toxic) of carbamazepine in children than in adults
- The upper boundary of the reference range for carbamazepine-10,11-epoxide is 9 μmol/L
- The conversion factor from mg to μmol is 3.96 (i.e., 1 mg/L = 3.96 μmol/L)
- The reference range of carbamazepine in plasma is considered to be the same for children and adults, although no data are available to support this clinical practice
- Carbamazepine can be monitored by use of saliva, which is a measure of the free non-protein-bound plasma concentration and is pharmacologically relevant

Other Warnings/Precautions
- Patients should be monitored carefully for signs of unusual bleeding or bruising, mouth sores, infections, fever, or sore throat, as the risk of aplastic anemia and agranulocytosis with carbamazepine use is five to eight times greater than in the general population (risk in the untreated general population is 6 patients per 1 million per year for agranulocytosis and 2 patients per 1 million per year for aplastic anemia)
- Because carbamazepine has a tricyclic chemical structure, it is not recommended to be taken with MAOIs, including 14 days after MAOIs are stopped; do not start an MAOI until 2 weeks after discontinuing carbamazepine
- May exacerbate narrow angle-closure glaucoma
- May need to restrict fluid intake because of risk of developing SIADH, hyponatremia, and its complications
- Use with caution in patients with mixed seizure disorders that include atypical absence seizures because carbamazepine has been associated with increased frequency of generalized convulsions in such patients

Do not Use
- If patient has a proven allergy to tricyclic compounds
- If patient has a proven allergy to carbamazepine, oxcarbazepine, or eslicarbazepine acetate
- If patient has bone marrow suppression
- If patient is taking an MAOI

C

Special Populations
Renal Impairment
- Carbamazepine is renally secreted, therefore, the dose may need to be lowered
- Because carbamazepine can be removed by hemodialysis, patients receiving hemodialysis may require supplemental doses of carbamazepine

Hepatic Impairment
- Carbamazepine is extensively metabolized in the liver and consequently lower doses may be required

Children
- Children have an increased metabolic capacity and consequently higher doses on an mg/kg basis are usually required to achieve the equivalent therapeutic plasma levels seen in adults
- Pharmacokinetic interactions in children are usually of a greater magnitude than that seen in adults

Elderly
- Elderly patients are more susceptible to adverse effects and therefore may not tolerate higher doses
- Because of an age-related reduction in renal and hepatic function, lower initial and target carbamazepine doses are appropriate
- Elderly patients are often prescribed concurrent drug therapies for comorbidities and therefore may be at greater risk for pharmacokinetic and pharmacodynamic interactions; the risk of pharmacokinetic interactions with carbamazepine is substantial

Pregnancy
- Specialist advice should be given to women who are of childbearing potential; they should be informed about the teratogenicity of all AEDs and the importance of avoiding an unplanned pregnancy; the AED treatment regimen should be reviewed when a woman is planning to become pregnant
- Rapid discontinuation of AEDs should be avoided as this may lead to breakthrough seizures, which could have serious consequences for the woman and the unborn child
- Carbamazepine was previously classified by the US FDA as risk category D (positive evidence of risk to human fetus; potential benefits may still justify its use during pregnancy); the current FDA Pregnancy and Lactation Rule has eliminated pregnancy risk category labels
- Use during first trimester may raise risk of neural tube defects (e.g., spina bifida) or other congenital anomalies
- Use in women of childbearing potential requires weighing potential benefits to the mother against the risks to the fetus

SPECIAL POPULATIONS

C

- If drug is to be continued, start on folate 1 mg/day before a planned pregnancy in all women of childbearing potential to reduce risk of neural tube defects
- Use with other AEDs in combination may cause a higher risk for teratogenic effects than carbamazepine monotherapy
- Taper drug if discontinuing
- Vitamin K-deficient hemorrhagic disease in newborns of mothers treated with carbamazepine can be prevented by administration of vitamin K to the mother before delivery
- Seizures, even mild seizures, may cause harm to the embryo/fetus
- Data on the pharmacokinetic changes of carbamazepine during pregnancy are conflicting; carbamazepine clearance can increase by up to 20% during pregnancy, accompanied by a decrease in the total plasma concentration of up to 42% and a 22% decrease in the free (pharmacologically active) concentration

Breast Feeding
- Breast milk: carbamazepine: 10–30% of maternal plasma levels; carbamazepine-10,11-epoxide: 50% of maternal plasma levels
- Breastfed infants: carbamazepine plasma levels are 10–20% of maternal plasma levels
- If drug is continued while breast feeding, infant should be monitored for possible adverse effects, including hematological effects
- Recommend bottle feeding if infant shows signs of irritability or sedation
- Some cases of neonatal seizures, respiratory depression, vomiting, and diarrhea have been reported in infants whose mothers received carbamazepine during pregnancy

The Overall Place of Carbamazepine in the Treatment of Epilepsy

Carbamazepine is particularly effective for the treatment of focal epilepsies (idiopathic or symptomatic) with or without secondary generalized tonic–clonic seizures. Carbamazepine is considered to be the drug of choice in nocturnal frontal lobe epilepsies, especially the channelopathy autosomal dominant nocturnal frontal lobe epilepsy. It is also effective in primary generalized tonic–clonic seizures, although may aggravate other generalized seizures types frequently seen in idiopathic or symptomatic generalized epilepsy syndromes, including absence, atypical absence, myoclonic, or tonic seizure types. Comparative studies show that carbamazepine is superior to most other older AEDs (e.g., phenytoin, phenobarbital, primidone, and valproate), and amongst the newer AEDs, levetiracetam may have similar efficacy, although several newer drugs are more tolerable and safer, including gabapentin, lamotrigine, and levetiracetam. However, carbamazepine is ineffective

CARBAMAZEPINE

C

in neonatal or febrile seizures and is contraindicated and ineffective in idiopathic generalized epilepsies and epileptic encephalopathies.

Primary Seizure Types
• Focal epilepsies of any type (idiopathic or symptomatic) with or without secondary generalized tonic–clonic seizures
• Primary generalized tonic–clonic seizures

Secondary Seizure Types
• None

Potential Advantages
• Carbamazepine is a particularly good AED for the treatment of focal epilepsies of any type (idiopathic or symptomatic) with or without secondary generalized tonic–clonic seizures
• Also effective in primary generalized tonic–clonic seizures
• In numerous comparative studies, no other AED showed better efficacy than carbamazepine in focal seizures, although some of the new AEDs are better tolerated
• Contrary to previous studies, a recent pregnancy register found that the risk of teratogenicity is small – monotherapy serious malformation rates are 2.3% versus 2.4% for no AED

Potential Disadvantages
• Idiosyncratic and other adverse effects
• Requires frequent blood testing and close monitoring
• Pharmacokinetics are not linear due to autoinduction
• Associated with significant pharmacokinetic interactions and usually acts as an inducer of drug metabolism
• Potential teratogen

Suggested Reading

Callaghan N, Kenny RA, O'Neil B, Crowley M, Goggin T. A prospective study between carbamazepine, phenytoin and sodium valproate as monotherapy in previously untreated and recently diagnosed patients with epilepsy. *Journal of Neurology, Neurosurgery, and Psychiatry* 1985; **48**: 639–644.

Chen P, Lin JJ, Lu CS, et al. Carbamazepine-induced toxic effects and HLA-B*1502 screening in Taiwan. *New England Journal of Medicine* 2011; **364**: 1126–1133.

Johannessen Landmark C, Patsalos PN. Drug interactions involving the new second- and third-generation antiepileptic drugs. *Expert Reviews in Neurotherapeutics* 2010; **10**: 119–140.

Marson AG, Al-Kharusi AM, Alwaidh M, et al. SANAD Study group. The SANAD study of effectiveness of carbamazepine, gabapentin, lamotrigine, oxcarbazepine, or topiramate for treatment of partial epilepsy: an unblinded randomised controlled trial. *Lancet* 2007; **369**: 1000–1015.

Mattson RH, Cramer JA, Collins JF. A comparison of valproate with carbamazepine for the treatment of complex partial seizures and secondarily generalized tonic-clonic seizures in adults. The Department of Veterans Affairs Epilepsy Cooperative Study. *New England Journal of Medicine* 1992; **327**: 765–771.

McCormack M, Alfirevic A, Bourgeois S, et al. HLA-A*3101 and carbamazepine-induced hypersensitivity reactions in Europeans. *New England Journal of Medicine* 2011; **364**: 1134–1143.

Misra A, Aggarwal A, Singh O, Sharma S. Effect of carbamazepine therapy on vitamin D and parathormone in epileptic children. *Pediatric Neurology* 2010; **43**: 320–324.

Patsalos PN. *Antiepileptic drug interactions – a clinical guide*, 3rd edition. Springer, London, UK; 2016.

Patsalos PN, Berry DJ, Bourgeois BFD, Cloyd JC, Glauser TA, Johannessen SI, Leppik IE, Tomson T, Perucca E. Antiepileptic drugs – best practice guidelines for therapeutic drug monitoring: a position paper by the Subcommission on Therapeutic Drug Monitoring, ILAE Commission on Therapeutic Strategies. *Epilepsia* 2008; **49**: 1239–1276.

Patsalos PN, Froscher W, Pisani F, van Rijn CM. The importance of drug interactions in epilepsy therapy. *Epilepsia* 2002; **43**: 365–385.

Patsalos PN, Perucca E. Clinically important interactions in epilepsy: general features and interactions between antiepileptic drugs. *Lancet Neurology* 2003; **2**: 347–356.

Patsalos PN, Perucca E. Clinically important interactions in epilepsy: interactions between antiepileptic drugs and other drugs. *Lancet Neurology* 2003; **2**: 473–481.

Powell G, Saunders M, Rigby A, Marson AG. Immediate-release versus controlled-release carbamazepine in the treatment of epilepsy. *Cochrane Database Systematic Review* 2016; **12**:CD007124.

Rambeck B, Salke-Treumann A, May T, Boenigh HE. Valproic acid induced carbamazepine-10,11-epoxide toxicity in children and adolescents. *European Neurology* 1990; **30**:79–83.

CARBAMAZEPINE

CLOBAZAM

Therapeutics

Chemical Name and Structure

Clobazam, 7-chloro-1-methyl-5-phenyl-1,5-benzodiazepine-2, 4-dione, is a white crystalline powder, with a molecular weight of 300.74 and an empirical formula of $C_{16}H_{13}O_2O_2$.

Brand Names
- Asabium
- Castilium; Clarmyl; Clobamax; Clobazan; Clopax
- Frisium
- Grifoclobam
- Karidium
- Lucium
- Noiafren
- Onfi
- Perizam
- Sederlona
- Tapclob
- Urbadan; Urbanil; Urbanol; Urbanyl

Generics Available
- Yes

Licensed Indications for Epilepsy
- Adjunctive intermittent therapy of partial or generalized seizures (UK SPC)
- Non-convulsive status epilepticus (UK SPC)
- Adjunctive treatment of seizures associated with Lennox–Gastaut syndrome in patients aged 2 years or older (FDA PI)
- Monotherapy for catamenial seizures (UK SPC)

Licensed Indications for Non-epilepsy Conditions
- Anxiolytic (UK SPC)
- Adjunctive treatment of schizophrenic or other psychotic illnesses (UK SPC)

C

Non-licensed Use for Epilepsy
• Reading epilepsy
• Febrile seizures
• Startle epilepsy
• Alcohol withdrawal seizures
• Benign childhood partial epilepsies

Non-licensed Use for Non-epilepsy Conditions
• There are none

Ineffective (Contraindicated)
• Data on seizure contraindications are not available

Mechanism of Action
• Binds to benzodiazepine receptors at the gamma-aminobutyric acid (GABA$_A$) ligand-gated chloride channel complex
• Enhances the inhibitory effects of GABA
• Boosts chloride conductance through GABA-regulated channels

Efficacy Profile
• Clobazam is commonly combined with other AEDs for the treatment of seizures
• The goals of treatment are to achieve complete seizure remission when possible, or at least improved frequency and severity of seizures, while also minimizing adverse effects and improving patient quality of life
• Onset of action may occur within the first few days
• Continue treatment until all symptoms are gone or until improvement is stable and then continue treating indefinitely as long as improvement persists
• Continue treatment indefinitely to avoid recurrence of seizures
• If clobazam is ineffective or only partially effective, it can be replaced by or combined with another AED that is appropriate for the patient's seizure type or epilepsy syndrome

CLOBAZAM

Pharmacokinetics
Absorption and Distribution
• Oral bioavailability: >95%
• Food co-ingestion: does not affect the extent of absorption but does slow the rate of absorption
• Tmax: 1–3 hours
• Time to steady state: 2–7 days (7–10 days if the pharmacologically active *N*-desmethylclobazam metabolite is included)
• Pharmacokinetics: linear
• Protein binding: 85%

C

- Volume of distribution: 0.87–1.83 L/kg
- Salivary concentrations: clobazam and N-desmethylclobazam are secreted into saliva and concentrations are similar to the unbound levels seen in plasma

Metabolism
- Metabolized in the liver, primarily by desmethylation, to N-desmethylclobazam, which is pharmacologically active
- Clobazam also undergoes metabolism by hydroxylation to form other metabolites, namely 4-hydroxyclobazam and 4-hydroxy desmethylclobazam
- N-desmethylclobazam undergoes further metabolism via the action of CYP2C19
- In patients who are poor CYP2C19 metabolizers, levels of N-desmethylclobazam increase
- The N-desmethylclobazam metabolite is pharmacologically active and contributes substantially to the efficacy of clobazam and also to its adverse-effect profile
- Autoinduction is not a feature of clobazam metabolism

Elimination
- Elimination half-life values for clobazam in adults are 10–30 hours
- Elimination half-life values for N-desmethylclobazam in adults are 36–46 hours
- In children clobazam half-life values are ~16 hours
- In the elderly clobazam half-life values are 30–48 hours
- Renal excretion: the excreted unchanged clobazam in urine is insignificant

Drug Interaction Profile
Pharmacokinetic Drug Interactions
- Interactions between AEDs: effects on clobazam:
  - Carbamazepine, perampanel, phenobarbital, and phenytoin can *increase* the clearance of clobazam and *decrease* clobazam plasma levels; concurrently N-desmethylclobazam plasma levels may also be increased
  - Felbamate can *decrease* the clearance of clobazam and *increase* clobazam plasma levels; concurrently N-desmethylclobazam plasma levels are also increased
  - Stiripentol can *decrease* the clearance of clobazam and, more potently, of N-desmethylclobazam and *increases* clobazam plasma levels and N-desmethylclobazam plasma levels

C

– Sulthiame can *decrease* the clearance of N-desmethylclobazam and *increases* N-desmethylclobazam plasma levels; clobazam plasma levels are unaffected
• Interactions between AEDs: effects by clobazam:
– Clobazam can *increase* plasma levels of phenytoin, primidone, stiripentol, and valproic acid
– Clobazam can *increase* the plasma levels of carbamazepine; concurrently carbamazepine-epoxide plasma levels are also increased
• Interactions between AEDs and non–AED drugs: effects on clobazam:
– Atkins diet (modified) can *decrease* clobazam and N-desmethylclobazam plasma levels
– Cimetidine can *increase* clobazam plasma levels but has no effect on N-desmethylclobazam plasma levels
– Etravirine, ketoconazole, miconazole, and omeprazole can *increase* clobazam plasma levels and also N-desmethylclobazam plasma levels
• Interactions between AEDs and non–AED drugs: effects by clobazam:
– Clobazam can *increase* plasma levels of dextromethorphan
– Clobazam can *decrease* plasma levels of tolbutamide

Pharmacodynamic Drug Interactions
• Clobazam can potentiate the effects of CNS depressants such as alcohol, barbiturates, and neuroleptics

Hormonal Contraception
• Clobazam does not enhance the metabolism of oral contraceptives so as to decrease plasma levels of hormonal contraceptives and, therefore, does not compromise contraception control

Adverse Effects
How Drug Causes Adverse Effects
• Same mechanism for adverse effects as for therapeutic effects – namely due to excessive actions at benzodiazepine receptors
• Long-term adaptations in benzodiazepine receptors may explain the development of dependence, tolerance, and withdrawal
• Adverse effects are generally immediate, but immediate adverse effects often disappear in time
• Major metabolite (N-desmethylclobazam) may contribute to the adverse effects observed

Common Adverse Effects
• Sedation (sometimes intolerably severe)
• Drowsiness, fatigue
• Hyposalivation, dryness of mouth
• Loss of appetite, constipation
• Behavioral and cognitive impairment
• Restlessness, aggressiveness, coordination disturbances

C

- Severe aggressive outbursts, hyperactivity, insomnia, and depression with suicidal ideation may occur, particularly in children
- Physical dependence characterized by a withdrawal syndrome when the drug is withdrawn – physical dependence develops more rapidly with larger doses

Life-threatening or Dangerous Adverse Effects
- Withdrawal syndrome in chronic use
- Respiratory depression, especially at high doses and when taken with CNS depressants in overdose
- Serious skin reaction may occur, including Stevens–Johnson syndrome and toxic epidermal necrosis

Rare and not Life-threatening Adverse Effects
- Amnesia accompanied by inappropriate behavior
- Hallucination, nightmare
- Unsteadiness of gait
- Nystagmus
- Loss of libido

Weight Change
- Not common

What to do About Adverse Effects
- Discuss common and severe adverse effects with patients or parents before starting medication, including symptoms that should be reported to the physician
- Lower the dose
- Somnolence may be partly prevented by administering the drug in small doses 1 hour before sleep

Dosing and Use
Usual Dosage Range
- Adults and children over 12 years of age: 20–40 mg/day
- Children under 12 years of age: 0.4–1.0 mg/kg/day

Available Formulations
- Tablets: 10 mg
- Capsules: 10 mg
- Oral suspension: 150 mL (1 mg/mL), 150 mL (2 mg/mL), 120 mL (2.5 mg/mL)

How to Dose
- When initiating clobazam treatment start with a low dose and titrate slowly so as to minimize adverse effects.

C

- *For adults and children over 12 years of age:* start treatment with 5–10 mg/day at night and increase at weekly intervals in increments of 5 mg/day up to a total of 40 mg/day
- *Children under 12 years of age:* start treatment with 0.25 mg/kg/day and increase at weekly intervals, as tolerated, in increments of 0.25 mg/kg/day up to a total of 1.0 mg/kg/day; doses of up to 2.0 mg/kg/day may be helpful and are usually well tolerated

Dosing Tips
- Administer as adjunctive therapy in all drug-resistant epilepsies at a dose of 20–30 mg nocte – half this dose in children <5 years old
- Using the oral suspension is particularly helpful for the low initial doses in younger children
- Twice-a-day dosing is fine – smaller dose should be ingested in the day with the larger dose just before sleep
- Tolerance may develop but more than a third of patients do not develop tolerance
- When clobazam is effective, most patients continue to benefit for years without drug dependence or unwanted adverse effects

How to Withdraw Drug
- May need to adjust dosage of concurrent medications as clobazam is being discontinued, because plasma levels of other drugs may change (see Pharmacokinetic Drug Interactions section)
- Withdrawal should be very slow, occurring over 4–6 months
- Rapid discontinuation often leads to withdrawal symptoms, seizures, and status epilepticus

Overdose
- To date, there have been no cases of overdose reported with clobazam
- The stomach should be emptied immediately by lavage or by induction of emesis
- Treatment of overdose consists of supportive care and the administration of the benzodiazepine receptor antagonist flumazenil
- It is not known whether hemodialysis removes clobazam from blood and, therefore, would serve as a useful procedure in cases of overdose

Tests and Therapeutic Drug Monitoring
- During treatment: periodic liver tests and blood counts may be prudent
- Therapeutic drug monitoring:
  - Optimum seizure control in patients on monotherapy is most likely to occur at clobazam plasma concentrations of 0.03–0.30 mg/L (0.1–1.0 μmol/L)
  - The conversion factor from mg/L to μmol/L is 3.33 (i.e., 1 mg/L = 3.33 μmol/L)
  - The reference range for N-desmethylclobazam is 0.30–3.00 mg/L (1–10 μmol/L)

C

- The conversion factor from mg/L to μmol/L is 3.49 (i.e., 1 mg/L = 3.49 μmol/L)
- The reference ranges of clobazam and *N*-desmethylclobazam in plasma are considered to be the same for children and adults, although no data are available to support this clinical practice
- Clobazam and *N*-desmethylclobazam can be monitored by use of saliva, which is a measure of the free non-protein-bound plasma concentration and is pharmacologically relevant

Other Warnings / Precautions
- Use with caution in patients with pulmonary disease; rare reports of death after initiation of benzodiazepines in patients with severe pulmonary impairment
- Use only with extreme caution if patient has obstructive sleep apnea
- Some depressed patients may experience a worsening of suicidal ideation
- Some patients may exhibit abnormal thinking or behavioral changes similar to those caused by other CNS depressants (i.e., either depressant actions or disinhibiting actions)
- Clobazam is a Schedule IV drug and the risk of dependence may increase with dose and duration of treatment

Do not Use
- If patient has respiratory depression
- If patient has acute pulmonary insufficiency
- If patient has sleep apnea syndrome
- If patient has marked neuromuscular respiratory weakness, including unstable myasthenia gravis
- If patient has severe liver disease
- If there is a proven allergy to clobazam or any other benzodiazepine
- Because some formulations contain lactose, patients with rare hereditary problems of galactose intolerance, Lapp lactose deficiency, or glucose–galactose malabsorption should not take this medicine

Special Populations
Renal Impairment
- Clobazam is renally secreted, so the dose may need to be lowered

Hepatic Impairment
- Clobazam is extensively metabolized in the liver and consequently lower doses may be required

Children
- Children have an increased metabolic capacity and consequently higher doses on an mg/kg basis are usually required to achieve the equivalent therapeutic plasma levels seen in adults

SPECIAL POPULATIONS

47

C

- Pharmacokinetic interactions in children are usually of a greater magnitude than that seen in adults

Elderly
- Elderly patients are more susceptible to adverse effects, and therefore may not tolerate higher doses
- Because of an age-related reduction in renal and hepatic function, lower clobazam doses are appropriate
- Elderly patients are often prescribed concurrent drug therapies for comorbidities and therefore may be at greater risk for pharmacokinetic and pharmacodynamic interactions; the risk of pharmacokinetic interactions with clobazam is moderate

Pregnancy
- Specialist advice should be given to women who are of childbearing potential; they should be informed about the teratogenicity of all AEDs and the importance of avoiding an unplanned pregnancy; the AED treatment regimen should be reviewed when a woman is planning to become pregnant
- Rapid discontinuation of AEDs should be avoided as this may lead to breakthrough seizures, which could have serious consequences for the woman and the unborn child
- Clobazam was previously classified by the US FDA as risk category C (some animal studies show adverse effects, no controlled studies in humans); the current FDA Pregnancy and Lactation Rule has eliminated pregnancy risk category labels
- Possible increased risk of birth defects when benzodiazepines are taken during pregnancy
- Infants whose mothers received a benzodiazepine late in pregnancy may experience withdrawal effects
- Neonatal flaccidity has been reported in infants whose mothers took a benzodiazepine during pregnancy
- Use in women of childbearing potential requires weighing potential benefits to the mother against the risks to the fetus
- If drug is continued, start on folate 1 mg/day early in pregnancy to reduce risk of neural tube defects
- Use with other AEDs in combination may cause a higher prevalence of teratogenic effects than clobazam monotherapy
- Taper drug if discontinuing
- Seizures, even mild seizures, may cause harm to the embryo/fetus
- Data on the pharmacokinetic changes of clobazam during pregnancy have not been identified

Breast Feeding
- Breast milk: clobazam plus *N*-desmethylclobazam: 13–36% of maternal plasma levels

CLOBAZAM

C

- Breastfed infants: it is not known what plasma clobazam and *N*-desmethylclobazam concentrations are achieved in breastfed infants compared with the levels of their mothers
- If drug is continued while breast feeding, infant should be monitored for possible adverse effects, including sedation and poor suckling
- Recommend bottle feed particularly if infant shows signs of sedation

The Overall Place of Clobazam in the Treatment of Epilepsy

Clobazam should be tried as adjunctive medication in all drug-resistant epilepsies, although it is less effective in symptomatic than in focal epilepsies. It is much less effective than clonazepam in myoclonic jerks and absences. Probably only 1 of 10 patients will have a clinically significant improvement, but this may be very dramatic and render the patient seizure-free. Clobazam has comparable effectiveness to carbamazepine and phenytoin as first-line monotherapy in children with newly diagnosed partial epilepsy. Its relatively wide spectrum of efficacy makes clobazam particularly suitable for the various types of seizures and epilepsy syndromes encountered in younger children, in whom the availability of an oral suspension facilitates the administration.

Primary Seizure Types
- All drug-resistant epilepsies

Secondary Seizure Types
- Reading epilepsy
- Febrile seizures
- Catamenial epilepsy
- Lennox–Gastaut syndrome
- Startle epilepsy
- Alcohol withdrawal seizures
- Benign childhood partial epilepsies

Potential Advantages
- Although tolerance may develop, more than 30% of patients do not develop tolerance
- When clobazam is effective, most patients continue to benefit for years without drug dependence or unwanted adverse effects
- Some patients (20%) experience dramatic seizure reduction and even become seizure-free

Potential Disadvantages
- Sedation
- Development of tolerance
- Associated with significant pharmacokinetic interactions and usually its metabolism is induced or inhibited
- Potential teratogen, but not more than most other AEDs

THE OVERALL PLACE OF CLOBAZAM

C

Suggested Reading

Anonymous. Clobazam has equivalent efficacy to carbamazepine and phenytoin as monotherapy for childhood epilepsy: Canadian Study Group for Childhood Epilepsy. *Epilepsia* 1998; **39**: 952–959.

Conry JA, Ng YT, Paolicchi JM, Kernitsky L, Mitchell WG, Ritter FJ, Collins SD, Tracy K, Kormany WN, Abdulnabi R, Riley B, Stolle J. Clobazam in the treatment of Lennox–Gastaut syndrome. *Epilepsia* 2009; **50**: 1158–1166.

Feely M, Gibson J. Intermittent clobazam for catamenial epilepsy: tolerance avoided. *Journal of Neurology, Neurosurgery, and Psychiatry* 1984; **47**: 1279–1282.

Kinoshita M, Ikeda A, Begum T, Terada K, Shibashaki H. Efficacy of low-dose, add-on therapy of clobazam (CLB) is produced by its major metabolite, *N*-desmethyl-CLB. *Journal of Neurological Sciences* 2007; **263**: 44–48.

Mechndiratta MM, Krishnamurthy M, Rajesh KN, Singh G. Clobazam monotherapy in drug naive adult patients with epilepsy. *Seizure* 2003; **12**: 226–228.

Ng YT, Collins SD. Clobazam. *Neurotherapeutics* 2007; **4**: 138–144.

Patsalos PN. *Antiepileptic drug interactions – a clinical guide*, 3rd edition. Springer, London, UK; 2016.

Patsalos PN, Zugman M, Lake C, James A, Ratnaraj N, Sander JW. Serum protein binding of 25 antiepileptic drugs in a routine clinical setting: a comparison of free non-protein-bound concentrations. *Epilepsia*, 2017; **58**: 1234–1243.

Riss J, Cloyd J, Gates J, Collins S. Benzodiazepines in epilepsy: pharmacology and pharmacokinetics. *Acta Neurologica Scandinavica* 2008; **118**: 69–86.

Sennoune S, Mesdjian E, Bonneton J, Genton P, Dravet C, Roger J. Interactions between clobazam and standard antiepileptic drugs in patients with epilepsy. *Therapeutic Drug Monitoring* 1992; **14**: 269–274.

Silva RC, Montenegro MA, Guerreiro CA, Guerreiro MM. Clobazam as add-on therapy in children with epileptic encephalopathy. *Canadian Journal of Neurological Sciences* 2006; **33**: 209–213.

CLOBAZAM

CLONAZEPAM

C

Therapeutics

Chemical Name and Structure

Clonazepam, 5-(2-chlorophenol)-1,3-dihydro-7-nitro-2H-1,4 benzo-diazepin-2-one, is a light yellow crystalline powder, with a molecular weight of 315.71 and an empirical formula of $C_{15}H_{10}ClN_3O_3$.

Brand Names

- Adnil; Almac; Alrest; Amotril; Antelepsin; Anxrea; Azpax
- Calmnir; Catier DT; Cleps; Clez; CLH MD; Cloam; Clon; Clonapax; Clonapik; Clonapilep; Clonark; Clonasig; Clonatrac; Clonatryl; Clonax; Clonaxyl; Clonazepamum; Cloneepam; Clonex; Clonix; Clonoasig; Clonopam; Clonotril; Clonzy; Clopam; Closed; Closis; Clotas; Clotweet; Cloze; Clozep DT; Clozer; Clozipam; Clozorix; Convaclon; Coquan; Cozil
- E–Cloz; Easyfeel; Eminaz; Epcon; Epicloz; Epilong; Epitril; Epizam
- Iktorivil
- Jasoclam
- Kenoket; Klonopin; Klopam; Kriadex
- Lansden; Logen MD; Lonazep; Lonin; Lonipax; Lozep
- MD Calm; Meloprax; Melzap
- Nazee; Neuryl; Nexclo; Norep; Nozim; Nupam
- Onapil; Ozepam
- Paxam; Petril; Povanil
- QP-Zep
- Ravotril; Repam; Revozip; Riklona; Rivatril; Rivotril
- Sezolan; Sezolep; Somnotril
- Ubitpam
- Xenotril SL
- Zaar; Zeficlar; Zepam; Zepamax; Zepanc; Zeptril; Zicam; Zolpidox; Zozep; Zymanta

C

Generics Available
• Yes

Licensed Indications for Epilepsy
• All of its licenses in the UK are for individuals of all ages
• Absence seizures (UK SPC; FDA PI)
• Akinetic seizures (FDA PI)
• Tonic seizures (UK SPC)
• Tonic–clonic seizures (UK SPC)
• Lennox–Gastaut syndrome (FDA PI)
• Myoclonic seizures (UK SPC; FDA PI)
• Partial (focal) seizures with or without secondary generalization (UK SPC)
• Status epilepticus (UK SPC)

Licensed Indications for Non-epilepsy Conditions
• Panic disorder (FDA PI)

Non-licensed Use for Epilepsy
• Acquired epileptic aphasia (Landau–Kleffner syndrome)
• Infantile spasms (West syndrome)
• Neonatal seizures
• Nocturnal spasms

Non-licensed Use for Non-epilepsy Conditions
• Insomnia
• Myoclonus (both cortical and subcortical)
• Parasomnias
• Periodic limb movement disorder
• Spasticity (short-term relief)
• Tic disorders

Ineffective (Contraindicated)
• Because of its sedation, problems during withdrawal, and hypersalivation, clonazepam is not indicated as first-line therapy for any type of seizures
• Tonic status epilepticus can be worsened by clonazepam
• Generalized tonic–clonic seizures can be exacerbated by clonazepam

Mechanism of Action
• Binds to benzodiazepine receptors at the $GABA_A$ ligand-gated chloride channel complex
• Enhances the inhibitory effects of GABA
• Boosts chloride conductance through GABA-regulated channels

CLONAZEPAM

Efficacy Profile
- Clonazepam is commonly combined with other AEDs for the treatment of seizures and usually only when better-tolerated adjunctive AEDs have not been helpful
- The goals of treatment are to achieve complete seizure remission when possible, or at least improved frequency and severity of seizures, while also minimizing adverse effects and improving patient quality of life
- Onset of action may occur within the first few days
- Effective against partial and generalized seizures: especially absence and myoclonic seizures
- Effective in the treatment of convulsive or non-convulsive status epilepticus, although its use as a second-line drug has been superseded in many centers by diazepam, midazolam, and lorazepam
- Continue treatment indefinitely to avoid recurrence of seizures
- If clonazepam is ineffective or only partially effective, it can be replaced by or combined with another AED that is appropriate for the patient's seizure type or epilepsy syndrome

Pharmacokinetics

Absorption and Distribution
- Oral bioavailability: >80%
- Food co-ingestion: it is not known whether food co-ingestion delays the rate of absorption or the extent of absorption
- Tmax: 1–4 hours (adults); 2–3 hours (children)
- Time to steady state: 2–10 days (adults); 5–7 days (children)
- Pharmacokinetics: linear
- Protein binding: 86%
- Volume of distribution: 1.5–4.4 L/kg
- Salivary concentrations: it is not known whether clonazepam is secreted into saliva and whether such concentrations are similar to the unbound levels seen in plasma

Metabolism
- Clonazepam is metabolized in the liver, primarily by CYP3A4, to 7-amino-clonazepam
- 7-amino-clonazepam is in turn metabolized by acetylation, by means of N-acetyl-transferase, to form 7-acetamido-clonazepam
- Clonazepam is also hydroxylated (isoenzymes not identified) to form 3-hydroxyclonazepam

C

PHARMACOKINETICS

- The 7-amino-clonazepam metabolite retains some pharmaco-logical activity; none of the other metabolites of clonazepam are pharmacologically active
- Autoinduction is not a feature of clonazepam metabolism

Elimination
- In healthy adult subjects half-life values are 17–56 hours
- In adult patients with enzyme-inducing AEDs half-life values are 12–46 hours
- In children half-life values are 22–33 hours
- In neonates half-life values are 22–81 hours
- Renal excretion: <1% of an administered dose is excreted unchanged in urine

Drug Interaction Profile
Pharmacokinetic Drug Interactions
- Interactions between AEDs: effects on clonazepam:
  - Carbamazepine, lamotrigine, phenobarbital, phenytoin, and primidone can *increase* the clearance of clonazepam and *decrease* clonazepam plasma levels
  - Felbamate can *decrease* the clearance of clonazepam and *increase* clonazepam plasma levels
- Interactions between AEDs: effects by clonazepam:
  - Clonazepam can *increase* or *decrease* the clearance of phenytoin and *decrease* or *increase* phenytoin plasma levels
- Interactions between AEDs and non-AED drugs: effects on clonazepam:
  - Amiodarone can *increase* clonazepam plasma levels
- Interactions between AEDs and non-AED drugs: effects by clonazepam:
  - Clonazepam can *decrease* the clearance of lithium and *increase* lithium plasma levels

Pharmacodynamic Drug Interactions
- Clonazepam can potentiate the effects of CNS depressants such as alcohol, barbiturates, neuroleptics, and sodium oxybate
- In combination with valproate, clonazepam is associated with pharmacodynamic synergism in patients with absence seizures resulting in enhanced seizure control

Hormonal Contraception
- Clonazepam does not enhance the metabolism of oral contraceptives so as to decrease plasma levels of hormonal contraceptives and, there-fore, does not compromise contraception control

C

Adverse Effects

How Drug Causes Adverse Effects
- Same mechanism for adverse effects as for therapeutic effects – namely due to excessive actions at benzodiazepine receptors
- Long-term adaptations in benzodiazepine receptors may explain the development of dependence, tolerance, and withdrawal
- Adverse effects are generally immediate, but immediate adverse effects often disappear in time

Common Adverse Effects
- Sedation, drowsiness, fatigue, depression
- Dizziness, ataxia, slurred speech, nystagmus
- Forgetfulness, confusion
- Hyperexcitability, nervousness
- Hypersalivation, dry mouth

Life-threatening or Dangerous Adverse Effects
- Withdrawal syndrome in chronic use
- Respiratory depression, especially when taken with CNS depressants in overdose
- Rare hepatic dysfunction, renal dysfunction, blood dyscrasias

Rare and not Life-threatening Adverse Effects
- Impotence
- Loss of libido
- Nausea, gastrointestinal symptoms
- Pruritus
- Urinary incontinence
- Urticaria

Weight Change
- Not common; weight gain reported but not expected

What to do About Adverse Effects
- Discuss common and severe adverse effects with patients or parents before starting medication, including symptoms that should be reported to the physician
- Lower the dose
- Take largest dose at bedtime to avoid sedative effects during the day

Dosing and Use

Usual Dosage Range
- Adults and children over 12 years of age: 4–10 mg/day
- Children up to 12 years of age: 0.1–0.2 mg/kg/day

C

Available Formulations
- Tablets: 0.5 mg, 1 mg, 2 mg
- Disintegrating wafer: 0.125 mg, 0.25 mg, 0.5 mg, 1 mg, 2 mg
- Liquid formulation: 1 mg/mL for dilution before iv injection
- Oral solution: 0.5 mg/5mL, 2 mg/mL

How to Dose
- When initiating clonazepam treatment start with a low dose and titrate slowly so as to minimize adverse effects.
  - *For adults and children over 12 years of age:* start treatment with 0.25 mg/day at night and increase at weekly intervals in increments of 0.25 mg/day; maintenance dose generally 4–10 mg/day; at doses > 4 mg/day some patients may require twice-a-day dosing.
  - *Children up to 12 years of age:* start treatment with 0.01–0.02 mg/kg/day and slowly increase up to 0.1–0.2 mg/kg/day
  - *Status epilepticus:* the usual preparation for emergency treatment is a 1-mL ampoule containing 1 mg clonazepam. For the treatment of early status epilepticus, clonazepam is usually given as a 1-mg iv bolus injection over 1 minute in adults, whereas 0.25–0.5 mg may be used in children. These doses can be repeated three times over a period of 3 hours. For established status epilepticus a short iv infusion may be used – clonazepam is constituted in a dextrose (5%) or 0.9% sodium chloride (normal saline) solution (1–2 mg in 250 mL)

Dosing Tips
- Doses much higher than 2 mg/day are associated with increased risk of dependence
- Frequency of dosing in practice is often greater than predicted from half-life, as duration of biological activity is often shorter than the pharmacokinetic terminal half-life
- Clonazepam accumulates during prolonged infusion, leading to hypotension, sedation, and finally, respiratory arrest. Too rapid an infusion may lead to severe hypotension and syncope, and continuous infusion should be avoided if possible

How to Withdraw Drug
- May need to adjust dosage of concurrent medications as clonazepam is being discontinued, because plasma levels of other drugs may change (see Pharmacokinetic Drug Interactions section)
- Withdrawal should be undertaken with caution
- Withdrawal at a rate of 0.25 mg per month will minimize withdrawal symptoms
- Typical withdrawal symptoms if withdrawal is abrupt include: rebound seizures, anxiety, tremor, insomnia, and, in some patients, psychotic episodes

C

Overdose
- Rarely fatal in monotherapy: symptoms include sedation, confusion, coma, diminished reflexes
- A fatality has been reported in a patient who overdosed with oxycodone and clonazepam
- If indicated the stomach should be emptied by lavage or by induction of emesis
- Treatment of overdose consists of supportive care and the administration of the benzodiazepine receptor antagonist flumazenil
- Hemodialysis removes clonazepam from blood and, therefore, serves as a useful procedure in cases of overdose

Tests and Therapeutic Drug Monitoring
- During treatment: periodic liver tests and blood counts may be prudent
- Therapeutic drug monitoring:
  - Optimum seizure control in patients on monotherapy is most likely to occur at clonazepam plasma concentrations of 0.013–0.070 mg/L (0.041–0.222 μmol/L)
  - The conversion factor from mg/L to μmol/L is 3.17 (i.e., 1 mg/L = 3.17 μmol/L)
  - The reference range of clonazepam in plasma is considered to be the same for children and adults, although no data are available to support this clinical practice
  - There are no data indicating the usefulness of monitoring clonazepam by use of saliva

Other Warnings / Precautions
- Use with caution in patients with pulmonary disease; there have been rare reports of death after initiation of benzodiazepines in patients with severe pulmonary impairment
- Use only with extreme caution if patient has untreated obstructive sleep apnea
- Some depressed patients may experience a worsening of suicidal ideation
- Some patients may exhibit abnormal thinking or behavioral changes similar to those caused by other CNS depressants (i.e., either depressant actions or disinhibiting actions)
- Clonazepam is a Schedule IV drug and the risk of dependence may increase with dose and duration of treatment

Do not Use
- If patient has respiratory depression
- If patient has acute pulmonary insufficiency
- If patient has untreated obstructive sleep apnea syndrome
- If patient has marked neuromuscular respiratory weakness, including unstable myasthenia gravis
- If patient has severe liver disease

C

CLONAZEPAM

- If there is a proven allergy to clonazepam or any other benzodi-azepine or to any of the excipients: tablets contain lactose
- Because formulation contains lactose, patients with rare hereditary problems of galactose intolerance, Lapp lactose deficiency, or glucose–galactose malabsorption should not take this medicine

Special Populations

Renal Impairment
- Clonazepam is renally secreted, so the dose may need to be lowered
- Because clonazepam can be removed by hemodialysis, patients receiving hemodialysis may require supplemental doses of clonazepam

Hepatic Impairment
- Clonazepam is extensively metabolized in the liver and consequently lower doses may be required

Children
- Children have an increased metabolic capacity and consequently higher doses on a mg/kg basis are usually required to achieve the equivalent therapeutic plasma levels seen in adults
- Long-term effects of clonazepam on children/adolescents are unknown
- Pharmacokinetic interactions in children are usually of a greater mag-nitude than that seen in adults

Elderly
- Elderly patients are more susceptible to adverse effects and therefore may not tolerate higher doses
- Because of an age-related reduction in renal and hepatic function, lower initial and target clonazepam doses are appropriate
- Elderly patients frequently receive concurrent drug therapies for comorbidities and therefore may be at greater risk for pharmacokinetic and pharmacodynamic interactions; the risk of pharmacokinetic interactions with clonazepam is moderate

Pregnancy
- Specialist advice should be given to women who are of childbearing potential; they should be informed about the teratogenicity of all AEDs and the importance of avoiding an unplanned pregnancy; the AED treatment regimen should be reviewed when a woman is planning to become pregnant
- Rapid discontinuation of AEDs should be avoided as this may lead to breakthrough seizures, which could have serious consequences for the woman and the unborn child
- Clonazepam was previously classified by the US FDA as risk category D (positive evidence of risk to human fetus; potential benefits may still justify its use during pregnancy); the current FDA Pregnancy and Lactation Rule has eliminated pregnancy risk category labels

- Possible increased risk of birth defects when benzodiazepines are taken during pregnancy
- Infants whose mothers received a benzodiazepine late in pregnancy may experience withdrawal effects
- Neonatal flaccidity has been reported in infants whose mothers took a benzodiazepine during pregnancy
- Seizures, even mild seizures, may cause harm to the embryo/fetus
- During pregnancy clonazepam pharmacokinetics change slightly so that clonazepam clearance increases by 17% but plasma concentrations remain approximately the same throughout pregnancy; a change in clonazepam dose is not expected to be required

Breast Feeding
- Breast milk: 13–33% of maternal plasma levels
- Breastfed infants: it is not known what plasma clonazepam concentrations are achieved in breastfed infants compared with the levels of their mothers
- If drug is continued while breast feeding, infant should be monitored for possible adverse effects, including sedation and apnea
- If adverse effects are observed, recommend bottle feeding

The Overall Place of Clonazepam in the Treatment of Epilepsy
Clonazepam, primarily as adjunctive therapy but also as monotherapy, is the most effective AED in the treatment of myoclonic jerks (superior to valproate), and is also effective in absences (although not as effective as valproate and ethosuximide). It is a drug of choice for reading epilepsy (superior to valproate) and is particularly effective in juvenile myoclonic epilepsy if the myoclonic jerks are not controlled by other AEDs. It has proven efficacy in tonic–clonic, partial, and absence status.

Primary Seizure Types
- Myoclonic jerks
- Absences
- Juvenile myoclonic epilepsy
- Status epilepticus
- Reading epilepsy

Secondary Seizure Types
- Acquired epileptic aphasia (Landau–Kleffner syndrome)
- Infantile spasms (West syndrome)
- Neonatal seizures

Potential Advantages
- Can be used as an adjunct or as monotherapy
- Generally used as second-line treatment for absence seizures if valproate or ethosuximide is ineffective

C

- Rapid onset of action
- Less sedation than some other benzodiazepines
- Longer duration of action than some other benzodiazepines (e.g., diazepam and midazolam)
- Availability of oral disintegrating wafer
- Easier to taper than some other benzodiazepines because of long half-life
- May have less abuse potential than some other benzodiazepines
- May cause less depression, euphoria, or dependence than some other benzodiazepines

Potential Disadvantages
- Development of tolerance may require dose increases
- Risk of dependence and/or tolerance, particularly for treatment periods longer than 12 weeks
- Potential for accumulation on prolonged infusion
- Respiratory arrest, hypotension, sedation, and thrombophlebitis
- Associated with significant pharmacokinetic interactions and usually its metabolism is induced or inhibited
- Potential teratogen

CLONAZEPAM

Suggested Reading

Dreifuss FE, Penry JK, Rose SW, Kupferberg HJ, Dyken P, Sato S. Serum clonazepam concentrations in children with absence seizures. *Neurology* 1975; **23**: 255–258.

Greenblatt DJ, Miller LG, Shader RI. Clonazepam pharmacokinetics, brain uptake, and receptor interactions. *Journal of Clinical Psychiatry* 1987; **48** (Suppl): 4–11.

Hakeem VF, Wallace SJ. EEG monitoring of therapy for neonatal seizures. *Developmental Medicine and Child Neurology* 1990; **32**: 858–864.

Mireles R, Leppik IL. Valproate and clonazepam comedication in patients with intractable epilepsy. *Epilepsia* 1985; **26**: 122–126.

Patsalos PN. *Antiepileptic drug interactions: a clinical guide*, 3rd edition. Springer, London, UK; 2016.

Patsalos PN, Zugman M, Lake C, James A, Ratnaraj N, Sander JW. Serum protein binding of 25 antiepileptic drugs in a routine clinical setting: a comparison of free non-protein-bound concentrations. *Epilepsia*, 2017; **58**: 1234–1243.

Sironi VA, Miserocchi G, DeRiu PL. Clonazepam withdrawal syndrome. *Acta Neurologica* 1984; **6**: 134–139.

Tomson T, Lindbom U, Hasselstrom J. Plasma concentrations of ethosuximide and clonazepam during pregnancy. *Journal of Epilepsy* 1990; **3**: 91–95.

DIAZEPAM

D

Therapeutics
Chemical Name and Structure
Diazepam, 7-chloro-1,3-dihydro-1-methyl-5-phenyl-2H-1,4 benzo-diazepin-2-one, is a yellowish crystalline powder, with a molecular weight of 284.7 and an empirical formula of $C_{16}H_{13}ClN_2O$.

Brand Names
- Aliseum; Anlin; Ansiolin; Antenex; Apaurin; Apo-Diazepam; Apozepam; Assival; Azepan
- Benzopin
- Calmpose; Cercine; Ceregulart; Compaz; Condition
- D-Pam; Dialag; Diano; Diapam; Diapin; Diapine; Diapo; Diastat; Diaz; Diazem; Diazemuls; Diazepam; Diazepam Desitin; Diazepam RecTubes; Diazepam-Eurogenerics; Diazepam-Lipuro; Diazepam-Ratiopharm; Diazepan; Diazer; Diazerekt; Dipaz; Dipezona; Doval; Ducene; Dupin; DZP
- Elcion CR; Euphorin
- Gewacalm
- Horizon
- Ifa Fonal
- Kratium; Kratium 2
- Lembrol
- Melode
- Nivalen; Nixtensyn; Noan; Normabel
- Ortopsique (MX)
- Paceum; Pacitran; Pax; Paxum; Placidox; Plidan; Propam; Psychopax
- Radizepam; Rectubes; Relanium; Relsed; Renborin
- Seduxen; Serenzin; Sipam; Stesolid; Stesolid Rectal Tube; Sunzepam
- Tranquirit
- Valaxona; Valdimex; Valiquid; Valisanbe; Valium; Valiuzam; Valpam; Vanconin; Vatran; Volclair

THERAPEUTICS

D

Generics Available
- Yes

Licensed Indications for Epilepsy
- Status epilepticus: injection only (UK SPC; FDA PI)
- Febrile convulsions (UK SPC)
- Seizure control for bouts of repetitive seizures/cluster seizures; rectal gel formulation only (FDA PI)
- Adjunctive use in seizure disorders (FDA PI)

Licensed Indications for Non-epilepsy Conditions
- Anxiolytic (UK SPC; FDA PI)
- Skeletal muscle relaxant (UK SPC; FDA PI)
- Perioperative sedative and analgesic (UK SPC; FDA PI)
- Management of alcohol withdrawal symptoms (UK SPC; FDA PI)
- Management of cerebral spasticity (UK SPC; FDA PI)
- Management of night terrors and somnambulism in children (UK SPC)
- Controlling tension and irritability in cerebral spasticity in children (UK SPC)
- Treatment of insomnia in children (UK SPC)

Non-licensed Use for Epilepsy
- To abort/terminate prolonged (i.e., >5 minute duration) generalized tonic–clonic seizures in a home/outpatient setting, and/or when parenteral access is not available; rectal gel formulation only

Non-licensed Use for Non-epilepsy Conditions
- There are none

Ineffective (Contraindicated)
- Can induce status epilepticus in patients with Lennox–Gastaut syndrome
- Should not be used as a long-term AED

Mechanism of Action
- Binds to benzodiazepine receptors at the $GABA_A$ ligand-gated chloride channel complex
- Boosts chloride conductance through GABA-regulated channels

Efficacy Profile
- Diazepam is the most widely used benzodiazepine in epilepsy
- It is the drug of first choice for the treatment of the premonitory stages of status epilepticus, for early status epilepticus, for serial seizures, for prolonged seizures, and for the prophylaxis of serial seizures

D

Pharmacokinetics

Absorption and Distribution
- Oral bioavailability: 100%
- Tmax: 30–90 minutes (tablets); 10–60 minutes (rectal solution); 30–60 minutes (rectal gel)
- Time to steady state: 6–11 days (diazepam); 15–20 days (N-desmethyldiazepam) – applies to adults on non-enzyme-inducing AEDs
- Pharmacokinetics: linear, but accumulation occurs following repeat administration
- Protein binding: 97–99%
- Volume of distribution: 1.1 L/kg
- Salivary concentrations: it is not known whether diazepam is secreted into saliva and whether such concentrations are similar to the unbound levels seen in plasma

Metabolism
- Diazepam is metabolized by desmethylation in the liver to desmethyldiazepam primarily by CYP2C19 but CYP3A4 also contributes
- N-desmethyldiazepam is in turn metabolized by hydroxylation, by means of CYP2C19, to form oxazepam, which is either excreted unchanged or undergoes sequential metabolism to a glucuronide conjugate
- Diazepam is also hydroxylated, by CYP3A4, to form temazepam, which in turn is demethylated to oxazepam or excreted unchanged
- N-desmethyldiazepam, along with the oxazepam and temazepam metabolites, is pharmacologically active
- N-desmethyldiazepam accumulates in blood to concentrations sevenfold higher than diazepam and contributes significantly to the pharmacological effect of diazepam
- A complication of diazepam metabolism is that it undergoes enterohepatic circulation, which can result in increased plasma levels and recurrence of drowsiness after 6–8 hours due to absorption from the gastrointestinal tract after excretion in the bile
- Autoinduction is not a feature of diazepam metabolism

Elimination
- Plasma concentrations decline rapidly with an initial half-life of ~1 hour
- In healthy adult subjects half-life values for diazepam are 28–54 hours, whereas for N-desmethyldiazepam values are 72–96 hours
- In adult patients with enzyme-inducing AEDs half-life values for diazepam are 31–41 hours
- In children half-life values are 14–20 hours
- In neonates half-life values are 29–33 hours
- In the elderly half-life values for diazepam are 80–100 hours, whereas for N-desmethyldiazepam values are 91–211 hours

PHARMACOKINETICS

- In patients with hepatic insufficiency half-life values for diazepam are 59–116 hours, whereas for *N*-desmethyldiazepam values are 68–148 hours
- Renal excretion: <5% of an administered dose is excreted unchanged in urine

Drug Interaction Profile
Pharmacokinetic Drug Interactions
- Interactions between AEDs: effects on diazepam:
  - Carbamazepine, phenytoin, phenobarbital, and primidone can *increase* the clearance of diazepam and *N*-desmethyldiazepam and *decrease* diazepam and *N*-desmethyldiazepam plasma levels
  - Valproic acid can displace diazepam from its plasma protein-binding sites and also inhibit its metabolism so that unbound diazepam levels are *increased* whereas *N*-desmethyldiazepam levels are *decreased*
- Interactions between AEDs: effects by diazepam:
  - To date, there have been no reports of diazepam affecting the clearance of other AEDs and affecting their plasma levels
- Interactions between AEDs and non-AED drugs: effects on diazepam:
  - Cimetidine, erythromycin, fluconazole, fluvoxamine, grapefruit juice, itraconazole, omeprazole, pantoprazole, sertraline, and voriconazole can *increase* diazepam plasma levels
- Interactions between AEDs and non-AED drugs: effects by diazepam:
  - Diazepam can *decrease* ibuprofen plasma levels

Pharmacodynamic Drug Interactions
- Diazepam depressive effects may be increased when taken with other CNS depressants

Hormonal Contraception
- Diazepam does not enhance the metabolism of oral contraceptives so as to decrease plasma levels of hormonal contraceptives and, therefore, does not compromise contraception control

Adverse Effects
How Drug Causes Adverse Effects
- Same mechanism for adverse effects as for therapeutic effects – namely due to actions at benzodiazepine receptors
- Long-term adaptations in benzodiazepine receptors may explain the development of dependence, tolerance, and withdrawal
- Adverse effects are generally immediate, but immediate adverse effects often disappear in time

D

Common Adverse Effects
• Sedation, fatigue, depression
• Dizziness, ataxia, slurred speech, weakness
• Forgetfulness, confusion
• Hyperexcitability, nervousness
• Hypersalivation, dry mouth
• Pain at injection site, phlebitis, venous thrombosis

Life-threatening or Dangerous Adverse Effects
• Respiratory depression, especially when taken with CNS depressants in overdose
• Rare hepatic dysfunction, renal dysfunction, blood dyscrasias
• Rare hypotension

Rare and not Life-threatening Adverse Effects
• Jaundice
• Urinary retention, incontinence
• Libido reduced, gynecomastia

Weight Change
• Not common; weight gain reported but not expected

What to do About Adverse Effects
• Discuss common and severe adverse effects with patients or parents before starting medication, including symptoms that should be reported to the physician
• Lower the dose

Dosing and Use
Usual Dosage Range
• In status epilepticus/acute repetitive, and/or cluster seizures, or to terminate prolonged generalized tonic–clonic seizure:
  – iv bolus (undiluted) 10–20 mg – adults; 0.2–0.3 mg/kg – children; rate not to exceed 2–5 mg/min and this can be repeated
  – rectal administration 10–30 mg – adults; 0.5–0.75 mg/kg – children; this can be repeated after 15 minutes if necessary

Available Formulations
• Tablets: 2 mg, 5 mg, 10 mg
• Liquid solution for injection: 5 mg/5 mL
• Liquid emulsion for injection: 5 mg/5 mL
• Oral solution: 2 mg/5 mL, 25 mg/5 mL (Intensol)
• Oral suspension: 2 mg/5 mL
• Rectal tubes (solution): 2.5 mg/1.25 mL, 5 mg/2.5 mL, 10 mg/ 2.5 mL
• Rectal solution: 5 mg/2.5 mL, 10 mg/2.5 mL
• Rectal suppositories: 10 mg
• Rectal gel (5 mg/mL): 2.5 mg, 5 mg, 10 mg, 15 mg, 20 mg

DOSING AND USE

D

How to Dose

Solutions need to be freshly prepared because diazepam is absorbed by polyvinylchloride plastics; typically fresh solutions should be made up within 6 hours

- Infusions should be carefully mixed so that 20 mg (Valium) should not be dissolved in less than 250 mL of solvent (4% dextrose, 0.18% sodium chloride) as there is a danger of precipitation at higher concentrations
- Diazemuls can be diluted in 5% or 10% dextrose solution to a maximum concentration of 200 mg in 500 mL and Stesolid to a maximum 10 mg in 200 mL of dextrose-saline
- Liquid formulation should be mixed with water or fruit juice, apple sauce, or pudding
- Because of risk of respiratory depression, rectal diazepam treatment should not be given more than once in 5 days or more than twice during treatment course, especially for alcohol withdrawal or status epilepticus

Dosing Tips

- Only benzodiazepine with a formulation specifically for rectal administration
- One of the few benzodiazepines available in an oral liquid formulation
- One of the few benzodiazepines available in an injectable formulation
- Diazepam injection is intended for acute use; patients who require long-term treatment should be switched to the oral formulation
- Diazepam is a Schedule IV drug and the risk of dependence may increase with dose and duration of treatment

How to Withdraw Drug

- Since diazepam is primarily used for the emergency treatment of seizure and not for chronic treatment, drug withdrawal is not a consideration

Overdose

- Fatalities can occur: symptoms include hypotension, tiredness, ataxia, confusion, coma
- The stomach should be emptied immediately by lavage or by induction of emesis
- Treatment of overdose consists of supportive care and the administration of the benzodiazepine receptor antagonist flumazenil
- Hemodialysis does not removes diazepam from blood and, therefore, is not a useful procedure in cases of overdose

Tests and Therapeutic Drug Monitoring

- During treatment: periodic liver tests and blood counts may be prudent

DIAZEPAM

D

- Therapeutic drug monitoring:
  - Diazepam plasma levels are not routinely used to guide patient management
  - The minimum plasma level required to suppress seizures probably depends on seizure type, duration of therapy, and other clinical factors but ranges from 200 to 600 ng/mL (702–2106 nmol/L) in most emergency settings
  - For initial seizure control plasma levels of 550 ng/mL (1930 nmol/L) are suggested
  - For maintenance of seizure control plasma levels of 150–300 ng/mL (526–1053 nmol/L) are suggested
  - The conversion factor from ng/mL to nmol/L is 3.17 (i.e., 1 ng/mL = 3.51 nmol/L)
  - The reference ranges highlighted above are considered to be the same for children and adults, although no data are available to support this clinical practice
  - There are no data indicating the usefulness of monitoring diazepam by use of saliva

Other Warnings/Precautions
- Use with caution in patients with pulmonary disease; rare reports of death after initiation of benzodiazepines in patients with severe pulmonary impairment
- Some depressed patients may experience a worsening of suicidal ideation
- Some patients may exhibit abnormal thinking or behavioral changes similar to those caused by other CNS depressants (i.e., either depressant actions or disinhibiting actions)

Do not Use
- If patient has respiratory depression
- If patient has acute pulmonary insufficiency
- If patient has untreated sleep apnea syndrome
- If patient has neuromuscular respiratory weakness, including unstable myasthenia gravis
- If patient has severe liver disease
- If there is a proven allergy to diazepam or any other benzodiazepine
- Avoid adjunctive benzodiazepine use in patients who are already receiving concomitant medications such as opioids or sodium oxybate that could lead to a further increased risk of respiratory depression

Special Populations
Renal Impairment
- Diazepam is renally secreted, so the dose may need to be lowered

Hepatic Impairment
- Diazepam is extensively metabolized in the liver and consequently lower doses may be required
- Initial dose is 2–2.5 mg, one–two times/day; increase gradually as needed

Children
- Children have an increased metabolic capacity and consequently higher doses on an mg/kg basis are usually required to achieve the equivalent therapeutic plasma levels seen in adults
- Neonates and infants have deceased hydroxylation and glucuronidation capacity, which may result in a decreased clearance of diazepam
- 6 months and up: initial 1–2.5 mg, three–four times/day; increase gradually as needed
- Parenteral administration should only be undertaken in children 30 days or older
- Rectal administration should only be undertaken in children 2 years or older
- Long-term effects of diazepam in children/adolescents are unknown; should generally receive lower doses and be more closely monitored

Elderly
- Elderly patients are more susceptible to adverse effects and, therefore, may not tolerate higher doses
- Because of an age-related reduction in renal and hepatic function, lower diazepam doses are appropriate
- Initial 2–2.5 mg, one–two times/day; increase gradually as needed

Pregnancy
- Specialist advice should be given to women who are of childbearing potential; they should be informed about the teratogenicity of all AEDs and the importance of avoiding an unplanned pregnancy; the AED treatment regimen should be reviewed when a woman is planning to become pregnant, in addition to recommendations for additional barrier contraceptives and folic acid 1,000 mg daily in all women of childbearing potential
- Rapid discontinuation of AEDs should be avoided as this may lead to breakthrough seizures, which could have serious consequences for the woman and the unborn child
- Diazepam was previously classified by the US FDA as risk category D (positive evidence of risk to human fetus; potential benefits may still justify its use during pregnancy); the current FDA Pregnancy and Lactation Rule has eliminated pregnancy risk category labels
- Pregnant women should be counseled about the increased risk of birth defects if benzodiazepines are to be taken during pregnancy
- Infants whose mothers received a benzodiazepine late in pregnancy may experience withdrawal effects

- Neonatal flaccidity has been reported in infants whose mothers took a benzodiazepine during pregnancy
- Seizures, even mild seizures, may cause harm to the embryo/fetus

Breast Feeding
- Breast milk: some drug is found in mothers' breast milk
- Breastfed infants: it is not known what plasma diazepam concentrations are achieved in breastfed infants compared with the levels of their mothers
- Recommend either to discontinue drug or initiate bottle feeding
- Effects on infant have been observed and include feeding difficulties, sedation, and weight loss

The Overall Place of Diazepam in the Treatment of Epilepsy

Diazepam is a widely used benzodiazepine in epilepsy treatment. It is a drug of first choice in the management of acute repetitive seizures, cluster seizures, and to abort acute prolonged generalized tonic–clonic seizures in home or when parenteral access is not available, when administered in the rectal gel formulation (Diastat). Diazepam also may be effective as an adjunctive oral agent in a wide range of established status types. While diazepam still carries an indication for use in status epilepticus in some countries, evidence clearly favors lorazepam (instead of diazepam) as the first drug of choice in the initial parenteral treatment of status epilepticus. However, diazepam rectal gel formulation may be preferentially used for seizure termination, including status epilepticus, when iv access is unavailable (i.e., in the home by caregivers, or in out-of-hospital settings prior to arrival of paramedics or emergency medicine personnel).

Primary Seizure Types
- Abortive therapy for the outpatient treatment/at-home management of prolonged generalized tonic–clonic seizures (in rectal gel formulation, i.e., Diastat)

Secondary Seizure Types
- Acute repetitive seizures (parenteral therapy, or as Intensol concentrate oral solution formulation)

Potential Advantages
- Ease of administration by rectal or oral routes in the management of prolonged generalized tonic–clonic seizures at home or when iv access is not available
- Rapid onset of action
- Multiple dosage formulations (oral, tablet, oral liquid, rectal gel, injectable) allow flexibility in administration

D

Potential Disadvantages
- Accumulates on repeated administration, with risk of sudden respiratory depression, sedation, and hypotension
- Pharmacologically active metabolite (N-desmethyldiazepam) which accumulates at concentrations manifold higher than that of diazepam
- Potential teratogen

Suggested Reading

Agurell S, Berlin A, Ferngren H, Hellstrom B. Plasma levels of diazepam after parenteral and rectal administration. *Epilepsia* 1975; **16**: 277–283.

Dhillon S, Richens A. Valproic acid and diazepam interaction in vivo. *British Journal of Clinical Pharmacology* 1982; **13**: 553–560.

Klotz U, Antonin KH, Brugel H, Bieck JR. Disposition of diazepam and its major metabolite desmethyldiazepam in patients with liver disease. *Clinical Pharmacology and Therapeutics* 1977; **21**: 430–436.

Meberg A, Langslet A, Bredesen JE, Lunde PKM. Plasma concentration of diazepam and N-desmethyldiazepam in children after a single rectal or intramuscular dose. *European Journal of Clinical Pharmacology* 1978; **12**: 273–276.

Norris E, Marzouk O, Nunn A, McIntyre J, Choonari I. Respiratory depression in children receiving diazepam for acute seizures: a prospective study. *Developmental Medicine and Neurology* 1999; **41**: 340–343.

Prensky AL, Raff MC, Moore MS, Schwab RS. Intravenous diazepam in the treatment of prolonged seizure activity. *New England Journal of Medicine* 1967; **276**: 779–886.

Schwartz MA, Koechlin BA, Postma E, Palmer S, Krol G. Metabolism of diazepam in rat, dog and man. *Journal of Pharmacology and Experimental Therapeutics* 1965; **149**: 423–435.

Shorvon S. *Status epilepticus: its clinical features and treatment in children and adults.* Cambridge University Press, Cambridge; 1994.

ESLICARBAZEPINE ACETATE

Therapeutics

Chemical Name and Structure

Eslicarbazepine acetate, (S)-10-acetoxy-10,11-dihydro-5H-dibenz[b,f] azepine-5-carboxamide, is a white to off-white crystalline powder, with a molecular weight of 296.32 and an empirical formula of $C_{17}H_{16}N_2O_3$.

Brand Names
- Aptiom
- Exalief
- Stedesa
- Zebinix

Generics Available
- No

Licensed Indications for Epilepsy
- Adjunctive treatment of focal (partial)-onset seizures with or without secondary generalization in patients with epilepsy aged 16 years and older (UK SPC)
- Adjunctive treatment of focal (partial)-onset seizures with or without secondary generalization in patients with epilepsy aged 18 years and older (FDA PI)

Licensed Indications for Non-epilepsy Conditions
- There are none

Non-licensed Use for Epilepsy
- There are none

Non-licensed Use for Non-epilepsy Conditions
- Bipolar disorder
- Cranial neuralgia

- Headache
- Neuropathic pain
- Trigeminal neuralgia

Ineffective (Contraindicated)
- The efficacy of eslicarbazepine acetate in primary generalized seizures has not been determined and therefore its use is not recommended in these patients

Mechanism of Action
- Acts as a use-dependent blocker of voltage-sensitive sodium channels resulting in stabilization of hyperexcitable neuronal membranes
- An effect on glutamate release may also occur

Efficacy Profile
- The goals of treatment are to achieve complete seizure remission when possible, or at least improved frequency and severity of seizures, while also minimizing adverse effects and improving patient quality of life
- Efficacy should be apparent within 4 weeks of treatment initiation
- If it is not producing clinical benefits within 6–8 weeks, it may require a dosage increase or it may not work at all
- If eslicarbazepine acetate is ineffective or only partially effective, it can be replaced by or combined with another AED that is appropriate for the patient's seizure type or epilepsy syndrome

Pharmacokinetics
Absorption and Distribution (All Values Refer to Eslicarbazepine)
- Oral bioavailability: >90%
- Food co-ingestion: neither delays the rate of absorption nor decreases the extent of absorption
- Tmax: 2–3 hours
- Time to steady state: 4–5 days
- Pharmacokinetics: linear
- Protein binding: 30%; blood cell-bound fraction: 46%
- Volume of distribution: 2.7 L/kg
- Salivary concentrations: it is not known whether eslicarbazepine is secreted into saliva and whether such concentrations are similar to the unbound levels seen in plasma. However, because eslicarbazepine is the same molecule as the pharmacologically active metabolite of oxcarbazepine, 10-hydroxycarbazepine, it can be expected that its transfer will be similar to that observed for 10-hydroxycarbazepine

Metabolism
- Eslicarbazepine acetate is rapidly metabolized (hydrolysis) in the liver to its pharmacologically active metabolite, eslicarbazepine (also known as S-licabazepine and 10-hydroxycarbazepine), by esterases (91%)
- Other minor metabolites, which are pharmacologically active, include R-licabazepine (~5%) and oxcarbazepine (~1%)
- Eslicarbazepine (33%) is subsequently metabolized by conjugation with glucuronic acid
- Although the metabolites of eslicarbazepine are pharmacologically active, they contribute to <5% of activity
- Autoinduction is not a feature of eslicarbazepine acetate metabolism

Elimination
- Half-life of eslicarbazepine acetate is <2 hours; thus eslicarbazepine acetate is a prodrug rapidly converted to its eslicarbazepine metabolite
- In healthy volunteers, half-life values for eslicarbazepine are 9–18 hours
- In the absence of enzyme-inducing AEDs, half-life values for eslicarbazepine in patients with epilepsy are 20–24 hours
- In the presence of enzyme-inducing AEDs, half-life values for eslicarbazepine are 13–20 hours
- Renal excretion: 92% of an administered dose is excreted as eslicarbazepine metabolites in urine; 33% as a glucuronide conjugate of eslicarbazepine and 67% as unchanged eslicarbazepine; 8% of metabolites comprise (R)-licarbazepine and oxcarbazepine and glucuronide conjugates of eslicarbazepine acetate, eslicarbazepine, (R)-licarbazepine, and oxcarbazepine
- Renal excretion: <1% of an administered dose is excreted unchanged as eslicarbazepine acetate in urine

Drug Interaction Profile
Pharmacokinetic Drug Interactions
- Interactions between AEDs – effects on eslicarbazepine:
  - Carbamazepine, phenytoin, and topiramate can *increase* the clearance of eslicarbazepine and *decrease* eslicarbazepine plasma levels
- Interactions between AEDs – effects by eslicarbazepine:
  - Eslicarbazepine can *increase* plasma levels of phenytoin
  - Eslicarbazepine can *decrease* plasma levels of lamotrigine, topiramate, and valproic acid
- Interactions between AEDs and non-AED drugs – effects on eslicarbazepine:
  - To date, there have been no reports of other non-AED drugs affecting the clearance of eslicarbazepine and affecting eslicarbazepine plasma levels
- Interactions between AEDs and non-AED drugs – effects by eslicarbazepine:

E

E

- Eslicarbazepine can *decrease* plasma levels of digoxin, metformin, simvastatin, and S-warfarin

Pharmacodynamic Drug Interactions
- Concurrent treatment with carbamazepine can be associated with a greater incidence of diplopia, abnormal coordination, and dizziness

Hormonal Contraception
- Eslicarbazepine acetate enhances the metabolism of oral contraceptives so as to decrease plasma levels of hormonal contraceptives and to reduce their effectiveness, leading to breakthrough bleeding and contraceptive failure; medium- or high-dose oral contraceptive preparations are indicated in patients taking eslicarbazepine acetate; in addition to recommendations for additional barrier contraceptives and folic acid 1,000 mg daily in all women of childbearing potential

Adverse Effects
How Drug Causes Adverse Effects
- CNS adverse effects may be due to excessive actions at voltage-sensitive sodium channels

Common Adverse Effects
- Dizziness, headache, abnormal coordination, somnolence, tremor, disturbance in attention
- Diplopia, blurred vision
- Vertigo
- Nausea, vomiting, diarrhea
- Rash
- Fatigue, gait disturbance
- Hyponatremia

Life-threatening or Dangerous Adverse Effects
- Increases PR interval, therefore patients with known second- or third-degree atrioventricular block may be at risk of myocardial infarction or heart failure
- Particular caution should be exercised with the elderly as they may be at an increased risk of cardiac disorders and prescribed Class I antiarrhythmic drugs and also may be co-prescribed AEDs (e.g., carbamazepine, lacosamide, lamotrigine, and pregabalin) that are known to be associated with PR prolongation
- Increased risk of suicidal ideation and behavior
- Rare adverse reactions, including Stevens–Johnson syndrome, bone marrow depression, serious cardiac arrhythmias, or systemic lupus erythematosus have not been observed but as they can be a feature of oxcarbazepine treatment, caution needs to be exercised with eslicarbazepine acetate

Rare and not Life-threatening Adverse Effects
• Constipation
• Nasopharyngitis

Weight Change
• Not common

What to do About Adverse Effects
• Discuss common and severe adverse effects with patients or parents before starting medication, including symptoms that should be reported to the physician
• Risk of adverse effects is greatest in the first few months of treatment
• Common adverse effects such as nausea often abate after a few months

Dosing and Use
Usual Dosage Range
• Adults: 800–1200 mg/day

Available Formulations
• Tablets: 400 mg, 800 mg
• Suspension: 60 mg/mL

How to Dose
• When initiating eslicarbazepine acetate treatment, start with a low dose and titrate slowly so as to minimize adverse effects
  – *For adults of age 16 years or older:* start treatment with 400 mg once daily for 1–2 weeks; increase by 400 mg/day at bi-weekly intervals; maximum dose 1200 mg/day, given once daily

Dosing Tips
• Titration of dose should be undertaken based on individual tolerability and response to the drug
• Concomitant use with oxcarbazepine should be avoided because it may result in overexposure to the pharmacologically active metabolites of both drugs

How to Withdraw Drug
• May need to adjust dosage of concurrent medications as eslicarbazepine acetate is being discontinued, since plasma levels of other drugs may change (see Pharmacokinetic Drug Interactions section)
• Taper: a gradual dose reduction over a minimum of a 1-week period should be undertaken
• Rapid discontinuation may increase the risk of seizures

Overdose
- Following accidental overdose vertigo, walking instability, and hemi-paresis have occurred
- The stomach should be emptied immediately by lavage or by induc-tion of emesis
- Hemodialysis removes eslicarbazepine and its metabolites from blood and therefore may be a useful procedure in case of overdose; two dia-lysis sessions may be necessary to virtually eliminate eslicarbazepine and its metabolites

Tests and Therapeutic Drug Monitoring
- Before starting: liver and kidney function tests, HLA-B★1502 in patients of Han Chinese, Thai, and other Southeastern Asian origin
- During treatment: liver and kidney function tests every 12 months
- Because eslicarbazepine acetate can alter vitamin D metabolism and affect bone mass, 25-hydroxyvitamin D levels should be monitored in all patients, and vitamin D supplementation should be prescribed as needed
- Therapeutic drug monitoring:
  - Optimum seizure control in patients on monotherapy is most likely to occur at eslicarbazepine plasma concentrations of 3–35 mg/L (12–139 µmol/L), which is based on that for racemic 10-hydroxycarbazepine derived from oxcarbazepine
  - The conversion factor from mg/L to µmol/L is 3.96 (i.e., 1 mg/L = 3.96 µmol/L)
  - Although there are no data indicating the usefulness of monitoring eslicarbazepine by use of saliva per se, given that eslicarbazepine is the same molecule as the pharmacologically active metabolite of oxcarbazepine, 10-hydroxycarbazepine, it can be expected that saliva monitoring would be similarly applicable

Other Warnings/Precautions
- Use cautiously in patients who have demonstrated hypersensitivity to carbamazepine and/or oxcarbazepine
- Eslicarbazepine acetate can cause dizziness and somnolence, which could increase the occurrence of accidental injury or falls
- Because eslicarbazepine acetate has a tricyclic chemical structure, it is not recommended to be taken with MAOIs
- In patients with pre-existing renal conditions associated with low sodium or in patients treated with sodium-lowering medications (e.g., diuretics, desmopressin, non-steroidal anti-inflammatory drugs (e.g., indometacin)) blood sodium levels should be measured prior to initi-ating treatment with eslicarbazepine acetate; thereafter, sodium levels should be measured after ~2 weeks and then at monthly intervals for the first 3 months or according to clinical need
- Usually hyponatremia (sodium levels <125 mmol/L) is asymptomatic and dose adjustment is not necessary; however if it becomes clinically significant (typically occurs in <1% of patients), it can be reversed

by either restricting fluid intake or a reduction in eslicarbazepine acetate dose

Do not Use
- If patient has a proven allergy to eslicarbazepine acetate or to any of the excipients
- Hypersensitivity to other carboxamide derivatives (e.g., carbamazepine and oxcarbazepine)
- If patient is taking an MAOI
- If patient has conduction problems or severe cardiac disease such as a history of myocardial infarction or heart failure

Special Populations
Renal Impairment
- Eslicarbazepine and its metabolites are renally excreted
- Mild to moderate renal impairment (CrCl >30 – <60 mL/min) results in a 40–80% decrease in clearance; an initial dose of 400 mg every other day for 2 weeks followed by a once-daily dose of 400 mg is recommended
- Severe renal impairment (CrCl <30 mL/min) results in a 90% decrease in clearance; eslicarbazepine acetate is not recommended for these patients
- Because eslicarbazepine can be removed by hemodialysis, patients receiving hemodialysis may require supplemental doses of eslicarbazepine acetate

Hepatic Impairment
- Eslicarbazepine acetate undergoes significant first-pass metabolism (91%) in the liver, and in patients with moderate hepatic impairment (Child–Pugh B) a slight increase in eslicarbazepine plasma levels occurs but a dose adjustment is not considered necessary

Children
- Eslicarbazepine acetate is not licensed for use in children
- Nevertheless, preliminary data show that for children, all of whom have an increased metabolic capacity, higher doses on an mg/kg basis are required in order to achieve the equivalent therapeutic plasma levels seen in adults
- Children may benefit from twice-daily dosing
- Pharmacokinetic interactions in children are usually of a greater magnitude than that seen in adults

Elderly
- Elderly patients are more susceptible to adverse effects and therefore may not tolerate higher doses

- Because of an age-related reduction in renal function, lower eslicarbazepine acetate doses are appropriate
- Because eslicarbazepine acetate is associated with dizziness and imbalance, the elderly may be at increased risk of falls
- The elderly with pre-existing renal conditions, and who may be taking sodium-lowering medications or non-steroidal anti-inflammatory drugs, have an increased risk of developing symptomatic hyponatremia
- Elderly patients are often prescribed concurrent drug therapies for comorbidities and therefore may be at greater risk for pharmacokinetic and pharmacodynamic interactions; the risk of pharmacokinetic interactions with eslicarbazepine acetate is minimal

Pregnancy
- Specialist advice should be given to women who are of childbearing potential; they should be informed about the teratogenicity of all AEDs and the importance of avoiding an unplanned pregnancy; the AED treatment regimen should be reviewed when a woman is planning to become pregnant
- Rapid discontinuation of AEDs should be avoided as this may lead to breakthrough seizures, which could have serious consequences for the woman and the unborn child
- Eslicarbazepine acetate has yet to be classified by the US FDA; if it was to be classified it would probably be in risk category C (some animal studies show adverse effects, no controlled studies in humans); the current FDA Pregnancy and Lactation Rule has eliminated pregnancy risk category labels
- Use in women of childbearing potential requires weighing potential benefits to the mother against the risks to the fetus
- Use with other AEDs in combination may cause a higher risk for teratogenic effects than eslicarbazepine acetate monotherapy
- Seizures, even mild seizures, may cause harm to the embryo/fetus. Data on the pharmacokinetic changes of eslicarbazepine during pregnancy are not available

Breast Feeding
- Breast milk: it is not known whether eslicarbazepine acetate or eslicarbazepine is excreted in breast milk
- Breastfed infants: it is not known what plasma eslicarbazepine acetate or eslicarbazepine concentrations are achieved in breastfed infants compared to the levels of their mothers
- If drug is continued while breast feeding, the infant should be monitored for possible adverse effects
- If adverse effects are observed, recommend bottle feeding

E

The Overall Place of Eslicarbazepine Acetate in the Treatment of Epilepsy

Eslicarbazepine acetate is structurally related to carbamazepine and oxcarbazepine and is licensed for use as adjunctive treatment of partial (focal)-onset seizures, with or without secondary generalization in patients with epilepsy aged 16 years and older. Because of its relatively recent introduction, it is too early to ascertain the place of eslicarbazepine acetate in the treatment of patients with epilepsy.

Primary Seizure Types
• Partial (focal) seizures with or without secondary generalization

Secondary Seizure Types
• None

Potential Advantages
• Its structural similarity to carbamazepine and oxcarbazepine results in an AED with a well-validated mode of action
• Not associated with the problematic pharmacologically active metabolite (carbamazepine-10,11-epoxide) that occurs with carbamazepine
• Dosing schedule is once per day

Potential Disadvantages
• Particular caution is warranted when prescribed with carbamazepine or oxcarbazepine as adverse effects associated with the latter drugs may be exacerbated
• In Europe only an 800-mg tablet formulation has been licensed and thus tablet cutting will be needed so as to achieve the recommended clinically effective dose range
• Potential teratogen

SUGGESTED READING

Suggested Reading

Almeida L, Falcao A, Maia J, Mazur D, Gellert M, Soares-da-Silva P. Single-dose and steady-state pharmacokinetics of eslicarbazepine acetate (BIA 2–093) in healthy elderly and young subjects. *Journal of Clinical Pharmacology* 2005; **45**: 1062–1066.

Almeida L, Potgieter JH, Maia J, Potgieter MA, Moto F, Soares-da-Silva P. Pharmacokinetics of eslicarbazepine acetate in patients with moderate hepatic impairment. *European Journal of Clinical Pharmacology* 2008; **64**: 267–273.

Almeida L, Soares-da-Silva P. Eslicarbazepine acetate (BIA-2-093). *Neurotherapeutics* 2007; **4**: 88–96.

Elger C, Halasz P, Maia J, Almeida L, Soares-da-Silva P, on behalf of the BIA-2093–301 Investigators Study Group. Efficacy and safety of eslicarbazepine acetate as adjunctive treatment in adults with refractory partial-onset seizures: a randomized, double-blind,

E

ESLICARBAZEPINE ACETATE

placebo controlled, parallel-group phase III study. *Epilepsia* 2009; **50**: 454–463.

Falcão A, Fuseau E, Nunes T, Almeida L, Soares-da-Silva P. Pharmacokinetics, drug interactions and exposure-response relationship of eslicarbazepine acetate in adult patients with partial-onset seizures: population pharmacokinetic and pharmacokinetic/pharmacody-namic analyses. *CNS Drugs* 2012; **26**: 79–91.

Gil-Nagel A, Elger C, Ben-Menachem E, Halász P, Lopes-Lima J, Gabbai AA, Nunes T, Falcão A, Almeida L, da-Silva PS. Efficacy and safety of eslicarbazepine acetate as add-on treatment in patients with focal-onset seizures: integrated analysis of pooled data from double-blind phase III clinical studies. *Epilepsia* 2013; **54**: 98–107.

Gil-Nagel A, Lopes-Lima J, Almeida L, Maia J, Soares-da-Silva P, on behalf of the BIA-2093–303 Investigators Study Group. Efficacy and safety of 800 and 1200 mg eslicarbazepine acetate as adjunctive treatment in adults with refractory partial-onset seizures. *Acta Neurologica Scandinavica* 2009; **120**: 281–287.

Johannessen Landmark C, Patsalos PN. Drug interactions involving the new second- and third-generation antiepileptic drugs. *Expert Reviews in Neurotherapeutics* 2010; **10**: 119–140.

Meis J, Almeida L, Falcao A, Soares E, Mota F, Potgieter MA, Potgieter JH, Soares-da-Silva P. Effect of renal impairment on the pharmacokinetics of eslicarbazepine acetate. *International Journal of Clinical Pharmacology and Therapeutics* 2008; **463**: 119–130.

Nunes T, Rocha JF, Falcão A, Almeida L, Soares-da-Silva P. Steady-state plasma and cerebrospinal fluid pharmacokinetics and tolerability of eslicarbazepine acetate and oxcarbazepine in healthy volunteers. *Epilepsia* 2013; **54**: 108–116.

Patsalos PN. *Antiepileptic drug interactions: a clinical guide*, 3rd edition. Springer, London, UK; 2016.

Patsalos PN, Berry DJ. Pharmacotherapy of the third-generation AEDs: lacosamide, retigabine and eslicarbazepine acetate. *Expert Opinion in Pharmacotherapy* 2012; **13**:699–715.

Perucca E, Elger C, Halász P, Falcão A, Almeida L, Soares-da-Silva P. Pharmacokinetics of eslicarbazepine acetate at steady-state in adults with partial-onset seizures. *Epilepsy Research* 2011; **96**: 132–1329.

Villanueva V, Bermejo P, Montoya J, Toledo M, Gómez-Ibáñez A, Garcés M, Vilella L, López-González FJ, Rodriguez-Osorio X, Campos D, Martínez P, Giner P, Zurita J, Rodríguez-Uranga J, Ojeda J, Mauri JA, Camacho JL, Ruiz-Giménez J, Poza JJ, Massot-Tarrús A, Galiano ML, Bonet M. EARLY-ESLI study: long-term experience with eslicarbazepine acetate after first monotherapy failure. *Acta Neurologica Scandinavica* 2017; **136**: 254–264.

ETHOSUXIMIDE

Therapeutics

Chemical Name and Structure

Ethosuximide, 2-ethyl-2-methylsuccinimide, is a white crystalline powder, with a molecular weight of 141.7 and an empirical formula of $C_7H_{11}NO_2$.

Brand Names
- Asamid
- Emeside; Ethymal; Etomal; Etosuximida
- Fluozoid
- Petimid; Petnidan; Petinimid
- Ronton
- Suxilep; Suximal; Suxinutin
- Zarondan; Zarontin

Generics Available
- Yes

Licensed Indications for Epilepsy
- As monotherapy for absence seizures (UK SPC)
- Control of absence (petit mal) epilepsy (FDA PI)

Licensed Indications for Non-epilepsy Conditions
- There are none

Non-licensed Use for Epilepsy
- Atypical absence seizures
- Myoclonic seizures
- Astatic seizures (drop attacks)

Non-licensed Use for Non-epilepsy Conditions
- There are none

Ineffective (Contraindicated)
- Generalized tonic–clonic seizures
- Partial-onset seizures

Mechanism of Action
- No single unifying mechanism of action of ethosuximide has been identified
- The prevailing hypothesis is that thalamic low-threshold calcium channels (T for "transient" or "tiny" channels) are involved. It has been demonstrated that ethosuximide, at therapeutic concentrations, can either reduce the number or reduce the conductance of these channels
- Ethosuximide also inhibits so-called noninactivating sodium currents and calcium-dependent potassium channels, but not low-threshold calcium channels of thalamocortical neurons

Efficacy Profile
- Goal of therapy in typical absence seizures is not only full seizure control without adverse effects, but also normalization of EEG. However, for many patients optimum seizure control with minimal tolerated adverse effects is more realistic
- Onset of action may occur within the first few days
- Once chronic therapy is initiated, it is usually continued for at least 2 years following the last seizure
- Myoclonic seizures associated with various epileptic syndromes, such as Lennox–Gastaut syndrome, severe myoclonic epilepsy of infancy, juvenile myoclonic epilepsy, and myoclonic astatic epilepsy, may also at times respond to ethosuximide
- If partially effective, consider co-prescribing with lamotrigine or valproic acid, or switch to valproic acid, lamotrigine, levetiracetam, acetazolamide, topiramate, or zonisamide

Pharmacokinetics
Absorption and Distribution
- Oral bioavailability: >90%, both for capsules and liquid formulations
- Food co-ingestion: it is not known whether food co-ingestion delays the rate of absorption or decreases the extent of absorption
- Tmax: ~1–4 hours, slightly longer for capsules than for syrup
- Time to steady state: 8–12 days (adults); 6–8 days (children)
- Volume of distribution: 0.7 L/kg (for all age groups)
- Pharmacokinetics: linear
- Protein binding: 0%
- Salivary concentrations: ethosuximide is secreted into saliva and concentrations are similar to the unbound levels seen in plasma

Metabolism
- Ethosuximide is metabolized in the liver by hydroxylation to form isomers of 2-(1-hydroxyethyl)-2-methylsuccinimide, of which at least 40% are glucuronide conjugates

- Metabolism is primarily mediated by CYP3A and to a lesser extent by CYP2E and CYP2B/C
- The metabolites of ethosuximide are not pharmacologically active
- Autoinduction is not a feature of ethosuximide metabolism

Elimination
- Half-life values of ethosuximide are 40–60 hours in adults and 30–40 hours in children
- In patients co-prescribed enzyme-inducing AEDs half-life values are 20–40 hours
- Renal excretion: ~20% of an administered dose is excreted unchanged in urine

Drug Interaction Profile
Pharmacokinetic Drug Interactions
- Interactions between AEDs: effects on ethosuximide:
  - Carbamazepine, phenobarbital, phenytoin, and primidone can *increase* the clearance of ethosuximide and *decrease* ethosuximide plasma levels
  - Stiripentol and valproic acid can *decrease* the clearance of ethosuximide and *increase* ethosuximide plasma levels
- Interactions between AEDs: effects by ethosuximide:
  - Ethosuximide can *decrease* plasma levels of valproic acid
  - Ethosuximide can *increase* plasma levels of primidone
- Interactions between AEDs and non-AED drugs: effects on ethosuximide:
  - Rifampicin can *decrease* ethosuximide plasma levels
  - Isoniazid can *increase* ethosuximide plasma levels
- Interactions between AEDs and non-AED drugs: effects by ethosuximide:
  - To date, there have been no reports of ethosuximide affecting the clearance of other non-AED drugs and affecting their plasma levels

Pharmacodynamic Drug Interactions
- The combination of ethosuximide with valproic acid can lead to a favorable pharmacodynamic interaction which may allow control of absence seizures in patients not responsive to monotherapy with either drug

Hormonal Contraception
- Ethosuximide does not enhance the metabolism of oral contraceptives so as to decrease plasma levels of hormonal contraceptives and, therefore, does not compromise contraception control

Adverse Effects
How Drug Causes Adverse Effects
• The mechanism by which ethosuximide causes adverse effects has not been established

Common Adverse Effects
• Abdominal discomfort
• Vomiting, diarrhea
• Hiccups
• Headaches
• Sedation, drowsiness, fatigue

Life-threatening or Dangerous Adverse Effects
• Dose-related reversible granulocytopenia
• More severe bone marrow reactions with granulocytopenia, thrombocytopenia, or pancytopenia
• Systemic lupus erythematosus
• Stevens–Johnson syndrome

Rare and not Life-threatening Adverse Effects
• Behavioral disturbances: nervousness, irritability, depression, hallucinations, and even psychosis
• Psychosis has been found to occur in conjunction with eradication of seizure activity, a phenomenon for which the term "forced normalization" has been coined
• Extrapyramidal reactions, such as dyskinesia

Weight Change
• Weight loss consequent to anorexia, nausea, vomiting, and diarrhea may occur

What to do About Adverse Effects
• Discuss common and severe adverse effects with patients or parents before starting medication, including symptoms that should be reported to the physician
• Gastrointestinal adverse effects can improve when the medication is taken at the end of a meal
• Gastrointestinal adverse effects can be minimized by undertaking a slow titration
• Clinical alertness to possible signs and symptoms is likely to be more effective in recognizing hematological adverse effects than routine monitoring of the blood count

Dosing and Use

Usual Dosage Range
• Adults, the elderly and children over 6 years of age: 500–1500 mg/day
• Children under 6 years of age: 20–30 mg/kg/day

Available Formulations
• Capsules (liquid-filled): 250 mg
• Syrup: 250 mg/5 mL

How to Dose
• When initiating ethosuximide treatment start with a low dose and titrate slowly so as to minimize adverse effects, particularly gastro-intestinal disturbances
  – *For adults and children over 6 years of age:* start treatment with 500 mg/day and increase at 5–7-day intervals in increments of 250 mg up to a total of 1000–1500 mg/day, in two or three daily doses. Occasionally 2000 mg/day in divided doses may be necessary
  – *Children under 6 years of age:* start treatment with 5–10 mg/kg/day and slowly increase at 5–7-day intervals in increments of 10 mg/kg/day up to a total of 20–30 mg/kg/day

Dosing Tips
• Ethosuximide should be ingested preferably after meals so as to minimize gastrointestinal symptoms
• If the patient's weight requires an increment of 125 mg, the capsules can be frozen and then easily cut in half
• The total daily dose can be divided into two daily doses, or also into three daily doses if this makes it easier for the child to take the medication or if it can be shown to improve gastrointestinal adverse effects
• When treatment of absence seizures is considered or reconsidered in patients above the age of 10 years, a drug with the appropriate broader spectrum of activity should be used, such as valproate or lamotrigine; alternatively ethosuximide should be combined with another drug that does provide protection against generalized tonic–clonic seizures

How to Withdraw Drug
• May need to adjust dosage of concurrent medications as ethosuximide is being discontinued, because plasma levels of other drugs may change (see Pharmacokinetic Drug Interactions section)
• Rapid discontinuation may increase the risk of seizures
• Dose can be decreased linearly at weekly intervals over a period of 1–3 months
• Because recurrence of absence seizures may be subtle clinically, or because significant subclinical spike-and-wave discharges may require reintroduction of therapy, it is good practice to repeat an EEG 1–3 months after ethosuximide has been discontinued

E

Overdose
- Usually not fatal: symptoms include nausea, vomiting, stupor, coma, respiratory depression
- If indicated the stomach should be emptied by lavage or by induction of emesis
- Hemodialysis removes ethosuximide from blood (~50% over a 6-hour dialysis interval) and, therefore, serves as a useful procedure in cases of overdose

Tests and Therapeutic Drug Monitoring
- Before starting: full blood count
- There are no clear guidelines regarding the need to monitor blood counts for the rare occurrence of bone marrow suppression, and clinical education and observation are likely to provide the best probability of early detection; blood count can be determined after 2 months, then every 6 months
- Therapeutic drug monitoring:
  - Optimum seizure control in patients on monotherapy is most likely to occur at ethosuximide plasma levels of 40–100 mg/L (300–700 μmol/L), but levels below 40 mg/L may be fully effective, and levels as high as 150 mg/L may be necessary and well tolerated
  - The conversion factor from mg/L to μmol/L is 7.06 (i.e., 1 mg/L = 7.06 μmol/L)
  - Once the patient is doing well clinically, there is no need to determine blood levels routinely
  - The reference range of ethosuximide in plasma is considered to be the same for children and adults, although no data are available to support this clinical practice
  - Ethosuximide can be monitored by use of saliva which is a measure of the free non-protein-bound plasma concentration and is pharmacologically relevant

Other Warnings / Precautions
- Patients should be monitored carefully for signs of unusual bleeding or bruising

Do not Use
- In patients with generalized tonic–clonic seizures unless they also take a medication that is known to be effective against tonic–clonic seizures

Special Populations
Renal Impairment
- Approximately 20% of the ethosuximide dose is not metabolized and renally secreted, therefore, the dose may need to be lowered

ETHOSUXIMIDE

- Because ethosuximide can be removed by hemodialysis, patients receiving hemodialysis may require supplemental doses of ethosuximide

Hepatic Impairment
- Ethosuximide is extensively metabolized in the liver and consequently lower doses may be required

Children
- Children have an increased metabolic capacity and consequently higher doses on a mg/kg/day basis are usually required to achieve the equivalent therapeutic plasma levels
- Pharmacokinetic interactions in children are usually of a greater magnitude than that seen in adults

Elderly
- Ethosuximide is used only very rarely in the elderly
- Elderly patients are more susceptible to adverse effects (especially somnolence) and, therefore, often do better at lower doses
- Because of an age-related reduction in renal and hepatic function, lower ethosuximide doses are appropriate
- Elderly patients are often prescribed concurrent drug therapies for comorbidities and therefore may be at greater risk for pharmacokinetic and pharmacodynamic interactions; the risk of pharmacokinetic interactions with ethosuximide is moderate

Pregnancy
- Specialist advice should be given to women who are of childbearing potential; they should be informed about the teratogenicity of all AEDs and the importance of avoiding an unplanned pregnancy; the AED treatment regimen should be reviewed when a woman is planning to become pregnant
- Rapid discontinuation of AEDs should be avoided as this may lead to breakthrough seizures, which could have serious consequences for the woman and the unborn child
- Ethosuximide was previously classified by the US FDA as risk category C (some animal studies show adverse effects, no controlled studies in humans); the current FDA Pregnancy and Lactation Rule has eliminated pregnancy risk category labels
- Use with other AEDs in combination may cause a higher prevalence of teratogenic effects than ethosuximide monotherapy
- Use in women of childbearing potential requires weighing potential benefits to the mother against the risks to the fetus
- Taper drug if discontinuing
- Seizures, even mild seizures, may cause harm to the embryo/fetus
- Data on the pharmacokinetic changes of ethosuximide during pregnancy are conflicting; ethosuximide clearance can increase accompanied by a decrease in plasma ethosuximide concentrations

E

ETHOSUXIMIDE

Breast Feeding
- Breast milk: 50–80% of maternal plasma levels
- Breastfed infants: ethosuximide plasma levels are 30–50% of maternal plasma levels
- If drug is continued while breast feeding, infant should be monitored for possible adverse effects
- If adverse effects are observed, recommend bottle feeding

The Overall Place of Ethosuximide in the Treatment of Epilepsy

Ethosuximide is the drug of first choice for the treatment of typical childhood absence seizures and is associated with a 70% seizure-free success rate as monotherapy. Ethosuximide should be considered as initial monotherapy only in those children with childhood absence epilepsy who have never experienced a generalized tonic–clonic seizure, against which ethosuximide has no protective effect and which it indeed may exacerbate.

Primary Seizure Types
- Typical childhood absence seizures

Secondary Seizure Types
- Atypical absence seizures
- Myoclonic seizures
- Astatic seizures (drop attacks)

Potential Advantages
- Ethosuximide is among the best AEDs for the treatment of childhood absence epilepsy
- It has a mostly benign adverse effect profile and severe adverse reactions are extremely rare
- Linear pharmacokinetics with a moderate interaction potential

Potential Disadvantages
- Narrow spectrum of seizure protection, limited mostly to absence seizures
- Abrupt withdrawal in patients with absences may precipitate absence status epilepticus
- Potential teratogen

Suggested Reading

Brigo F, Igwe SC. Ethosuximide, sodium valproate or lamotrigine for absence seizures in children and adolescents. *Cochrane Database Systematic Review* 2017 Feb 14; 2: CD003032. doi: 10.1002/14651858.CD003032.pub3.

Callaghan N, O'Hare J, O'Driscoll D, O'Neill B, Dally M. Comparative study of ethosuximide and sodium valproate in the treatment of typical absence seizures (petit mal). *Developmental Medicine and Child Neurology* 1982; **24**: 830–836.

Capovilla G, Beccaria F, V eggiotti P, Rubboli G, Meletti S, Tassinari CA. Ethosuximide is effective in the treatment of epileptic negative myoclonus in childhood partial epilepsy. *Journal of Child Neurology* 1999; **14**: 395–400.

Giaccone M, Bartoli A, Gatti G, Marchiselli R, Pisani F, Latella MA, Perucca E. Effect of enzyme-inducing anticonvulsants on ethosuximide pharmacokinetics in epileptic patients. *British Journal of Clinical Pharmacology* 1996; **41**: 575–579.

Glauser TA, Cnaan A, Shinnar S, Hirtz DG, Dlugos D, Masur D, Clark PO, Capparelli EV, Adamson PC. For the Childhood Absence Epilepsy Study Group. Ethosuximide, valproic acid, and lamotrigine in childhood absence epilepsy. *New England Journal of Medicine* 2010; **362**: 790–799.

Mattson RH, Cramer JA. Valproic acid and ethosuximide interaction. *Annals of Neurology* 1980; **7**: 583–584.

Panayiotopoulos CP. Treatment of typical absence seizures and related epileptic syndromes. *Paediatric Drugs* 2001; **3**: 379–403.

Patsalos PN. *Antiepileptic drug interactions – a clinical guide*, 3rd edition. Springer, London, UK; 2016.

Patsalos PN, Zugman M, Lake C, James A, Ratnaraj N, Sander JW. Serum protein binding of 25 antiepileptic drugs in a routine clinical setting: a comparison of free non-protein-bound concentrations. *Epilepsia* 2017; **58**: 1234–1243.

Posner EB, Mohamed K, Marson AG. Ethosuximide, sodium valproate or lamotrigine for absence seizures in children and adolescents. *Cochrane Database of Systematic Reviews* 2005; **4**: CD003032.

Rowan AJ, Meiser JW, De-Beer-Pawlikowski N. Valproate-ethosuximide combination therapy for refractory absence seizures. *Archives of Neurology* 1983; **40**: 797–802.

Sato S, White BG, Penry JK, Dreifuss FE, Sackellares JC, Kupferberg HJ. Valproic acid versus ethosuximide in the treatment of absence seizures. *Neurology* 1982; **32**: 157–163.

Snead OC, Horsey L. Treatment of epileptic falling spells with ethosuximide. *Brain Development* 1987; **9**: 602–604.

F

FELBAMATE

Therapeutics

Chemical Name and Structure

Felbamate, 2-phenyl-1,3-propanediol dicarbamate, is an off–white crystalline powder, with a molecular weight of 238.24 and an empirical formula of $C_{11}H_{14}N_2O_4$.

Brand Names
- Felbamyl; Felbatol
- Taloxa

Generics Available
- No

Licensed Indications for Epilepsy
- Monotherapy or adjunctive therapy of partial and secondary generalized seizures in adults (FDA PI)
- Adjunctive therapy for the treatment of partial and generalized seizures associated with Lennox–Gastaut syndrome in children (FDA PI)
- Felbamate is recommended only in patients who responded inadequately to alternative treatments (FDA PI)

Licensed Indications for Non-epilepsy Conditions
- There are none

Non-licensed Use for Epilepsy
- Absence seizures
- Acquired epileptic aphasia (Landau–Kleffner syndrome)
- Infantile spasms (West syndrome)
- Juvenile myoclonic epilepsy

Non-licensed Use for Non-epilepsy Conditions
- There are none

Ineffective (Contraindicated)
- Because of its potentially serious adverse effects, felbamate is not indicated as first-line therapy for any type of seizure

Mechanism of Action
- Inhibits glycine-enhanced *N*-methyl-D-aspartate (NMDA)-induced intracellular calcium currents
- Potentiates GABA responses at high felbamate concentrations
- Inhibits excitatory NMDA responses at high felbamate concentrations
- Effects use-dependent inhibition of NMDA currents (at therapeutic levels of 50–300 µmol)

Efficacy Profile
- The goals of treatment are to achieve complete seizure remission when possible, or at least improved frequency and severity of seizures, while also minimizing adverse effects and improving patient quality of life
- Onset of efficacy occurs mostly within the first 2 weeks of treatment
- Once chronic therapy is initiated, it is usually continued for at least 2 years following the last seizure
- If felbamate does not provide significant seizure control within 2–3 months, it should be discontinued because of the associated risk of severe adverse effects
- If felbamate is ineffective or only partially effective, it can be replaced by or combined with another AED that is appropriate for the patient's seizure type or epilepsy syndrome

Pharmacokinetics
Absorption and Distribution
- Oral bioavailability: >90%
- Food co-ingestion: neither delays the rate of absorption nor decreases the extent of absorption
- Tmax: 2–6 hours
- Time to steady state: 3–5 days
- Pharmacokinetics: linear
- Protein binding: 25%
- Volume of distribution: 0.76 L/kg (adults); 0.91 L/kg (children)
- Salivary concentrations: it is not known whether felbamate is secreted into saliva and whether such concentrations are similar to the unbound levels seen in plasma

Metabolism
- Only 50% of an administered dose is metabolized in the liver, by CYP3A4 and CYP2E1, to form two hydroxylated metabolites (*para*-hydroxyfelbamate and 2-hydroxyfelbamate – 10–15%) and a

variety of other unidentified polar metabolites, some of them being glucuronides or sulfate esters
- There is evidence to suggest that in humans the formation of several other metabolites, including atropaldehyde (2-phenylpropenal) may contribute to the cytotoxicity seen in some patients treated with felbamate
- The metabolites of felbamate are not pharmacologically active
- Autoinduction is not a feature of felbamate metabolism

Elimination
- In adult volunteers felbamate half-life values are 16–22 hours
- In patients co-prescribed enzyme-inducing AEDs felbamate half-life values are 10–18 hours
- Renal excretion: ~50% of an administered dose is excreted unchanged in urine

Drug Interaction Profile

Pharmacokinetic Drug Interactions
- Interactions between AEDs: effects on felbamate:
  - Carbamazepine and phenytoin can *increase* the clearance of felbamate and *decrease* felbamate plasma levels
  - Gabapentin and valproic acid can *decrease* the clearance of felbamate and *increase* felbamate plasma levels
- Interactions between AEDs: effects by felbamate:
  - Felbamate can *increase* the plasma levels of carbamazepine-10, 11-epoxide, clobazam, N-desmethyl-clobazam, clonazepam, lamotrigine, methsuximide, phenobarbital, phenytoin, and valproic acid
  - Felbamate can *decrease* the plasma levels of carbamazepine and vigabatrin
- Interactions between AEDs and non-AED drugs: effects on felbamate:
  - To date, there have been no reports of other non-AED drugs affecting the clearance of felbamate and affecting felbamate plasma levels
- Interactions between AEDs and non-AED drugs: effects by felbamate:
  - Felbamate can *increase* plasma levels of warfarin

Pharmacodynamic Drug Interactions
- To date, none have been reported

Hormonal Contraception
- Felbamate enhances the metabolism of oral contraceptives so as to decrease plasma levels of hormonal contraceptives and to reduce their effectiveness, leading to breakthrough bleeding and contraceptive failure; medium- or high-dose oral contraceptive preparations are indicated in patients taking felbamate, with additional recommendations for use of barrier methods and supplemental folic acid 1000 mg in all women of childbearing potential

F

Adverse Effects
How Drug Causes Adverse Effects
• Some metabolites, including atropaldehyde (2-phenylpropenal), are considered to contribute to the cytotoxicity associated with felbamate

Common Adverse Effects
• Nausea, vomiting, anorexia, dyspepsia
• Insomnia, irritability
• Dizziness, somnolence, diplopia
• Headache

Life-threatening or Dangerous Adverse Effects
• Aplastic anemia (risk may be >100 times above risk for general population; ~30–40% are fatal)
• Hepatic failure (~50% fatal)

Rare and not Life-threatening Adverse Effects
• Choreoathetosis
• Dystonia
• Kidney stones

Weight Change
• Weight loss commonly occurs

What to do About Adverse Effects
• Discuss common and severe adverse effects with patients or parents before starting medication, including symptoms that should be reported to the physician
• Do not use felbamate in patients with a history of blood dyscrasia or hepatic dysfunction
• Obtain CBC and transaminases at baseline, then at the latest 1 month after initiation of felbamate, then at least every 3 months
• There is no evidence that such monitoring will allow detection of bone marrow suppression before aplastic anemia occurs
• Clinical alertness to possible signs and symptoms is likely to be more effective in recognizing hematological adverse effects than routine monitoring of the blood count
• The common adverse effects have a higher incidence in antiepileptic polytherapy than in monotherapy
• Risk factors for aplastic anemia may include: age 18 years or above, female gender, cytopenia with previous AEDs, polytherapy, and clinical or serological evidence of a concomitant immune disorder
• If felbamate shows no effectiveness within 2–3 months in any given patient, discontinue its use
• Serious adverse effects have occurred mostly within the first 6 months of treatment, and are much less likely after 18 months of treatment

ADVERSE EFFECTS

Dosing and Use

Usual Dosage Range
- Adults and children over 12 years of age: 2400–5000 mg/day
- Children under 12 years of age: 30–60 mg/kg/day

Available Formulations
- Tablets: 400 mg, 600 mg
- Suspension: 600 mg/5 mL

How to Dose
- *For adults and children over 12 years of age:* start treatment with 1200 mg/day, twice daily, for 1 week; during the second week, increase to 2400 mg/day; during the third week of treatment, if necessary and if tolerated, the dose is to be increased to 3600 mg/day. If felbamate is introduced in a patient who is not taking an enzyme-inducing AED, a slower titration is recommended; in adults doses of 5000–6000 mg/day have been commonly used
- *Children under 12 years of age:* start treatment with 15 mg/kg/day, twice daily, for 1 week; during the second week, increase to 30 mg/kg/day; during the third week of treatment, if necessary and if tolerated, the dose is to be increased to 45 mg/kg/day. If felbamate is introduced in a patient who is not taking an enzyme-inducing AED, a slower titration is recommended; maintenance doses may often safely exceed 45 mg/kg/day

Dosing Tips
- Do not use felbamate in patients with a history of blood dyscrasia or hepatic dysfunction
- To decrease adverse effects, the daily dose of concomitant AEDs should be decreased by approximately one-fifth to one-third when felbamate is introduced
- Slow dose titration may delay onset of therapeutic action but enhance tolerability to sedating effects
- Whenever possible, try to achieve monotherapy with felbamate

How to Withdraw Drug
- May need to adjust dosage of concurrent medications as felbamate is being discontinued, because plasma levels of other drugs may change (see Pharmacokinetic Drug Interactions section)
- Rapid discontinuation may increase the risk of seizures
- Dose can be decreased at weekly intervals over a period of 1–3 months

Overdose
- No serious adverse reactions have been reported at up to 12,000 mg in 12 hours
- May cause crystalluria and even renal failure
- If indicated the stomach should be emptied by lavage or by induction of emesis

- It is not known whether hemodialysis removes felbamate from blood and, therefore, can serve as a useful procedure in cases of overdose

Tests and Therapeutic Drug Monitoring
- Obtain CBC and transaminases at baseline, then at the latest 1 month after initiation of felbamate, then at least every 3 months
- Therapeutic drug monitoring:
  - Optimum seizure control in patients on monotherapy is most likely to occur at felbamate plasma levels of 30–60 mg/L (125–250 μmol/L)
  - The conversion factor from mg/L to μmol/L is 4.20 (i.e., 1 mg/L = 4.20 μmol/L)
  - The reference range of felbamate in plasma is considered to be the same for children and adults, although no data are available to support this clinical practice
  - It is not known whether felbamate can be monitored by use of saliva, which is a measure of the free non-protein-bound plasma concentration and is pharmacologically relevant

Other Warnings/Precautions
- Patients should be monitored carefully for signs of unusual bleeding or bruising
- Obtain liver function test in cases of symptoms suggestive of felbamate hepatotoxicity, which include nausea, vomiting, anorexia, lethargy, jaundice, and at times loss of seizure control

Do not Use
- In patients with a history of blood dyscrasia or hepatic dysfunction
- Because of its potentially serious adverse effects, felbamate is not indicated as first-line therapy for any type of seizure
- If patient has a proven allergy to felbamate or to any of the excipients – tablets contain lactose
- Because the tablet formulation contains lactose, patients with rare hereditary problems of galactose intolerance, Lapp lactose deficiency, or glucose–galactose malabsorption should not take this formulation

Special Populations
Renal Impairment
- Felbamate is renally excreted (~50%) and, therefore, the dose may need to be lowered

Hepatic Impairment
- Felbamate undergoes moderate metabolism (~50%) in the liver and consequently lower doses may be required

Children
- Children have an increased metabolic capacity and consequently higher doses on a mg/kg/day basis are usually required to achieve the equivalent therapeutic plasma levels
- Pharmacokinetic interactions in children are usually of a greater magnitude than that seen in adults
- Risk of fatal hepatotoxicity is similar for all age groups
- Fatal aplastic anemia has not been reported in any patient younger than 18 years

Elderly
- No systematic studies in elderly patients have been conducted
- Elderly patients are more susceptible to adverse effects of AEDs (especially somnolence) and, therefore, often do better at lower doses
- Because of an age-related reduction in renal and hepatic function, lower felbamate doses may be appropriate
- Elderly patients are often prescribed concurrent drug therapies for comorbidities and therefore may be at greater risk for pharmacokinetic and pharmacodynamic interactions; the risk of pharmacokinetic interactions with felbamate is moderate

Pregnancy
- Specialist advice should be given to women who are of childbearing potential; they should be informed about the teratogenicity of all AEDs and the importance of avoiding an unplanned pregnancy; the AED treatment regimen should be reviewed when a woman is planning to become pregnant
- Rapid discontinuation of AEDs should be avoided as this may lead to breakthrough seizures, which could have serious consequences for the woman and the unborn child
- Felbamate was previously classified by the US FDA as risk category C (some animal studies show adverse effects, no controlled studies in humans); the current FDA Pregnancy and Lactation Rule has eliminated pregnancy risk category labels
- Use in women of childbearing potential requires weighing potential benefits to the mother against the risks to the fetus
- Taper drug if discontinuing
- Seizures, even mild seizures, may cause harm to the embryo/fetus
- There are no data on the pharmacokinetic changes of felbamate during pregnancy

Breast Feeding
- Breast milk: felbamate has been detected in human breast milk
- Breastfed infants: it is not known what plasma felbamate concentrations are achieved in breastfed infants compared with the levels of their mothers

F

- If drug is continued while breast feeding, infant should be monitored for possible adverse effects
- If adverse effects are observed, recommend bottle feeding

The Overall Place of Felbamate in the Treatment of Epilepsy

The clinical use of felbamate has been significantly compromised consequent to its association with a high incidence of aplastic anemia and hepatic failure which resulted in several fatalities. Presently, felbamate is never considered as a first-line therapy for any seizure type and should only be prescribed to patients who respond inadequately to alternative AEDs and whose epilepsy is so severe that a substantial risk of aplastic anemia and/or liver failure is deemed acceptable in light of the benefits conferred by its use. In this setting, felbamate can be considered in combination therapy or in monotherapy for the treatment of Lennox–Gastaut syndrome and of partial (focal) seizures with or without secondary generalization.

Primary Seizure Types
- Partial (focal) seizures with or without secondary generalization
- Lennox–Gastaut syndrome

Secondary Seizure Types
- Myoclonic seizures
- Infantile spasms (West syndrome)

Potential Advantages
- Felbamate probably has a broad spectrum of seizure protection
- Felbamate may be one of the more effective drugs in the treatment of Lennox–Gastaut syndrome

Potential Disadvantages
- Relatively high incidence of two potentially life-threatening adverse effects: aplastic anemia and liver failure
- Requires frequent blood testing and close monitoring
- Associated with significant pharmacokinetic interactions and usually acts as an inhibitor of hepatic metabolism
- Potential teratogen

Suggested Reading

Faught E, Sachdeo RC, Remler MP, Chayasirisobhon S, Iraqui-Madoz VJ, Ramsay RE, Sutula TP, Kanner A, Harner RN, Kuzniecki R. Felbamate monotherapy for partial-onset seizures: an active-control trial. *Neurology* 1993; **43**: 688–692.

French J, Smith M, Faught E, Brown L. The use of felbamate in the treatment of patients with intractable epilepsy: practice advisory. *Neurology* 1999; **52**: 1540–1545.

Harden CL, Trifiletti R, Kutt H. Felbamate levels in patients with epilepsy. *Epilepsia* 1996; **37**: 280–283.

Hurst DL, Rolan TD. The use of felbamate to treat infantile spasms. *Journal of Child Neurology* 1995; **10**: 134–136.

Johannessen Landmark C, Patsalos PN. Drug interactions involving the new second- and third-generation antiepileptic drugs. *Expert Reviews in Neurotherapeutics* 2010; **10**: 119–140.

Kaufman DW, Kelly JP, Anderson T, Harmon DC, Shapiro S. Evaluation of case reports of aplastic anemia among patients treated with felbamate. *Epilepsia* 1997; **38**: 1265–1269.

O'Neil MG, Perdun CS, Wilson MB, McGown ST, Patel S. Felbamate-associated fatal acute hepatic necrosis. *Neurology* 1996; **46**: 1457–1459.

Patsalos PN. *Antiepileptic drug interactions: a clinical guide*, 3rd edition. 2016, Springer, London, UK; 2016.

Pellock JM, Faught E, Leppik IE, Shinnar S, Zupanc ML. Felbamate: consensus of current clinical experience. *Epilepsy Research* 2006; **71**: 89–101.

Shah YD, Singh K, Friedman D, Devinsky O, Kothare SV. Evaluating the safety and efficacy of felbamate in the context of a black box warning: a single center experience. *Epilepsy and Behavior* 2016; **56**: 50–53.

The Felbamate Study Group in Lennox–Gastaut syndrome. Efficacy of felbamate in childhood epileptic encephalopathy (Lennox–Gastaut syndrome). *New England Journal of Medicine* 1993; **328**: 29–33.

Zupanc ML, Roell Werner R, Schwabe MS, O'Connor SE, Marcuccilli CJ, Hecox KE, Chico MS, Eggener KA. Efficacy of felbamate in the treatment of intractable pediatric epilepsy. *Pediatric Neurology* 2010; **42**: 396–403.

FOSPHENYTOIN

Therapeutics

Chemical Name and Structure

Fosphenytoin, a disodium phosphate ester of 3-hydroxymethyl-5,5-diphenylhydantoin, is a white powder, with a molecular weight of 406.24 and an empirical formula of $C_{16}H_{15}N_2O_6P$. It is an injectable prodrug of phenytoin.

Brand Names
- Cerebyx
- Fosolin; Fosphen
- Milorgen
- Prodilantin; Pro-Epanutin

Generics Available
- Yes

Licensed Indications for Epilepsy
- Control of generalized convulsive status epilepticus (UK SPC; FDA PI)
- Prevention of seizures occurring during neurosurgery and/or head trauma (UK SPC; FDA PI)
- As a substitute, short-term, for oral phenytoin if oral administration is not possible and/or contraindicated (UK SPC; FDA PI)

Licensed Indications for Non-epilepsy Conditions
- There are none

Non-licensed Use for Epilepsy
- im/iv loading dose administration in patients who are unconscious or if oral administration is not possible and/or contraindicated

Non-licensed Use for Non-epilepsy Conditions
- Acute relief of trigeminal neuralgia attacks

F

FOSPHENYTOIN

Ineffective (Contraindicated)
- im administration of fosphenytoin is contraindicated in the treatment of status epilepticus
- Because phenytoin is ineffective against absence seizures, if tonic–clonic seizures are present simultaneously with absence seizures, combined drug therapy is recommended
- Fosphenytoin is not used chronically in the treatment of epileptic seizures

Mechanism of Action
- Fosphenytoin is a prodrug of phenytoin, and therefore its anticonvulsant effects are those attributable to phenytoin
- Acts as a use-dependent blocker of voltage-sensitive sodium channels
- Interacts with the open-channel conformation of voltage-sensitive sodium channels
- Modulates sustained repetitive firing
- Regulates calmodulin and second messenger systems
- Inhibits calcium channels and calcium sequestration

Efficacy Profile
- Fosphenytoin is a valuable alternative to parenteral phenytoin
- It is for the treatment of status epilepticus and for the prophylaxis of serial seizures
- If fosphenytoin does not terminate seizures, the use of alternative AEDs should be considered

Pharmacokinetics
Absorption and Distribution
- Bioavailability: 100% (im administration)
- Tmax: fosphenytoin: at end of infusion following iv administration; ~0.5 hours following im administration
- Tmax: phenytoin: 0.5–1.0 hours following the start of iv infusion; 1.5–4 hours following im administration
- Time to steady state: 6–21 days (phenytoin)
- Pharmacokinetics: non-linear due to saturable metabolism so that clearance decreases with increasing dose
- Protein binding: fosphenytoin: 95–99%; phenytoin: 90%
- Volume of distribution: 0.04–0.13 L/kg

Metabolism
- Fosphenytoin undergoes hydrolysis by phosphatase enzymes, present in liver, red blood cells and other tissues, to form phenytoin and two metabolites, namely phosphate and formaldehyde
- Formaldehyde is subsequently converted to formate, which is further metabolized by means of folate-dependent pathways

- The half-life for conversion of fosphenytoin to phenytoin is 8–15 minutes
- The derived phenytoin undergoes metabolism in the same way as when phenytoin is administered as such (see Phenytoin section)

Elimination
- The derived phenytoin undergoes elimination in the same way as when phenytoin is administered as such (see Phenytoin section)
- Renal excretion: <4% of an administered dose is excreted as unchanged fosphenytoin in urine

Drug Interaction Profile
There are no drugs known to interfere with the conversion of fosphenytoin to phenytoin

Pharmacokinetic Drug Interactions
- Interactions between AEDs: effects on phenytoin:
  - Fosphenytoin can displace phenytoin from its plasma protein-binding sites and *increase* free non-protein-bound phenytoin levels
  - Drug interactions which may occur following the administration of fosphenytoin are those that are expected to occur with drugs known to interact with phenytoin (see Phenytoin section)
- Interactions between AEDs: effects by phenytoin:
  - Drug interactions which may occur following the administration of fosphenytoin are those that are expected to occur with drugs known to interact with phenytoin (see Phenytoin section)
- Interactions between AEDs and non-AED drugs: effects on phenytoin:
  - Drug interactions which may occur following the administration of fosphenytoin are those that are expected to occur with drugs known to interact with phenytoin (see Phenytoin section)
- Interactions between AEDs and non-AED drugs: effects by phenytoin:
  - Drug interactions which may occur following the administration of fosphenytoin are those that are expected to occur with drugs known to interact with phenytoin (see Phenytoin section)

Pharmacodynamic Drug Interactions
- To date, none have been identified

Hormonal Contraception
- Although it is not known whether or not fosphenytoin affects hormonal contraceptives, phenytoin enhances the metabolism of oral contraceptives so as to decrease plasma levels of hormonal contraceptives and to reduce their effectiveness, leading to break-through bleeding and contraceptive failure; medium- or high-dose oral contraceptive preparations are, therefore, indicated in patients

F

taking fosphenytoin; in addition to recommendations for additional barrier contraceptives and folic acid 1,000 mg daily in all women of childbearing potential

Adverse Effects

How Drug Causes Adverse Effects
• Fosphenytoin is a prodrug of phenytoin and, therefore, the mechanisms whereby adverse effects occur are those attributable to phenytoin (see Phenytoin section)

Common Adverse Effects
• Fosphenytoin is a prodrug of phenytoin and, therefore, its adverse effects are those attributable to phenytoin (see Phenytoin section)

Life-threatening or Dangerous Adverse Effects
• See Phenytoin section
• Fosphenytoin should be used with caution in patients with hypotension and severe myocardial insufficiency because severe cardiovascular reactions, including atrial and ventricular conduction depression and ventricular fibrillation, and sometimes fatalities, have occurred following fosphenytoin administration

Rare and not Life-threatening Adverse Effects
• See Phenytoin section
• In addition, pruritus may be seen, an adverse effect not typically seen with phenytoin that is attributed to the phosphorylated prodrug formulation; pruritus following fosphenytoin administrations may be confined to the genital region or other unusual body distribution and is often misdiagnosed as psychogenic

Weight Change
• See Phenytoin section

What to do About Adverse Effects
• Dosage reduction in cases of presumably dose-related adverse effects
• Hypotension may occur following iv administration of high doses and/or high infusion rates of fosphenytoin, even within recommended doses and rates; a reduction in the rate of administration or discontinuation of dosing may be necessary

Dosing and Use
Doses of fosphenytoin are always expressed as their phenytoin sodium equivalent (PE) to avoid the need to perform molecular weight-based adjustments when substituting fosphenytoin for phenytoin or vice versa; 1.5 mg of fosphenytoin is equivalent to 1 mg PE.

Usual Dosage Range
- In status epilepticus:
  - iv loading dose: 20 mg PE/kg and an infusion rate of 100–150 mg PE/min – adults; 15 mg PE/kg and an infusion rate of 2–3 mg PE/kg/min – children
  - iv or im maintenance dose: 4–5 mg PE/kg/day; iv infusion rate 50–100 mg PE/min – adults; 4–5 mg PE/kg/day; iv infusion rate 1–2 mg PE/kg/min – children
- In treatment or prophylaxis of seizures:
  - iv or im loading dose: 10–15 mg PE/kg and an infusion rate of 50–100 mg PE/min – adults; 10–15 mg PE/kg and an infusion rate of 1–2 mg PE/kg/min – children
  - iv or im maintenance dose: 4–5 mg PE/kg/day; iv infusion rate 50–100 mg PE/min – adults; 1–2 mg PE/kg/min – children

Available Formulations
- Solution for injection: 750 mg/10 mL (equivalent to 500 mg of phenytoin sodium and referred to as 500 mg PE))

How to Dose
- iv administration is essential for the management of status epilepticus whereby either iv or im administration can be used in the treatment or prophylaxis of seizures
- In status epilepticus:
  - *For adults:* start treatment with a loading dose of 20 mg PE/kg administered as a single dose by iv infusion; the recommended iv infusion rate is 100–150 mg PE/min and should not exceed 150 mg PE/min; maintenance dose is 4–5 mg PE/kg/day and may be administered by iv infusion or by im injection in one or two divided doses; iv infusion rate is 50–100 mg PE/min and should not exceed 100 mg PE/min
  - *Children 5 years and above:* start treatment with a loading dose of 20 mg PE/kg administered as a single dose by iv infusion; the recommended iv infusion rate is 2–3 mg/kg/min and should not exceed 3 mg PE/kg/min or 150 mg PE/min; maintenance dose is 4–5 mg PE/kg/day and may be administered by iv infusion in one or two divided doses; iv infusion rate is 1–2 mg PE/kg/min and should not exceed 100 mg PE/min
- In treatment or prophylaxis of seizures:
  - *For adults:* start treatment with a loading dose of 10–15 mg PE/kg administered as a single dose by iv infusion or by im injection; the recommended iv infusion rate is 100–150 mg PE/min and should not exceed 150 mg PE/min; maintenance dose is 4–5 mg PE/kg/day and may be administered by iv infusion or by im injection in one or two divided doses; iv infusion rate is 50–100 mg PE/min and should not exceed 100 mg PE/min
  - *Children 5 years and above:* start treatment with a loading dose of 10–15 mg PE/kg administered as a single dose by iv infusion; the

F

recommended iv infusion rate is 1–2 mg/kg/min and should not exceed 3 mg PE/kg/min or 150 mg PE/min; maintenance dose is 4–5 mg PE/kg/day and may be administered by iv infusion in one to four divided doses; iv infusion rate is one frequent maintenance dose −2 mg PE/kg/min and should not exceed 100 mg PE/min

Dosing Tips
• Before iv infusion fosphenytoin should be diluted in 5% glucose/dextrose or 0.9% saline so that the concentration ranges from 1.5 to 2.5 mg PE/mL
• Transient itching, burning, warmth, or tingling in the groin during and shortly after iv infusion of fosphenytoin can be avoided or minimized by using a slower rate of infusion or by temporarily stopping the infusion
• im administration should generally not be used in the treatment of status epilepticus because the attainment of peak fosphenytoin and phenytoin plasma levels is delayed, but may be considered if iv access is not attainable
• Because of the risk of hypotension, the recommended rate of administration by iv infusion in routine clinical settings is 50–100 mg PE/min and should not exceed 150 mg PE/min even in the emergency situation, as occurs with status epilepticus
• Cardiac resuscitation equipment should be available and continuous monitoring of electrocardiogram (ECG), blood pressure, and respiratory function for the duration of iv infusion is essential; the patient should also be observed throughout the period where maximum plasma phenytoin levels occur (~30 minutes after the end of infusion period); however, cardiac or hemodynamic monitoring is not essential during im administration

How to Withdraw Drug
• May need to adjust dosage of concurrent medications as fosphenytoin is being discontinued, because plasma levels of other drugs may change (see Pharmacokinetic Drug Interactions section)
• Taper: a gradual dose reduction over a period of many weeks should be undertaken
• Rapid discontinuation may induce withdrawal seizures and should only be undertaken if there are safety concerns (e.g., a rash with serious characteristics)

Overdose
• Initial symptoms of fosphenytoin toxicity are those associated with phenytoin and include ataxia, nystagmus, and dysarthria; subsequently the patient becomes comatose, the pupils are unresponsive, and hypotension occurs followed by respiratory depression and apnea; death is the consequence of respiratory and circulatory depression
• Hemodialysis removes phenytoin from blood and, therefore, serves as a useful procedure in cases of overdose

Tests and Therapeutic Drug Monitoring
- Therapeutic drug monitoring:
  - Fosphenytoin plasma levels are not necessary or helpful to guide patient management
  - Optimum seizure control is most likely to occur at plasma phenytoin concentrations of 10–20 mg/L (40–80 μmol/L); however, many patients in status epilepticus often require higher levels (usually dosing to above 20 mg/L and up to 30 mg/mL (120 μmol/L))
  - The conversion factor from mg/L to μmol/L is 3.96 (i.e., 1 mg/L = 3.96 μmol/L)

Other Warnings/Precautions
- Life-threatening rashes have developed in association with phenytoin use; fosphenytoin should generally be discontinued at the first sign of serious rash
- See Phenytoin section

Do not Use
- If patient has a proven allergy to fosphenytoin, phenytoin, or to any of the excipients

Special Populations
Renal Impairment
- Except in the treatment of status epilepticus, a lower loading dose and/or infusion rate and lower or less frequent maintenance dose may be required in renally impaired patients; a 10–25% reduction in dose or rate may be considered and clinical monitoring is essential
- The conversion rate of fosphenytoin to phenytoin may be increased
- Plasma unbound phenytoin levels may also be increased and patient management may best be guided by monitoring free non-protein-bound levels
- Because phenytoin can be removed by hemodialysis, patients receiving hemodialysis may require supplemental doses of fosphenytoin

Hepatic Impairment
- Except in the treatment of status epilepticus, a lower loading dose and/or infusion rate and lower or less frequent maintenance dose may be required in renally impaired patients; a 10–25% reduction in dose or rate may be considered and careful clinical monitoring is essential
- The conversion rate of fosphenytoin to phenytoin may be increased
- Plasma unbound phenytoin levels may also be increased and patient management may best be guided by monitoring free non-protein-bound levels

F

FOSPHENYTOIN

Children
- Children have an increased metabolic capacity and consequently higher doses on a mg/kg basis are usually required to achieve the equivalent therapeutic plasma levels seen in adults

Elderly
- Elderly patients are more susceptible to adverse effects and, therefore may not tolerate higher doses
- Because of an age-related reduction in hepatic function, a lower loading dose and/or infusion rate and a lower or less frequent maintenance dose may be required if fosphenytoin is being given in a non-urgent setting, i.e., outside of the indication of status epilepticus; a 10–25% reduction in dose or rate may be considered and careful clinical monitoring is essential

Pregnancy
- Specialist advice should be given to women who are of childbearing potential; they should be informed about the teratogenicity of all AEDs and the importance of avoiding an unplanned pregnancy; the AED treatment regimen should be reviewed when a woman is planning to become pregnant
- Fosphenytoin was previously classified by the US FDA as risk category D (positive evidence of risk to human fetus; potential benefits may still justify its use during pregnancy); the current FDA Pregnancy and Lactation Rule has eliminated pregnancy risk category labels
- Use in women of childbearing potential requires weighing potential benefits to the mother against the risks to the fetus
- Seizures, even mild seizures, may cause harm to the embryo/fetus
- It is not known whether the pharmacokinetics of fosphenytoin change during pregnancy, but the pharmacokinetics of phenytoin do change significantly (see Phenytoin section)

Breast Feeding
- Breast milk: it is not known whether fosphenytoin is excreted in breast milk; phenytoin – 10–60% of maternal plasma levels
- Breastfed infants: it is not known what plasma fosphenytoin concentrations are achieved in breastfed infants compared with the levels of their mothers
- If drug is continued while breast feeding, infant should be monitored for possible adverse effects (irritability or sedation)
- If adverse effects are observed, recommend bottle feeding

The Overall Place of Fosphenytoin in the Treatment of Epilepsy
Although phenytoin is an invaluable AED for the management of acute seizures and status epilepticus, its parenteral formulation has numerous

disadvantages, including toxicity and administration problems, given that phenytoin is water-insoluble and must be formulated in propylene glycol and alcohol and has a pH of 14. A major disadvantage of iv phenytoin is that, with extravasation, it may result in severe tissue reactions such as "purple glove syndrome," which causes purplish-black skin discoloration, edema, and pain, and may progress to compartment syndrome and in some cases requires amputation.

Fosphenytoin by contrast is water-soluble and has a physiological pH, and is easier and safer to administer iv. Since im fosphenytoin is also well tolerated and safe, it may allow expanded use in clinical settings where prompt administration is indicated but secure iv access and cardiac monitoring are not available. Fosphenytoin is a well-tolerated and effective alternative to parenteral phenytoin in the emergency and non-emergency management of acute seizures in children and adults. It is often considered the drug of choice for the management of established status epilepticus.

Primary Seizure Types
• Generalized tonic–clonic seizures

Secondary Seizure Types
• Focal/partial seizures

Potential Advantages
• A useful alternative to parenteral phenytoin, especially since when fosphenytoin is given via im administration, cardiac and hemodynamic monitoring is not required
• Better tolerated at the injection site and has a similar onset of therapeutic action as parenteral phenytoin with rapid infusion

Potential Disadvantages
• Phenytoin is the pharmacologically active metabolite of fosphenytoin and dosing needs to be guided by therapeutic drug monitoring (measurement of blood levels) of phenytoin
• Phenytoin pharmacokinetics are not linear due to saturable metabolism
• iv administration requires that cardiac resuscitation equipment is available and continuous monitoring of ECG, blood pressure, and respiratory function for the duration of an iv infusion is essential
• Dosing units (mg PE) can be confusing

Suggested Reading

Aweeka FT, Gottwald MD, Gambertoglio JG, Wright TL, Boyer TD, Pollock AS, Eldon MA, Kuglar AR, Alldredge BK. Pharmacokinetics of fosphenytoin in patients with hepatic or renal disease. *Epilepsia* 1999; **40**: 777–782.

F

SUGGESTED READING

F

Boucher BA, Bombassaro A, Rasmussen SN, Watridge CB, Achari R, Turlapaty P. Phenytoin prodrug 3-phosphoryloxy-methyl phenytoin (ACC-9653): pharmacokinetics in patients following intravenous and intramuscular administration. *Journal of Pharmacological Sciences* 1989; **78**: 923–932.

Eldon MA, Loewen GR, Voigtman RE, Holmes GB, Hunt TL, Sedman AJ. Safety, tolerance, and pharmacokinetics of intravenous fosphenytoin. *Clinical Pharmacology and Therapeutics* 1993; **53**: 212.

Leppik IE, Boucher BA, Wilder BJ, Murthy VS, Watridge C, Graves NM, Rask CA, Turlapaty P. Pharmacokinetics and safety of a phenytoin prodrug given IV in patients. *Neurology* 1990; **40**: 456–460.

Pryor FM, Gidal B, Ramsay RE, DeToledo J, Morgan RO. Fosphenytoin: pharmacokinetics and tolerance of intramuscular loading doses. *Epilepsia* 2001; **42**: 245–250.

Thomson A. Fosphenytoin for the treatment of status epilepticus: an evidence-based assessment of its clinical and economic outcomes. *Core Evidence* 2005; **1**: 65–75.

GABAPENTIN

G

Therapeutics

Chemical Name and Structure

Gabapentin, 1-(aminomethyl)-cyclohexaneacetic acid, is a crystalline substance, with a molecular weight of 171.23 and an empirical formula of $C_9H_{17}NO_2$.

Brand Names
- Alpentin
- Bapex; Blugat
- Calmpent
- Dineurin; Dobin
- Encentin; Engaba; Epiven; Epleptin
- Fanatrex; Fusepaq
- Gaba; Gabacent; Gabaciz; Gabadin; Gabahexal; Gabalep; Gabalept; Gabantin; Gabapenin; Gabapin; Gabapin SR; Gabarone; Gabastar; Gabata; Gabatin; Gabatine; Gabatol; Gabator; Gabax; Gabexol; Gabietal; Gabin; Gabix; Gabtin; Gaby; Ganin; Gantin; Gapatin; Gapridol; Gaty; Gentin; Goben; Gralise
- Horizant (gabapentin enacarbil)
- Kaptin
- Mygaba
- Neogaba; Nepatic; Nervibrain; Neupent; Neuril; Neuronti; Neurontin; Neuropentin; Neuropin; New-GABA; Nopatic; Nulex; Nupentin
- Pendine; Pengatine; Progaba
- Reinin; Rejunate; Rejuron
- Sologab
- Templer
- Vultin
- Zepentine
- Zintigo

Generics Available
- Yes

Licensed Indications for Epilepsy
- Adjunctive treatment of partial seizures with or without secondary generalization in adults and children aged 6 years and above (UK SPC)

THERAPEUTICS

- Adjunctive treatment of partial seizures with or without secondary generalization in adults and children aged 3 years and above (FDA PI)
- Monotherapy treatment of partial seizures with or without secondary generalization in adults and children aged 12 years and above (UK SPC)

Licensed Indications for Non-epilepsy Conditions
- Peripheral neuropathic pain such as painful diabetic neuropathy and postherpetic neuralgia in adults (UK SPC)
- Postherpetic neuralgia in adults (FDA PI)
- Moderate to severe restless legs syndrome in adults (gabapentin enacarbil only; FDA PI)

Non-licensed Use for Epilepsy
- Use as monotherapy in the treatment of adolescents and adults with newly diagnosed epilepsy with partial/focal onset or mixed seizures

Non-licensed Use for Non-epilepsy Conditions
- Anxiety
- Bipolar disorder
- Fibromyalgia
- Insomnia
- Migraine
- Neuropathic pain
- Phantom limb pain
- Pruritus
- Restless legs syndrome
- Social phobia
- Trigeminal neuralgia

Ineffective (Contraindicated)
- It is ineffective or may exaggerate primary generalized seizures of any type, e.g., absence, atypical absence, myoclonic jerks, generalized tonic–clonic seizures
- Should be used with caution in patients with mixed seizures, including absence

Mechanism of Action
- Binds to the α2-δ protein subunit of voltage-gated calcium channels
- This closes N and P/Q presynaptic calcium channels, diminishing excessive neuronal activity and neurotransmitter release
- Although structurally related to GABA, it does not directly act on GABA or its receptors

Efficacy Profile
- The goals of treatment are to achieve complete seizure remission when possible, or at least improved frequency and severity of seizures,

GABAPENTIN

G

DRUG INTERACTION PROFILE

while also minimizing adverse effects and improving patient quality of life
- Efficacy should be apparent within 2 weeks of treatment initiation
- If it is not producing clinical benefits within 6–8 weeks, it may require a dosage increase or it may not work at all
- If gabapentin is ineffective or only partially effective, it can be replaced by or combined with another AED that is appropriate for the patient's seizure type or epilepsy syndrome

Pharmacokinetics
Absorption and Distribution
- Oral bioavailability: <60%, decreases at increasing doses
- Food co-ingestion: decreases the extent of absorption (25–30%) and absorption is delayed by ~2.5 hours
- As a leucine analog, gabapentin is transported both into the blood from the gut and also across the blood–brain barrier into the brain from the blood by the L transport system (a sodium-independent transporter)
- Tmax: 2–3 hours
- Time to steady state: 1–2 days
- Pharmacokinetics: non-linear due to saturable absorption
- Protein binding: 0%
- Volume of distribution: 0.65–1.04 L/kg
- Salivary concentrations: gabapentin is secreted into saliva and concentrations are similar to the unbound levels seen in plasma

Metabolism
- Gabapentin is not metabolized

Elimination
- Following a single dose, half-life values are 5–9 hours
- The renal clearance of gabapentin is proportional to the CrCl
- Renal excretion: 100% of an administered dose is excreted unchanged in urine

Drug Interaction Profile
Pharmacokinetic Drug Interactions
- Interactions between AEDs: effects on gabapentin:
  - To date, there have been no reports of AEDs affecting the clearance of gabapentin and affecting gabapentin plasma levels
- Interactions between AEDs: effects by gabapentin:
  - Gabapentin can *increase* felbamate plasma levels
  - Gabapentin can *decrease* pregabalin plasma levels
- Interactions between AEDs and non-AED drugs: effects on gabapentin:

- Antacids (Maalox, aluminum hydroxide, magnesium hydroxide) can reduce oral bioavailability of gabapentin and *decrease* gabapentin plasma levels
  - Cimetidine can *increase* gabapentin plasma levels
  - Hydrocodone, morphine, and naproxen can enhance the absorption of gabapentin and *increase* gabapentin plasma levels
- Interactions between AEDs and non-AED drugs: effects by gabapentin:
  - To date, there have been no reports of gabapentin affecting the clearance of other non-AED drugs and affecting their plasma levels

Pharmacodynamic Drug Interactions
- Gabapentin can enhance the analgesic effect of morphine

Hormonal Contraception
- Gabapentin does not enhance the metabolism of oral contraceptives and therefore does not compromise contraception control

Adverse Effects
How Drug Causes Adverse Effects
- CNS adverse effects may be due to excessive blockade of voltage-sensitive calcium channels

Common Adverse Effects
- Somnolence, dizziness, ataxia, fatigue, nystagmus, tremor
- Vomiting, dyspepsia, diarrhea, constipation, anorexia, increased appetite, dry mouth
- Blurred vision, diplopia, vertigo
- Edema, weight gain, purpura, rash, pruritus, acne
- Impotence
- Additional effects in children under age 12 include: aggressive behavior, emotional lability, hyperkinesia, thought disorder, respiratory tract infections, otitis media, bronchitis

Life-threatening or Dangerous Adverse Effects
- Caution is recommended in patients with a history of psychotic illness
- Some patients may experience acute pancreatitis
- Patients on hemodialysis due to end-stage renal failure may develop myopathy with elevated creatinine kinase
- Rarely rash, leukopenia, EEG changes, and angina
- May unmask myasthenia gravis

Rare and not Life-threatening Adverse Effects
- To date, none have been reported

G

Weight Change
• Weight gain is common

What to do About Adverse Effects
• Discuss common and severe adverse effects with patients or parents before starting medication, including symptoms that should be reported to the physician
• Sedation is dose-related and can be problematic at high doses
• Sedation can subside with time, but may not at high doses
• Can consider dividing the total daily dosage into more frequent smaller individual doses, although adherence/compliance may then be difficult and decline
• Take more of the dose at night to reduce daytime sedation

Dosing and Use
Usual Dosage Range
• Adults and children over 12 years of age: 900–3600 mg/day
• Children 3–12 years of age: 25–40 mg/kg/day

Available Formulations
• Capsules: 100 mg, 300 mg, 400 mg
• Tablets: 600 mg, 800 mg
• Extended-release (gabapentin enacarbil) tablets: 300 mg, 600 mg
• Oral solution: 50 mg/L

How to Dose
• When initiating gabapentin treatment start with a low dose and titrate slowly so as to minimize adverse effects.
   – *For adults and children over 12 years of age:* start treatment with 300 mg/day on day 1; subsequently increase to 300 mg twice daily on day 2; subsequently increase to 300 mg thrice daily on day 3; increase subsequently according to response in steps of 300 mg in three divided doses; maintenance dose generally not greater than 3600 mg/day given in three equally divided doses
   – *Children: 6–12 years of age:* start treatment only as adjunctive therapy with 10–15 mg/kg daily in three divided doses; subsequently increase according to response over 3 days in steps of 10 mg/kg daily in three divided doses; maintenance dose is generally 25–35 mg/kg/day given in three equally divided doses
   – *Children: 3–5 years of age:* start treatment only as adjunctive therapy with 10–15 mg/kg daily in three divided doses; subsequently increase over 3 days to 40 mg/kg/day; maximum dose generally 50 mg/kg/day; time between any two doses should usually not exceed 12 hours

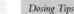

GABAPENTIN

Dosing Tips
- Titration of dose can be undertaken rapidly; usually maintenance dosages can be achieved within a week, and should be undertaken based on individual tolerability and response to the drug
- In patients with poor general health (e.g., low body weight, organ transplantation) the dose should be titrated more slowly, either by using smaller dosage strengths or longer intervals between dosage increases
- Co-administration of gabapentin with antacids containing aluminum and magnesium reduces gabapentin bioavailability by ~25% – this can be avoided by delaying gabapentin ingestion until at least 2 hours after antacid ingestion
- While generally best titrated over several days, in exceptional or urgent situations, gabapentin may be safely rapidly titrated, or even started at a maximal dosage of 3,600 mg daily

How to Withdraw Drug
- There is no need to adjust dosage of concurrent medications as gabapentin is being discontinued, because plasma levels of other drugs do not change (see Pharmacokinetic Drug Interactions section)
- Taper: a gradual dose reduction over a minimum of a 1-week period should be undertaken
- Rapid discontinuation may induce withdrawal seizures

Overdose
- In overdoses up to 49 g, life-threatening adverse effects have not been observed
- The most common adverse effects observed with gabapentin overdose include dizziness, double vision, slurred speech, drowsiness, lethargy, and mild diarrhea
- Reduced absorption of gabapentin at higher doses (due to saturable absorption) probably limits drug absorption and hence minimizes toxicity
- Overdoses of gabapentin in combination with other CNS-depressant medications may result in coma
- The stomach should be emptied immediately by lavage or by induction of emesis
- Hemodialysis removes gabapentin from blood (30–40% over 4 hours) and, therefore, may be a useful procedure in cases of overdose

Tests and Therapeutic Drug Monitoring
- Before starting: liver and kidney function tests
- Therapeutic drug monitoring:
  - Optimum seizure control in patients on monotherapy is most likely to occur at gabapentin plasma concentrations of 2–20 mg/L (12–117 μmol/L)
  - The conversion factor from mg/L to μmol/L is 5.84 (i.e., 1 mg/L = 5.84 μmol/L)

G

- The reference range of gabapentin in plasma is considered to be the same for children and adults, although no data are available to support this clinical practice
- Gabapentin can be monitored by use of saliva, which is a measure of the free non-protein-bound plasma concentration and is pharmacologically relevant
• Before giving a drug that can cause weight gain to an overweight or obese patient, consider determining whether the patient already has pre-diabetes (fasting plasma glucose 100–125 mg/dL), diabetes (fasting plasma glucose greater than 126 mg/dL), or dyslipidemia (increased total cholesterol, low-density lipoprotein (LDL) cholesterol, and triglycerides; decreased high-density lipoprotein (HDL) cholesterol), and treat or refer such patients for treatment, including nutrition and weight management, physical activity counseling, smoking cessation, and medical management
• Monitor weight and body mass index (BMI) during treatment

Other Warnings / Precautions
• Some diabetic patients who gain weight on gabapentin treatment may need to adjust their hypoglycemic medications
• Some patients may experience dizziness and somnolence and thus caution needs to be exercised if patient intends to drive or use machinery

Do not Use
• If patient has a proven allergy to gabapentin or pregabalin or to any of the excipients – capsules contain lactose
• Because the capsule formulation contains lactose, patients with rare hereditary problems of galactose intolerance, Lapp lactose deficiency, or glucose–galactose malabsorption should not take this formulation

Special Populations
Renal Impairment
• Gabapentin is renally excreted, so the dose needs to be adjusted according to CrCl as follows:
  - CrCl of ≥ 80 mL/min – total daily dose: 900–3600 mg/day taken three times a day
  - CrCl of 50–79 mL/min – total daily dose: 600–1800 mg/day taken three times a day
  - CrCl of 30–49 mL/min – total daily dose: 300–900 mg/day taken three times a day
  - CrCl of 15–29 mL/min – total daily dose: 150–600 mg/day taken as 300 mg every other day
  - CrCl of <15 mL/min – total daily dose: 150–300 mg/day taken as 300 mg every other day

- For patients with CrCl of <15 mL/min, the daily dose should be reduced in proportion to CrCl. For example, patients with a CrCl of 7.5 mL/min should receive half the daily dose that patients with a CrCl of 15 mL/min receive
- Because gabapentin can be removed by hemodialysis, patients receiving hemodialysis may require supplemental doses of gabapentin

Hepatic Impairment
- Because gabapentin is not metabolized and is excreted predominantly as unchanged drug in urine, dosage adjustment will not be necessary in patients with hepatic impairment

Children
- Children have an increased metabolic capacity and consequently higher doses on an mg/kg basis are usually required to achieve the equivalent therapeutic plasma levels seen in adults

Elderly
- Elderly patients are more susceptible to adverse effects and, therefore, tolerate lower doses better
- Because of an age-related reduction in renal function, lower gabapentin doses are appropriate and should be based on CrCl values. Because gabapentin is associated with dizziness, somnolence, and ataxia, the elderly are at increased risk of accidental injury (fall)
- The elderly have an increased risk of somnolence, peripheral edema, and asthenia
- Elderly patients are often prescribed concurrent drug therapies for comorbidities and therefore may be at greater risk for pharmacokinetic and pharmacodynamic interactions; as the risk of pharmacokinetic interactions with gabapentin is low or non-existent, gabapentin may be advantageous for use in the elderly

Pregnancy
- Specialist advice should be given to women who are of childbearing potential; they should be informed about the teratogenicity of all AEDs and the importance of avoiding an unplanned pregnancy; the AED treatment regimen should be reviewed when a woman is planning to become pregnant
- Rapid discontinuation of AEDs should be avoided as this may lead to breakthrough seizures, which could have serious consequences for the woman and the unborn child
- Gabapentin was previously classified by the US FDA as risk category C (some animal studies show adverse effects, no controlled studies in humans); the current FDA Pregnancy and Lactation Rule has eliminated pregnancy risk category labels; in humans, gabapentin has recently been found to be associated with a lower risk of major malformations compared to several other AEDs

- Use in women of childbearing potential requires weighing potential benefits to the mother against the risks to the fetus
- Use with other AEDs in combination may cause a higher prevalence of teratogenic effects than gabapentin monotherapy
- Taper drug if discontinuing
- Seizures, even mild seizures, may cause harm to the embryo/fetus
- Gabapentin pharmacokinetics do not change during pregnancy

Breast Feeding
- Breast milk: the milk/maternal blood concentration ratio is 0.7–1.3
- Breastfed infants: gabapentin plasma levels are 4–12% of maternal plasma levels
- If drug is continued while breast feeding, infant should be monitored for possible adverse effects (irritability or sedation), including hematological effects
- If adverse effects are observed, recommend bottle feeding

The Overall Place of Gabapentin in the Treatment of Epilepsy
Gabapentin is a narrow-spectrum AED whose role is limited to the management of partial (focal) seizures, although its efficacy is relatively weak compared with other AEDs. The number of patients who respond to gabapentin is disproportionately low even when higher doses are used, although some patients with severe focal epilepsies derive therapeutic benefit.

Primary Seizure Types
- Partial (focal)-onset seizures

Secondary Seizure Types
- None

Potential Advantages
- Gabapentin is generally well tolerated, with only mild adverse effects
- Not associated with any significant pharmacokinetic interactions

Potential Disadvantages
- Most studies have shown gabapentin to be less potent than pregabalin, although a recent head-to-head trial of flexibly titrated gabapentin 400–600 mg tid vs. pregabalin 200 mg tid showed no significant difference in efficacy between these drugs
- Exacerbates absences, myoclonic jerks, and generalized tonic–clonic seizures
- Requires tid dosing
- Pharmacokinetics are not linear due to saturable absorption
- Potential teratogen

G

Suggested Reading

Bergey GK, Morris HH, Rosenfeld W, Blume WT, Penovich PE, Morrell MJ, Leiderman DB, Crockatt JG, LaMoreaux L, Garofalo E, Pierce M. Gabapentin monotherapy: I. An 8-day, double-blind, dose-controlled, multicenter study in hospitalized patients with refractory complex partial or secondarily generalized seizures. The US Gabapentin Study Group 88/89. *Neurology* 1997; **49**: 739–745.

Costa J, Fareleira F, Ascenção R, Borges M, Sampaio C, Vaz-Carneiro A. Clinical comparability of the new antiepileptic drugs in refractory partial epilepsy: a systematic review and meta-analysis. *Epilepsia* 2011; **52**: 1280–1291.

Fink K, Dooley DJ, Meder WP, Suman-Chauhan N, Duffy S, Clusmann H, Gothert M. Inhibition of neuronal Ca(2+) influx by gabapentin and pregabalin in the human neocortex. *Neuropharmacology* 2002; **42**: 229–236.

French J, Glue P, Friedman D, Almas M, Yardi N, Knapp L, Pitman V, Posner HB. Adjunctive pregabalin vs gabapentin for focal seizures: interpretation of comparative outcomes. *Neurology* 2016; **87**: 1242–1249.

French JA, Kanner AM, Bautista J, et al. Efficacy and tolerability of the new antiepileptic drugs I: treatment of new onset epilepsy: report of the Therapeutics and Technology Assessment Subcommittee and Quality Standards Subcommittee of the American Academy of Neurology and the American Epilepsy Society. *Neurology* 2004; **62**: 1252–1260.

French JA, Kanner AM, Bautista J, et al. Efficacy and tolerability of the new antiepileptic drugs II: treatment of refractory epilepsy: efficacy and tolerability of the new antiepileptic drugs II: treatment of refractory epilepsy: report of the Therapeutics and Technology Assessment Subcommittee and Quality Standards Subcommittee of the American Academy of Neurology and the American Epilepsy Society. *Neurology* 2004; **62**: 1261–1273.

Fujii H, Goel A, Bernard N, Pistelli A, Yates LM, Stephens S, Han JY, Matsui D, Etwell F, Einarson TR, Koren G, Einarson A. Pregnancy outcomes following gabapentin use: results of a prospective comparative cohort study. *Neurology* 2013; **80**: 1565–1570.

Gidal BE, Radulovic LL, Kruger S, Rutecki P, Pitterle M, Bockbrader HN. Inter- and intra-subject variability in gabapentin absorption and absolute bioavailability. *Epilepsy Research* 2000; **40**: 123–127.

Johannessen Landmark C, Patsalos PN. Drug interactions involving the new second- and third-generation antiepileptic drugs. *Expert Reviews in Neurotherapeutics* 2010; **10**: 119–140.

Marson AG, Kadir ZA, Hutton JL, Chadwick DW. The new antiepileptic drugs: a systematic review of their efficacy and tolerability. *Epilepsia* 1997; **38**: 859–880.

McLean MJ, Gidal BE. Gabapentin dosing in the treatment of epilepsy. *Clinical Therapeutics* 2003; **25**: 1382–1406.

GABAPENTIN

Ohman I, Vitolis S, Tomson T. Pharmacokinetics of gabapentin during delivery, in the neonatal period and lactation. *Epilepsia* 2005; **46**: 1621–1624.

Patsalos PN. *Antiepileptic drug interactions: a clinical guide*, 3rd edition. Springer, London, UK; 2016.

Patsalos PN, Zugman M, Lake C, James A, Ratnaraj N, Sander JW. Serum protein binding of 25 antiepileptic drugs in a routine clinical setting: a comparison of free non-protein-bound concentrations. *Epilepsia* 2017; **58**: 1234–1243.

St. Louis EK. The art of managing conversions between antiepileptic drugs; maximizing patient tolerability and quality of life. *Pharmaceuticals* 2010; **3**: 2956–2969.

St. Louis EK, Gidal BE, Henry TR, Kaydanova Y, Krumholz A, McCabe PH, Montouris GD, Rosenfeld WE, Smith BJ, Stern JM, Waterhouse EJ, Schulz RM, Garnett WR, Bramley T. Conversions between monotherapies in epilepsy: expert consensus. *Epilepsy and Behavior* 2007; **11**: 222–234.

Vollmer KO, von Hodenberg A, Kolle EU. Pharmacokinetics and metabolism of gabapentin in rat, dog and man. *Arzneimittel Forschung Drug Research* 1988; **36**: 830–839.

Wolf SM, Shinner S, Kang H, Gil KB, Moshe SL. Gabapentin toxicity in children manifesting as behavioural changes. *Epilepsia* 1995; **36**: 1203–1205.

G

SUGGESTED READING

LACOSAMIDE

Therapeutics

Chemical Name and Structure

Lacosamide, (R)-2-acetamido-*N*-benzyl-3-methoxypropramide, is a white powder, with a molecular weight of 250.29 and an empirical formula of $C_{13}H_{18}N_2O_3$.

Brand Names
• Vimpat

Generics Available
• No

Licensed Indications for Epilepsy
• Adjunctive or monotherapy treatment of partial (focal)–onset seizures with or without secondary generalization in patients with epilepsy aged 16 years and older (UK SPC)
• Adjunctive treatment of partial (focal)–onset seizures with or without secondary generalization in patients with epilepsy aged 17 years and older. Injection is indicated as short-term replacement therapy when oral administration is not feasible in these patients. (FDA PI)
• Monotherapy in the treatment of partial (focal)–onset seizures in adults aged 17 years and older (FDA PI)
• Single loading dose administration option for all formulations aged 17 years and older (FDA PI)

Licensed Indications for Non-epilepsy Conditions
• There are none

Non-licensed Use for Epilepsy
• Monotherapy in newly diagnosed epilepsy in adults
• Status epilepticus (iv formulation)

Non-licensed Use for Non-epilepsy Conditions
• Neuropathic pain
• Restless legs syndrome

L

Ineffective (Contraindicated)
• Data on seizure contraindications are not available

Mechanism of Action
• Acts by enhancing slow inactivation of voltage-gated sodium channels, resulting in stabilization of hyperexcitable neuronal membranes

Efficacy Profile
• The goals of treatment are to achieve complete seizure remission when possible, or at least improved frequency and severity of seizures, while also minimizing adverse effects and improving patient quality of life
• Efficacy should be apparent within 4 weeks of treatment initiation
• If it is not producing clinical benefits within 6–8 weeks, it may require a dosage increase or it may not work at all
• If lacosamide is ineffective or only partially effective, it can be replaced by or combined with another AED that is appropriate for the patient's seizure type or epilepsy syndrome

Pharmacokinetics
Absorption and Distribution
• Oral bioavailability: 100%
• Food co-ingestion: neither delays the rate of absorption nor decreases the extent of absorption
• Tmax: 1–2 hours
• Time to steady state: 2–3 days
• Pharmacokinetics: linear
• Protein binding: <15%
• Volume of distribution: 0.6–0.7 L/kg
• Salivary concentrations: lacosamide is secreted into saliva and concentrations are similar to the unbound levels seen in plasma

Metabolism
• Metabolized in the liver, by demethylation, to O-desmethyl lacosamide (30%)
• CYP2C19 is considered to be primarily responsible for the formation of O-desmethyl lacosamide, although CYP2C9 and CYP3A4 contribute
• Other unidentified metabolites constitute a further 30% of metabolism
• The metabolites of lacosamide are not pharmacologically active
• Autoinduction is not a feature of lacosamide metabolism

Elimination
• The plasma half-life in healthy volunteers and in patients with epilepsy is 13 hours
• Renal excretion: 40% of an administered dose is excreted unchanged in urine

PHARMACOKINETICS

L

LACOSAMIDE

Drug Interaction Profile

Pharmacokinetic Drug Interactions
- Interactions between AEDs: effects on lacosamide:
  - Carbamazepine, phenobarbital, and phenytoin can *increase* the clearance of lacosamide and *decrease* lacosamide plasma levels
- Interactions between AEDs: effects by lacosamide:
  - Lacosamide can *decrease* plasma levels of 10-hydroxycarbazepine
- Interactions between AEDs and non-AED drugs: effects on lacosamide:
  - To date, there have been no reports of other non-AED drugs affecting the clearance of lacosamide and affecting lacosamide plasma levels
- Interactions between AEDs and non-AED drugs: effects by lacosamide:
  - To date, there have been no reports of lacosamide affecting the clearance of other non-AED drugs and affecting their plasma levels

Pharmacodynamic Drug Interactions
- Co-medication with carbamazepine: neurotoxicity may present as blurred vision, dizzy spells, and decreased alertness – this occurs in the absence of any change in lacosamide, carbamazepine, or carbamazepine-epoxide plasma levels
- Co-medication with lamotrigine: neurotoxicity may present – this occurs in the absence of any change in lacosamide or lamotrigine plasma levels
- Co-medication with oxcarbazepine: neurotoxicity may present as diplopia, ataxia, and vertigo – this occurs in the absence of any change in lacosamide or 10-hydroxycarbazepine plasma levels
- Co-medication with phenytoin: neurotoxicity may present as unsteadiness and diplopia – this occurs in the absence of any change in lacosamide or phenytoin plasma levels
- Hyperammonemic encephalopathy may occur in combination with valproic acid consequent to a pharmacodynamic interaction

Hormonal Contraception
- Lacosamide does not enhance the metabolism of oral contraceptives and therefore does not compromise contraception control

Adverse Effects

How Drug Causes Adverse Effects
- Not known

Common Adverse Effects
- Dizziness, headache, balance disorder, abnormal coordination, memory impairment, somnolence, tremor, nystagmus
- Diplopia, blurred vision

- Vertigo
- Nausea, vomiting, constipation, flatulence
- Pruritus
- Depression

Life-threatening or Dangerous Adverse Effects
- Increases PR interval, therefore, patients with known second- or third-degree atrioventricular block may be at risk of severe symptomatic bradycardia or syncope; particular caution is necessary in patients with a known history of cardiac conduction problems (e.g., atrioventricular block or sick sinus syndrome), myocardial ischemia, or heart failure
- Particular caution should be exercised with the elderly who are at an increased risk of cardiac disorders, patients receiving antiarrhythmic or AEDs (e.g., carbamazepine, lamotrigine, and pregabalin) that are associated with PR prolongation

Rare and not Life-threatening Adverse Effects
- To date, none have been reported

Weight Change
- No significant effect on weight is expected

What to do About Adverse Effects
- Discuss common and severe adverse effects with patients or parents before starting medication, including symptoms that should be reported to the physician
- Dosage reduction or considering dividing the total daily dosage into more frequent smaller doses (i.e., three or four times daily dosing) can be considered, but may cause difficulties with adherence/compliance
- Risk of adverse effects is greatest in the first few months of treatment
- Common adverse effects such as nausea often abate after a few months

Dosing and Use
Usual Dosage Range
- Adults: 200–400 mg/day

Available Formulations
- Tablets: 50 mg, 100 mg, 150 mg, 200 mg
- Syrup (strawberry-flavored): 15 mg/mL (200 mL/bottle and 465 mL/bottle)
- Solution: 10 mg/mL (20 mL/vial)

L

DOSING AND USE

L

How to Dose
- When initiating lacosamide treatment start with a low dose and titrate slowly so as to minimize adverse effects
  - *For adults of age 16 years or older:* start treatment with 50 mg twice daily for 1 week; increase by 100 mg/day in divided doses at weekly intervals; maximum dose 200 mg twice daily

Although dosage recommendations for children have not been provided, the following suggestions are based on general rules of dosage requirements in infants and children:

- In a *child less than 16 years:* start treatment with 1.5 mg/kg twice daily (3 mg/kg/day) for 1 week; increase by 3 mg/kg/day in divided doses as tolerated and as needed at weekly intervals; maximum dose 6 mg/kg twice daily (12 mg/kg/day)
- In an *infant:* start treatment with 2.0 mg/kg twice daily (4 mg/kg/day) for 1 week; increase by 4 mg/kg/day in divided doses as tolerated and as needed at weekly intervals; maximum dose 8 mg/kg twice daily (16 mg/kg/day)

Dosing Tips
- The solution for infusion and the tablets are bioequivalent and, therefore, can be used interchangeably
- When using infusion, administer iv over 15–30 minutes twice daily

How to Withdraw Drug
- May need to adjust dosage of concurrent medications as lacosamide is being discontinued, because plasma levels of other drugs may change (see Pharmacokinetic Drug Interactions section)
- Taper: reduce dose by 200 mg/week
- Rapid discontinuation may increase the risk of seizures

Overdose
- Following doses of more than 800 mg/day, dizziness, nausea, vomiting, and seizures have been reported
- In one case of lacosamide overdose (12 g) in conjunction with toxic doses of other AEDs, the subject was initially comatose and then fully recovered without permanent sequelae
- The stomach should be emptied immediately by lavage or by induction of emesis
- Hemodialysis removes ~50% of lacosamide from blood over 4 hours and, therefore, may be a useful procedure in cases of overdose

Tests and Therapeutic Drug Monitoring
- Before starting: liver and kidney function tests
- Consider ECG to rule out atrioventricular block
- During treatment: liver and kidney function tests every 12 months

- Therapeutic drug monitoring:
  - Optimum seizure control in patients on monotherapy is most likely to occur at lacosamide plasma concentrations of 10–20 mg/L (40–80 µmol/L)
  - The conversion factor from mg/L to µmol/L is 3.99 (i.e., 1 mg/L = 3.99 µmol/L)
  - The reference range of lacosamide in plasma is considered to be the same for children and adults, although no data are available to support this clinical practice
  - Lacosamide can be monitored by use of saliva, which is a measure of the free non-protein-bound plasma concentration and is pharmacologically relevant

Other Warnings/Precautions
- Lacosamide can cause dizziness and blurred vision which could increase the occurrence of accidental injury or falls

Do not Use
- If patient has conduction problems or severe cardiac disease such as a history of myocardial ischemia or heart failure
- If patient has a proven allergy to the active substance or to peanuts or soya or to any of its excipients
- If patient has hereditary problems of fructose intolerance (syrup formulation only)
- If patient suffers from phenylketonuria (syrup formulation only as it contains aspartame – a source of phenylalanine)

Special Populations
Renal Impairment
- Lacosamide and its metabolites are renally excreted
- Mild to moderate renal impairment (CrCl >30 – <80 mL/min) results in increased lacosamide AUC values of ~30%; a dosage reduction may be necessary in some patients
- Severe renal impairment (CrCl <30 mL/min) results in increased lacosamide AUC values of ~60%; a maximum dosage of 250 mg/day is recommended for these patients
- Because lacosamide can be removed by hemodialysis, patients receiving hemodialysis may require supplemental doses of lacosamide

Hepatic Impairment
- Lacosamide undergoes moderate metabolism (60%) in the liver and consequently lower doses may be required
- Moderate hepatic impairment (Child–Pugh B) can be associated with a 20% increase in lacosamide AUC values

Children

• Lacosamide is not licensed for use in children, but dosage suggestions are provided under "How to Dose"

Elderly

• Elderly patients are more susceptible to adverse effects and, therefore, tolerate lower doses better
• Because of an age-related reduction in hepatic and renal function, lower lacosamide doses are appropriate
• Elderly patients are often prescribed concurrent drug therapies for comorbidities and therefore may be at greater risk for pharmacokinetic and pharmacodynamic interactions; as the risk of pharmacokinetic interactions with lacosamide is low or non-existent, lacosamide may be advantageous for use in the elderly

Pregnancy

• Specialist advice should be given to women who are of childbearing potential; they should be informed about the teratogenicity of all AEDs and the importance of avoiding an unplanned pregnancy; the AED treatment regimen should be reviewed when a woman is planning to become pregnant
• Rapid discontinuation of AEDs should be avoided as this may lead to breakthrough seizures, which could have serious consequences for the woman and the unborn child
• Lacosamide was previously classified by the US FDA as risk category C (some animal studies show adverse effects); the current FDA Pregnancy and Lactation Rule has eliminated pregnancy risk category labels; in humans, lacosamide has been found to be associated with a lower risk of major malformations compared to several other AEDs
• Use in women of childbearing potential requires weighing potential benefits to the mother against the risks to the fetus
• Use with other AEDs in combination may cause a higher prevalence of teratogenic effects than lacosamide monotherapy
• Taper drug if discontinuing
• Seizures, even mild seizures, may cause harm to the embryo/fetus
• Data on the pharmacokinetic changes of lacosamide during pregnancy are not available

Breast Feeding

• Breast milk: it is not known whether lacosamide is excreted in breast milk
• Breastfed infants: it is not known what plasma lacosamide concentrations are achieved in breastfed infants compared with the levels of their mothers
• If drug is continued while breast feeding, infant should be monitored for possible adverse effects
• If adverse effects are observed, recommend bottle feeding

The Overall Place of Lacosamide in the Treatment of Epilepsy
Lacosamide is an effective option for the treatment of patients with partial (focal) epilepsy and has a prominent role as an adjunctive therapy in current practice, with an emerging role as a monotherapy choice or conversion to monotherapy. It has equally good efficacy in children and has the additional advantage of iv administration when necessary.

Primary Seizure Types
• Partial/focal seizures with or without secondary generalization

Secondary Seizure Types
• None

Potential Advantages
• Simple straightforward pharmacokinetics
• Not associated with any significant pharmacokinetic interactions

Potential Disadvantages
• The adverse effect of vomiting may compromise compliance
• Potential teratogen

Suggested Reading

Baulac M, Rosenow F, Toledo M, Terada K, Li T, De Backer M, Werhahn KJ, Brock M. Efficacy, safety, and tolerability of lacosamide monotherapy versus controlled-release carbamazepine in patients with newly diagnosed epilepsy: a phase 3, randomised, double-blind, non-inferiority trial. *Lancet Neurology* 2017; **16**: 43–54.

Ben-Menachem E, Biton V, Jatuzis D, Abdul-Khalil B, Doty P, Rudd GD. Efficacy and safety of oral lacosamide as adjunctive therapy in adults with partial-onset seizures. *Epilepsia* 2007; **48**: 1308–1317.

Beyreuther BK, Freitag J, Heers C, Krebsfanger N, Scharfenecker U, Stohr T. Lacosamide: a review of preclinical properties. *CNS Drug Reviews* 2007; **13**: 21–42.

Biton V, Rosenfeld WE, Whitesides J, Fountain NB, Vaiciene N, Rudd GD. Intravenous lacosamide as replacement of oral lacosamide in patients with partial-onset seizures. *Epilepsia* 2008; **49**: 418–424.

Halasz P, Kalviainen R, Mazurkiewicz-Beldzinska M, Rosenow F, Doty P, Hebert D, Sullivan T, on behalf of the SP755 Study Group. Adjunctive lacosamide for partial-onset seizures: efficacy and safety results from a randomized controlled study. *Epilepsia* 2009; **50**: 443–453.

Höfler J, Trinka E. Lacosamide as a new treatment option in status epilepticus. *Epilepsia* 2013; **53**: 393–404.

Kellinghaus C, Berning S, Besselmann M. Intravenous lacosamide as successful treatment for nonconvulsive status epilepticus after failure of first-line therapy. *Epilepsy and Behavior* 2009; **14**: 429–431.

L

SUGGESTED READING

L

Miro J, Toledo M, Santamarina E, Ricciardi AC, Villanueva V, Pato A, Ruiz J, Juvany R, Falip M. Efficacy of intravenous lacosamide as add-on treatment in refractory status epilepticus: a multicentric prospective study. *Seizure* 2013; **22**: 77–79.

Novy J, Pastsalos PN, Sander JW, Sisodiya SM. Lacosamide neurotoxicity associated with concomitant use of sodium channel-blocking antiepileptic drugs: a pharmacodynamic interaction? *Epilepsy and Behavior* 2011; **20**: 20–23.

Nunes VD, Sawer L, Neilson J, Sarri G, Cross JH. Profile of lacosamide and its long-term treatment of epilepsy: a prospective from the updated NICE guidelines. *Neuropsychiatric Disease and Treatment* 2013; **9**: 467–476.

Patsalos PN, Berry DJ. Pharmacotherapy of the third-generation AEDs: lacosamide, retigabine and eslicarbazepine acetate. *Expert Opinion in Pharmacotherapy* 2012; **13**: 699–715.

Verrotti A, Loiacono G, Pizzolorusso A, Parisi P, Bruni O, Luchetti A, Zamponi N, Cappanera S, Grosso S, Kluger G, Janello C, Franzoni E, Elia M, Spalice A, Coppola G, Striano P, Pavone P, Savasta S, Viri M, Romeo A, Aloisi P, Gobbi G, Ferretti A, Cusmai R, Curatolo P. Lacosamide in paediatric and adult patients: comparison of efficacy and safety. *Seizure* 2013; **22**: 210–216.

Vossler DG, Wechsler RT, Williams P, Byrnes W, Therriault S; ALEX-MT study group. Long-term exposure and safety of lacosamide monotherapy for the treatment of partial-onset (focal) seizures: results from a multicenter, open-label trial. *Epilepsia* 2016; **57**: 1625–1633.

Wechsler RT, Li G, French J, O'Brien TJ, D'Cruz O, Williams P, Goodson R, Brock M; ALEX-MT Study Group. Conversion to lacosamide monotherapy in the treatment of focal epilepsy: results from a historical-controlled, multicenter, double-blind study. *Epilepsia* 2014; **55**: 1088–1098.

LACOSAMIDE

LAMOTRIGINE

L

Therapeutics

Chemical Name and Structure

Lamotrigine, 3,5-diamino-6[2,3-dichlorophenyl]-1,2,4-triazine, is a white crystalline powder, with a molecular weight of 256.09 and an empirical formula of $C_9H_7Cl_2N_5$.

Brand Names

- Elmendos; Epitec; Epitic
- Gerolamic
- Labicitin; Labileno; Lagotran; Lamal; Lambipol; Lamdra; Lamepil; Lamepril; Lametec; Lamictal; Lamictal XR; Lamictin; Lamidus; Lanitor; Lamitrin; Lamodex; Lamogin; Lamogine; Lamonex; Lamo-Q; Lamorig; Lamosyn; Lamot; Lamotrigin; Lamotrigina; Lamotrigine; Lamotrine; Lamotrix; Lamozine; Laogine; Latrigine; Lemit; Lemogen; Logem; Lotrigine; Lyzin
- Medotrigin; Meganox; Mogine
- Neural; Neurium
- Pinral; Plexxo; Protalgine
- Reedos
- Seaze; Solaban; Symia
- Topepil; Tradox; Trigilab; Trigin; Triginet; Trizol
- Xebarin

Generics Available

- Yes

Licensed Indications for Epilepsy

- Monotherapy conversion from another AED (labeled conversions include carbamazepine, phenytoin, phenobarbital, primidone, and valproate) in adults and children over 16 years of age for the treatment of partial/focal seizures and primary and secondary generalized tonic–clonic seizures (FDA PI)
- Adjunctive therapy in adults and children over 2 years of age and treatment of partial/focal seizures and primary and secondary generalized tonic–clonic seizures and generalized seizures of Lennox–Gastaut syndrome (UK SPC; FDA PI)

THERAPEUTICS

L

- Adjunctive therapy in adults and children over 2 years of age of seizures associated with Lennox–Gastaut syndrome (UK SPC; FDA PI)
- Monotherapy of typical absence seizures (UK SPC)

Licensed Indications for Non-epilepsy Conditions
- Maintenance treatment of bipolar I disorder in adults (≥ 18 years of age) (FDA PI)
- Prevention of depressive episodes in patients with bipolar I disorder who experience predominantly depressive episodes (UK SPC)

Non-licensed Use for Epilepsy
- There are none

Non-licensed Use for Non-epilepsy Conditions
- Bipolar II disorders
- Cluster headaches
- Depersonalization disorder
- Migraine
- Neuropathic pain
- Peripheral neuropathy
- Psychosis
- Schizophrenia
- Trigeminal neuralgia
- Unipolar depression and other mood disorders

Ineffective (Contraindicated)
- Lamotrigine may aggravate myoclonic seizures and syndromes with predominantly myoclonic seizures (e.g., juvenile myoclonic epilepsy, Dravet syndrome, and progressive myoclonic epilepsy)

Mechanism of Action
- Acts as a use-dependent blocker of voltage-sensitive sodium channels
- Interacts with the open-channel conformation of voltage-sensitive sodium channels
- Interacts at a specific site of the alpha pore-forming subunit of voltage-sensitive sodium channels
- Inhibits release of glutamate

Efficacy Profile
- The goals of treatment are to achieve complete seizure remission when possible, or at least improved frequency and severity of seizures, while also minimizing adverse effects and improving patient quality of life
- Efficacy should be apparent within 2 weeks of treatment initiation
- If it is not producing clinical benefits within 6–8 weeks, it may require a dosage increase or it may not work at all
- If lamotrigine is ineffective or only partially effective, it can be replaced by or combined with another AED that is appropriate for the patient's seizure type or epilepsy syndrome

LAMOTRIGINE

Pharmacokinetics

Absorption and Distribution
- Oral bioavailability: >95%
- Food co-ingestion: causes a slight delay in the rate of absorption but the extent of absorption is unaffected
- Tmax: 1–3 hours
- Time to steady state: 3–7 days
- Pharmacokinetics: linear
- Protein binding: 55%
- Volume of distribution: 0.9–1.3 L/kg
- Salivary concentrations: lamotrigine is secreted into saliva and concentrations are similar to the unbound levels seen in plasma

Metabolism
- Lamotrigine undergoes extensive metabolism in the liver, by conjugation with glucuronic acid, to various metabolites, including 2-N-glucuronide (76% of dose) and 5-N-glucuronide (10% of dose), a 2-N-methyl metabolite (0.14% of dose), and other unidentified minor metabolites (4% of dose)
- Glucuronidation is by means of uridine diphosphate (UDP)-glucuronosyltransferases and the isoform that is responsible for the N-glucuronidation of lamotrigine is uridine glucuronyl transferase (UGT) 1A4
- The metabolites of lamotrigine are not pharmacologically active
- Lamotrigine undergoes autoinduction so that clearance can increase by 17–37% and this may require an upward dosage adjustment when prescribed as monotherapy

Elimination
- As a monotherapy, or in polytherapy in the absence of enzyme-inducing co-medications, half-life values for lamotrigine are 15–35 hours
- When co-administered with valproic acid, in the absence of enzyme-inducing co-medication, half-life values for lamotrigine are 30–90 hours
- In polytherapy including an enzyme-inducing co-medication, half-life values for lamotrigine are 8–20 hours
- In polytherapy with valproate together with an enzyme-inducing co-medication, half-life values for lamotrigine are 15–35 hours
- Renal excretion: ~90% of an administered dose is excreted as metabolites in urine; 2-N-glucuronide (76%), 5-N-glucuronide (10%), 2-N-methyl metabolite (0.14%), and other unidentified minor metabolites (4%)
- Renal excretion: approximately 10% of an administered dose is excreted as unchanged lamotrigine in urine

L

Drug Interaction Profile

Pharmacokinetic Drug Interactions
- Interactions between AEDs: effects on lamotrigine:
  - Carbamazepine, eslicarbazepine acetate, methsuximide, oxcarbazepine, perampanel, phenobarbital, phenytoin, primidone, and rufinamide can *increase* the clearance of lamotrigine and *decrease* lamotrigine plasma levels
  - Felbamate, sulthiame, and valproic acid can *decrease* the clearance of lamotrigine and *increase* lamotrigine plasma levels
- Interactions between AEDs: effects by lamotrigine:
  - Lamotrigine can *decrease* plasma levels of clonazepam, levetiracetam, and valproic acid
- Interactions between AEDs and non-AED drugs: effects on lamotrigine:
  - Oral contraceptives can *increase* the clearance of lamotrigine and *decrease* lamotrigine plasma levels
  - Isoniazid and sertraline can *increase* lamotrigine plasma levels
  - Acetaminophen, aripiprazole, atazanavir, Atkins diet (modified), ethambutol, lopinavir, olanzapine, orlistat, rifampicin, and ritonavir can *decrease* lamotrigine plasma levels
- Interactions between AEDs and non-AED drugs: effects by lamotrigine:
  - Lamotrigine can *increase* plasma levels of aripiprazole and atorvastatin
  - Lamotrigine can *decrease* plasma levels of lithium and quetiapine

Pharmacodynamic Drug Interactions
- Concomitant administration with valproic acid is associated with a probable pharmacodynamic interaction whereby small doses of lamotrigine are associated with significant (synergistic) efficacy; adverse effects (e.g., disabling tremor) may also be exacerbated
- Concomitant administration with carbamazepine has been associated with an increased risk of adverse effects (nausea, dizziness, headache, blurred vision, diplopia, and ataxia)
- Concomitant administration with lacosamide has been associated with an increased risk of neurotoxicity
- During combination therapy with phenytoin, a drug-induced chorea can occur consequent to a pharmacodynamic interaction
- Lamotrigine and topiramate in combination can have a synergistic anticonvulsant effect
- Lamotrigine and vigabatrin in combination can have a synergistic anticonvulsant effect

Hormonal Contraception
- Lamotrigine does not enhance the metabolism of the estrogen (ethinylestradiol) component of hormonal contraceptives and, therefore, does not compromise contraception control

- Lamotrigine can, however, enhance the metabolism of the progesterone (levonorgestrel) component of hormonal contraceptives and potentially lead to contraceptive failure when progesterone-only contraceptive formulations are used; medium- or high-dose progesterone oral contraceptive preparations are advisable in patients taking lamotrigine

Adverse Effects

How Drug Causes Adverse Effects
- CNS adverse effects theoretically due to excessive actions at voltage-sensitive sodium channels
- Rash hypothetically an allergic reaction

Common Adverse Effects
- Rash (typical drug eruption, ~10%)
- Diplopia, dizziness, ataxia
- Headache
- Tremor, asthenia, anxiety, drowsiness, insomnia
- Nausea, vomiting, diarrhea

Life-threatening or Dangerous Adverse Effects
- Serious rash, including Stevens–Johnson syndrome and toxic epidermal necrolysis (Lyell syndrome), can occur within 8 weeks of initiation of lamotrigine treatment or if medication is suddenly stopped then resumed at the normal dose – incidence in adults and children over 12 years old is 1 in 1000; risk of serious skin rash is comparable to other traditional AEDs, including carbamazepine, phenytoin, and phenobarbital
- Risk of serious rash is increased in pediatric patients, especially in children under 12 and in children taking valproate, from 1 in 100 to 1 in 300
- In children, the initial presentation of a rash can be mistaken for an infection; physicians should consider the possibility of a drug reaction if a child develops symptoms of rash and fever during the first 8 weeks of therapy
- Rash can occur as part of a hypersensitivity syndrome comprising a variable pattern of systemic symptoms, including fever, lymphadenopathy, facial edema, and abnormalities of the blood count and liver functions
- The value of screening for the HLA-B*15:02 allele as a predictor for serious rash in patients of Southeast Asian descent receiving lamotrigine (similar to its proven association and recommended testing in patients receiving carbamazepine or phenytoin) remains unclear, but may be considered; one recent meta-analysis suggested

that Han Chinese patients having the HLA-B*15:02 allele who were treated with lamotrigine had a higher risk of experiencing Stevens–Johnson syndrome or toxic epidermal necrolysis
• Rare hematological abnormalities may also occur independently without the full hypersensitivity syndrome, including neutropenia, leukopenia, anemia, thrombocytopenia, pancytopenia, and very rarely, aplastic anemia and agranulocytosis
• Rare hepatic dysfunction including hepatic failure
• Lamotrigine, through its action in blocking cardiac rapid delayed rectifier potassium ion current, may increase the risk of cardiac arrhythmia and in turn sudden unexplained deaths in epilepsy

Rare and not Life-threatening Adverse Effects
• Rare movement disorders such as tics and chorea have been reported
• Aseptic meningitis
• Sensitivity to sunlight (about 2%)

Weight Change
• Not common; weight gain reported but not expected

What to do About Adverse Effects
• Discuss common and severe adverse effects with patients or parents before starting medication, including symptoms that should be reported to the physician
• If patient develops signs of a rash as a typical drug eruption (i.e., a rash that peaks within days, settles in 10–14 days, is spotty, non-confluent, non-tender, has no systemic features, and laboratory tests are normal):
  – Advise patient to stop drug and contact physician if rash worsens or new symptoms emerge
  – Prescribe antihistamine and/or topical corticosteroid for pruritus
  – Monitor patient closely
• If patient develops signs of a rash with serious characteristics (i.e., a rash that is confluent and widespread, or purpuric or tender; with any prominent involvement of neck or upper trunk; any involvement of eyes, lips, mouth, etc.; or is associated with fever, malaise, pharyngitis, anorexia, lymphadenopathy, or abnormal laboratory tests for CBC, liver function, urea, creatinine):
  – Stop lamotrigine (and valproate if administered)
  – Monitor and investigate organ involvement (hepatic, renal, hematological)
  – Patient may require hospitalization for supportive care, observation, and hemodynamic monitoring

L

Dosing and Use

Usual Dosage Range

• Dosage range varies depending on whether lamotrigine is prescribed as monotherapy, as a co-medication with valproic acid, or with enzyme-inducing AEDs.
• For adults and children over 12 years:
  – *Monotherapy or adjunctive treatment with valproic acid:* maintenance dose generally 100–200 mg/day given either as a single dose or in two equally divided doses; some patients have required 500 mg/day to achieve the desired response
  – *Adjunctive treatment with enzyme-inducing AEDs:* maintenance dose generally 200–400 mg/day given in two equally divided doses; some patients have required up to 1000 mg/day in two divided doses to achieve the desired response, and in the setting of refractory epilepsy, it may also be helpful to monitor serum lamotrigine levels to achieve concentrations in the range of at least 10–20 μg/mL to ensure the dose of lamotrigine has been appropriately fully titrated
• Children aged 2–12 years:
  – *Monotherapy:* maintenance dose generally 2–8 mg/kg/day given either as a single dose or in two equally divided doses
  – *Adjunctive treatment with valproic acid:* maintenance dose generally 1–5 mg/kg/day given either as a single dose or in two equally divided doses
  – *Adjunctive treatment with enzyme-inducing AEDs:* maintenance dose generally 5–15 mg/kg/day in two equally divided doses

Available Formulations

• Tablets: 25 mg, 50 mg, 100 mg, 200 mg
• Dispersible chewable tablets: 2 mg, 5 mg, 25 mg, 100 mg

How to Dose

• Dosage and titration vary considerably depending on whether lamotrigine is prescribed as monotherapy, as a co-medication with valproic acid, or with enzyme-inducing AEDs
• For adults and children over 12 years:
  – *Monotherapy (or adjunctive treatment with drugs other than valproic acid or enzyme inducers):* start treatment with 25 mg/day for 2 weeks; subsequently increase to 50 mg/day for 2 weeks; thereafter, the dose should be increased by a maximum of 50–100 mg every 1–2 weeks until an optimum response is achieved; maintenance dose is generally 100–400 mg/day given either as a single dose, or in two equally divided doses
  – *Adjunctive treatment with valproic acid:* start treatment with 25 mg every other day for 2 weeks; subsequently increase to 25 mg/day for 2 weeks; thereafter, the dose should be increased by a maximum of 25–50 mg every 1–2 weeks until an optimum response

DOSING AND USE

is achieved; maintenance dose is generally 100–200 mg/day given either as a single dose, or in two equally divided doses
- *Adjunctive treatment with enzyme-inducing AEDs:* start treatment with 50 mg/day for 2 weeks; subsequently increase to 100 mg/day for 2 weeks; thereafter, the dose should be increased by a maximum of 100 mg every 1–2 weeks until an optimum response is achieved; maintenance dose is generally 200–500 mg/day given in two equally divided doses

• Children aged 2–12 years:
- *Monotherapy (or adjunctive treatment with drugs other than valproic acid or enzyme inducers):* start treatment with 0.4 mg/kg/day for 2 weeks; subsequently increase to 0.8 mg/kg/day for 2 weeks; thereafter, the dose should be increased by a maximum of 0.8 mg/kg every 1–2 weeks until an optimum response is achieved; maintenance dose is generally 2–8 mg/kg/day given either as a single dose or two equally divided doses; maximum dose is generally 300 mg/day
- *Adjunctive treatment with valproic acid:* start treatment with 0.15 mg/kg/day for 2 weeks; subsequently increase to 0.3 mg/kg/day for 2 weeks; thereafter, the dose should be increased by a maximum of 0.3 mg/kg every 1–2 weeks until an optimum response is achieved; maintenance dose is generally 1–5 mg/kg/day given either as a single dose or two equally divided doses; maximum dose is generally 200 mg/day
- *Adjunctive treatment with enzyme-inducing AEDs:* start treatment with 0.6 mg/kg/day given in two equally divided doses for 2 weeks; subsequently increase to 1.2 mg/kg/day for 2 weeks; thereafter, the dose should be increased by a maximum of 1.2 mg/kg every 1–2 weeks until an optimum response is achieved; maintenance dose is generally 5–15 mg/kg/day given either as two equally divided doses; maximum dose is generally 400 mg/day

Dosing Tips
• The dose should never be titrated faster than recommended in the package insert
• Very slow dose titration may reduce the incidence of skin rash and risk of other adverse effects
• If patient stops taking lamotrigine for 5 days or more, it may be necessary to restart the drug with the initial dose titration, as rashes have been reported on re-exposure
• Advise patient to avoid new medications, foods, or products during the first 3 months of lamotrigine treatment to decrease the risk of unrelated rash; patients should also not start lamotrigine within 2 weeks of a viral infection, rash, or vaccination
• Since valproate inhibits lamotrigine metabolism, if lamotrigine is added into a polytherapy regimen including valproate, lamotrigine titration rate and target dose should be reduced by 50% to reduce the risk of rash; conversely, if concomitant valproate is discontinued in

a patient receiving lamotrigine in stable doses, then the lamotrigine dose should be doubled gradually over 1 week following discontinuation of valproate so as to maintain a stable lamotrigine level, because the competitive inhibition of lamotrigine metabolism by valproate is immediately reversible and decreases only when the valproate dose is less than 250 mg/day
• Since valproate at doses as low as 250 mg/day immediately and maximally inhibits lamotrigine metabolism, if valproate is added into a polytherapy regimen including lamotrigine, lamotrigine dosage should be decreased by about 50% to prevent its level from doubling within 2–3 days
• Also, if concomitant enzyme-inducing AEDs (e.g., carbamazepine, phenobarbital, phenytoin, and primidone) are discontinued after lamotrigine dose is stabilized, then the lamotrigine dose should be maintained for 1 week following discontinuation of the other drug and then reduced by half over 2 weeks in equal decrements each week, because enzymatic induction is only slowly reversible
• Dispersible chewable tablets should only be administered as whole tablets; dose should be rounded down to the nearest whole tablet; these can be dispersed by adding the tablet to liquid (enough to cover the drug); after approximately 1 minute the solution should be stirred and then consumed immediately in its entirety

How to Withdraw Drug
• May need to adjust dosage of concurrent medications as lamotrigine is being discontinued, because plasma levels of other drugs may change (see Pharmacokinetic Drug Interactions section)
• Taper: a gradual dose reduction over a period of 2 weeks should be undertaken
• Rapid discontinuation may induce withdrawal seizures and should only be undertaken if there are safety concerns (e.g., serious rash)

Overdose
• Doses in excess of 10–20 times the maximum lamotrigine therapeutic dose have been ingested, and some fatalities have occurred
• Symptoms include ataxia, nystagmus, seizures, coma, and intraventricular conduction delay
• If indicated, the stomach should be emptied by lavage or by induction of emesis
• Hemodialysis removes lamotrigine from blood and, therefore, serves as a useful procedure in cases of overdose

Tests and Therapeutic Drug Monitoring
• Before starting: liver function test and CBC
• During treatment: liver function test and CBC every 12 months

DOSING AND USE

- Therapeutic drug monitoring:
  - Optimum seizure control in patients on monotherapy is most likely to occur at lamotrigine plasma concentrations of 3–15 mg/L (12–58 μmol/L)
  - The conversion factor from mg/L to μmol/L is 3.90 (i.e., 1 mg/L = 3.90 μmol/L)
  - The reference range of lamotrigine in plasma is considered to be the same for children and adults, although no data are available to support this clinical practice
  - Lamotrigine can be monitored by use of saliva, which is a measure of the free non-protein-bound plasma concentration and is pharmacologically relevant

Other Warnings/Precautions
- Life-threatening rashes have developed in association with lamotrigine use; lamotrigine should generally be discontinued at the first sign of a rash
- Risk of rash may be increased with higher doses, faster dose escalation, concomitant use of valproate, or in children under 12 years of age
- Patients should be instructed to report any symptoms of hypersensitivity immediately (fever; flu-like symptoms; rash; blisters on skin or in eyes, mouth, ears, nose, or genital areas; swelling of eyelids, conjunctivitis, lymphadenopathy)
- Caution is required when treating patients with a history of allergy or rash to other AEDs – the frequency of non-serious rash after treatment with lamotrigine is threefold greater
- Depressive effects may be increased by other CNS depressants (e.g., alcohol, MAOIs, other AEDs)
- A small number of patients may experience a worsening of seizures
- May cause photosensitivity
- Lamotrigine inhibits dihydrofolate reductase and may, therefore, reduce folate concentrations

Do not Use
- If patient has a proven allergy to lamotrigine or to any of the excipients

Special Populations
Renal Impairment
- Lamotrigine is renally secreted and thus the dose may need to be lowered in renally impaired patients
- Because lamotrigine can be removed by hemodialysis, patients receiving hemodialysis may require supplemental doses of lamotrigine

Hepatic Impairment
- Lamotrigine is extensively metabolized and consequently lower doses will be required in patients with hepatic impairment

- Dose may need to be reduced and titration may need to be slower, perhaps by 50% in patients with moderate impairment (Child–Pugh grade B) and 75% in patients with severe impairment (Child–Pugh grade C)

Children
- Children have an increased metabolic capacity and consequently higher doses in mg/kg are usually required to achieve the equivalent therapeutic plasma levels seen in adults
- Pharmacokinetic interactions in children are usually of a greater magnitude than that seen in adults

Elderly
- Elderly patients are more susceptible to adverse effects and may be unable to tolerate higher doses; slower titration to a lower initial target dosage should be considered
- Because of an age-related reduction in hepatic function, lower lamotrigine doses are appropriate
- Because lamotrigine is associated with dizziness and ataxia, the elderly may be at higher risk of falls
- Elderly patients are often prescribed concurrent drug therapies for comorbidities and therefore may be at greater risk for pharmacokinetic and pharmacodynamic interactions; the risk of pharmacokinetic interactions with lamotrigine is substantial

Pregnancy
- Specialist advice should be given to women who are of childbearing potential; they should be informed about the teratogenicity of all AEDs and the importance of avoiding an unplanned pregnancy; the AED treatment regimen should be reviewed when a woman is planning to become pregnant
- Rapid discontinuation of AEDs should be avoided as this may lead to breakthrough seizures, which could have serious consequences for the woman and the unborn child
- Lamotrigine was previously classified by the US FDA as risk category C (some animal studies show adverse effects); the current FDA Pregnancy and Lactation Rule has eliminated pregnancy risk category labels; in humans, lamotrigine has been found to be associated with a lower risk of major malformations than valproate, and comparable to or less than several other AEDs
- Use in women of childbearing potential requires weighing potential benefits to the mother against the risks to the fetus
- Use with other AEDs in combination may cause a higher risk for teratogenic effects than with lamotrigine monotherapy
- Taper drug if discontinuing
- Seizures, even mild seizures, may cause harm to the embryo/fetus
- During pregnancy lamotrigine pharmacokinetics change significantly; lamotrigine plasma concentrations decrease by 26–66% due

L

LAMOTRIGINE

to increased clearance consequent to enhanced glucuronidation; an increase in lamotrigine dose is often required to maintain steady plasma levels, so levels should be checked regularly, at least once per trimester; in the postpartum period, glucuronidation returns to baseline rates, and lamotrigine concentrations subsequently again increase, so dose reduction following delivery is necessary, and may be again guided by plasma levels

Breast Feeding
- Breast milk: 40–80% of maternal plasma levels
- Breastfed infants: lamotrigine plasma levels are 25–50% of maternal plasma levels
- If drug is continued while breast feeding, the infant should be monitored for possible adverse effects (irritability or sedation)
- If adverse effects are observed, recommend bottle feeding

The Overall Place of Lamotrigine in the Treatment of Epilepsy

Lamotrigine is an effective broad-spectrum AED for the treatment of all types of seizures except myoclonic seizures. It is useful in the treatment of all partial/focal or generalized, idiopathic, or symptomatic epileptic syndromes of adults, children, and neonates. In monotherapy, lamotrigine has comparable efficacy to carbamazepine in the management of partial/focal seizures and secondary generalized tonic–clonic seizures, and it is better tolerated. In polytherapy, lamotrigine is particularly efficacious with valproate, and this combination may be ideal for drug-resistant generalized epilepsies. However, against absence seizures, lamotrigine is less effective than ethosuximide and valproate.

Primary Seizure Types
- Partial (focal) seizures
- Generalized tonic–clonic seizures
- Lennox–Gastaut syndrome

Secondary Seizure Types
- Absence seizures

Potential Advantages
- Lamotrigine is a broad-spectrum drug with significant efficacy
- It is particularly efficacious with valproate as a result of pharmacodynamic synergism

Potential Disadvantages
- Lamotrigine is associated with significant pharmacokinetic interactions with other AEDs, which can be associated with

exacerbation of adverse effects, requiring complex dosing and titration protocols
• Very slow titration is required
• Risk of a serious skin rash is a major consideration, particularly in patients receiving rapid lamotrigine titration and/or high dosing, in younger children, and in those who are receiving concomitant valproate
• Rash related to lamotrigine may affect up to 10% of patients, but resolve rapidly with drug discontinuation
• Frequent dosage adjustments may be necessary before, during, and after pregnancy and hormonal contraception
• Potential teratogen, but less than several other AEDs

Suggested Reading

Barr PA, Buettiker VE, Antony JH. Efficacy of lamotrigine in refractory neonatal seizures. *Pediatric Neurology* 1999; **20**: 161–163.

Barron TF, Hunt SL, Hoban TF, Price ML. Lamotrigine monotherapy in children. *Pediatric Neurology* 2000; **23**: 160–163.

Baumann RJ, Fakhoury TA, Kustra RP, Vuong A, Hammer AE, Messenheimer JA. Conversion to lamotrigine monotherapy from valproate monotherapy in older adolescent patients with epilepsy. *Current Medical Research Opinion* 2007; **23**: 2461–2465.

Brodie MJ, Richens A, Yuen AW. Double-blind comparison of lamotrigine and carbamazepine in newly diagnosed epilepsy. UK Lamotrigine/Carbamazepine Monotherapy Trial Group. *Lancet* 1995; **345**: 476–479.

Brodie MJ, Yuen AW. Lamotrigine substitution study: evidence for synergism with sodium valproate? 105 Study Group. *Epilepsy Research* 1997; **26**: 423–432.

Campbell E, Kennedy F, Russell A, Smithson WH, Parsons L, Morrison PJ, Liggan B, Irwin B, Delanty N, Hunt SJ, Craig J, Morrow J. Malformation risks of antiepileptic drug monotherapies in pregnancy: updated results from the UK and Ireland Epilepsy and Pregnancy Registers. *Journal of Neurology Neurosurgery and Psychiatry* 2014; **85**: 1029–1034.

Cheung YK, Cheng SH, Chan EJ, Lo SV, Ng MH, Kwan P. HLA-B alleles associated with severe cutaneous reactions to antiepileptic drugs in Han Chinese. *Epilepsia* 2013; **54**: 1307–1314.

Cunnington MC, Weil JG, Messenheimer JA, Ferber S, Yerby M, Tennis P. Final results from 18 years of the International Lamotrigine Pregnancy Registry. *Neurology* 2011; **76**: 1817–1823.

Fitton A, Goa KL. Lamotrigine: an update of its pharmacology and therapeutic use in epilepsy. *Drugs* 1995; **50**: 691–713.

Frank LM, Enlow T, Holmes GL, Manesco P, Concannon S, Chen C, Womble G, Casale EJ. Lamictal (lamotrigine) monotherapy for typical absence seizures in children. *Epilepsia* 1999; **40**: 973–979.

French JA, Kanner AM, Bautista J, et al. Efficacy and tolerability of the new antiepileptic drugs I: treatment of new onset epilepsy: report of the Therapeutics and Technology Assessment Subcommittee and Quality Standards Subcommittee of the American Academy of Neurology and the American Epilepsy Society. *Neurology* 2004; **62**: 1252–1260.

French JA, Kanner AM, Bautista J, et al. Efficacy and tolerability of the new antiepileptic drugs II: treatment of refractory epilepsy: Efficacy and tolerability of the new antiepileptic drugs II: treatment of refractory epilepsy: report of the Therapeutics and Technology Assessment Subcommittee and Quality Standards Subcommittee of the American Academy of Neurology and the American Epilepsy Society. *Neurology* 2004; **62**: 1261–1273.

Gamble C, Williamson PR, Chadwick DW, Marson AG. A meta-analysis of individual patient responses to lamotrigine or carbamazepine monotherapy. *Neurology* 2006; **66**: 1310–1317.

Gidal BE, Sheth R, Parnell J, Maloney K, Sale M. Evaluation of VPA dose and concentration effects on lamotrigine pharmacokinetics: implications for conversion to lamotrigine monotherapy. *Epilepsy Research* 2003; **57**: 85–93.

Glauser TA, Cnaan A, Shinnar S, Hirtz DG, Dlugos D, Masur D, Clark PO, Capparelli EV, Adamson PC. for the Childhood Absence Epilepsy Study Group. Ethosuximide, valproic acid, and lamotrigine in childhood absence epilepsy. *New England Journal of Medicine* 2010; **362**: 790–799.

Guberman AH, Besag FM, Brodie MJ, Dooley JM, Duchowny MS, Pellock JM, Richens A, Stern RS, Trevathan E. Lamotrigine-associated rash: risk/benefit considerations in adults and children. *Epilepsia* 1999; **40**: 985–991.

Hernandez-Diaz S, Smith CR, Shen A, Mittendorf R, Hauser WA, Yerby M, Holmes LB. Comparative safety of antiepileptic drugs during pregnancy. *Neurology* 2012; **78**: 1692–1699.

Johannessen Landmark C, Patsalos PN. Drug interactions involving the new second- and third-generation antiepileptic drugs. *Expert Reviews in Neurotherapeutics* 2010; **10**: 119–140.

Kanner AM, Frey M. Adding valproate to lamotrigine: a study of their pharmacokinetic interaction. *Neurology* 2000; **55**: 588–591.

Marson AG, Al-Kharusi AM, Alwaid M, et al. SANAD Study Group. The SANAD study of effectiveness of carbamazepine, gabapentin, lamotrigine, oxcarbazepine, or topiramate for treatment of partial epilepsy: an unblinded randomized controlled trial. *Lancet* 2007; **369**: 1000–1015.

Patsalos PN. *Antiepileptic drug interactions: a clinical guide*, 3rd edition. Springer, London, UK; 2016.

Patsalos PN, Berry DJ, Bourgeois BFD, Cloyd JC, Glauser TA, Johannessen SI, Leppik IE, Tomson T, Perucca E. Antiepileptic drugs – best practice guidelines for therapeutic drug monitoring: a position paper by the Subcommission on Therapeutic Drug

Monitoring, ILAE Commission on Therapeutic Strategies. *Epilepsia* 2008; **49**: 1239–1276.

Patsalos PN, Berry DJ. Therapeutic drug monitoring of antiepileptic drugs by use of saliva. *Therapeutic Drug Monitoring* 2013; **35**: 4–29.

Pennell PB, Newport DJ, Stowe ZN, Helmers SL, Montgomery JQ, Henry TR. The impact of pregnancy and childbirth on the metabolism of lamotrigine. *Neurology* 2004; **62**: 292–295.

Sabers A, Ohman I, Christensen J, Tomson T. Oral contraceptives reduce lamotrigine plasma levels. *Neurology* 2003; **61**: 570–571.

Simms KM, Kortepeter C, Avigan M. Lamotrigine and aseptic meningitis. *Neurology* 2012; **78**: 921–927.

St. Louis EK. The art of managing conversions between antiepileptic drugs; maximizing patient tolerability and quality of life. *Pharmaceuticals* 2010; **3**: 2956–2969.

St. Louis EK, Gidal BE, Henry TR, Kaydanova Y, Krumholz A, McCabe PH, Montouris GD, Rosenfeld WE, Smith BJ, Stern JM, Waterhouse EJ, Schulz RM, Garnett WR, Bramley T. Conversions between monotherapies in epilepsy: expert consensus. *Epilepsy and Behavior* 2007; **11**: 222–2234.

Tomson T, Luef G, Sabers A, Pittschieler S, Ohman I. Valproate effects on kinetics of lamotrigine in pregnancy and treatment with oral contraceptives. *Neurology* 2006; **67**: 1297–1299.

Zupanc ML. Antiepileptic drugs and hormonal contraceptives in adolescent women with epilepsy. *Neurology* 2006; **66**(Suppl 3): S37–S45.

L

SUGGESTED READING

LEVETIRACETAM

L

Therapeutics

Chemical Name and Structure

Levetiracetam, (S)-alpha-ethyl-2 oxo-1-pyrrolidine acetamide, is a white to off-white crystalline powder, with a molecular weight of 170.21 and an empirical formula of $C_8H_{14}N_2O_2$.

Brand Names
- Ceumid
- Desitrend
- Epictal; Epifast
- Keppra; Keppra XR; Kopodex
- Lenerve; Levebon; Levecetam; Levepsy; Leveron; Levesam; Levetee; Levracet; Levroxa; Levtam; L-TAM
- Torleva

Generics Available
- Yes

Licensed Indications for Epilepsy
- Monotherapy of partial seizures with or without secondary generalization in patients aged 16 years and older (UK SPC)
- Adjunctive treatment of partial seizures with or without secondary generalization in adults, adolescents, children, and infants from 1 month of age (UK SPC)
- Adjunctive treatment of myoclonic seizures in adults and adolescents from 12 years of age with juvenile myoclonic epilepsy (UK SPC)
- Adjunctive treatment of primary generalized tonic–clonic seizures in adults and adolescents from 12 years of age with idiopathic generalized epilepsy (UK SPC)
- Adjunctive treatment of partial (focal)-onset seizures in patients 4 years and older (FDA PI)
- Adjunctive treatment of primary generalized tonic–clonic seizures in patients 6 years and older with idiopathic general epilepsies (FDA PI)
- Adjunctive treatment of myoclonic seizures in patients 12 years and older with juvenile myoclonic epilepsy (FDA PI)

LEVETIRACETAM

Licensed Indications for Non-epilepsy Conditions
• There are none

Non-licensed Use for Epilepsy
• Absence seizures
• Benign rolandic epilepsy
• Childhood occipital epilepsy – Gastaut type
• Febrile seizures
• Myoclonus (posthypoxic and postencephalitic)
• Neonatal seizures
• Progressive myoclonic epilepsy (Unverricht–Lundborg syndrome)
• Severe myoclonic epilepsy in infancy (Dravet syndrome)
• Status epilepticus

Non-licensed Use for Non-epilepsy Conditions
• Mania

Ineffective (Contraindicated)
• Levetiracetam is potentially effective against all seizure types and is not contraindicated for any seizure type or epilepsy
• Experience in neonatal seizures is increasing and appears to be a promising drug in this regard

Mechanism of Action
• The precise mechanism by which levetiracetam exerts its antiepileptic activity is unknown
• Levetiracetam does not share with other AEDs any of their three main mechanisms, such as sodium channel blockade, inhibition of calcium currents, or increase in GABAergic inhibitory responses
• Levetiracetam can oppose the activity of negative modulators of GABA- and glycine-gated currents, and can partially inhibit N-type calcium currents
• Binds to synaptic vesicle protein SV2A, which is involved in synaptic vesicle exocytosis

Efficacy Profile
• The goals of treatment are to achieve complete seizure remission when possible, or at least improved frequency and severity of seizures, while also minimizing adverse effects and improving patient quality of life
• Onset of efficacy occurs mostly within the first 2 weeks of treatment; there is evidence that onset of efficacy may actually begin within first day following initiation of treatment
• Levetiracetam can suppress interictal epileptiform activity in certain forms of epilepsy
• Levetiracetam appears to be as effective as carbamazepine against partial seizures

L

LEVETIRACETAM

- Levetiracetam can be effective in all types of primary (or idiopathic) generalized epilepsies
- If levetiracetam is ineffective or only partially effective, it can be replaced by or combined with another AED that is appropriate for the patient's seizure type or epilepsy syndrome

Pharmacokinetics

Absorption and Distribution
- Oral bioavailability: ≥95%
- Food co-ingestion: causes a slight delay in the rate of absorption but the extent of absorption is unaffected
- Tmax: 1–2 hours
- Time to steady state: 1–2 days
- Pharmacokinetics: linear
- Protein binding: 0%
- Volume of distribution: 0.5–0.7 L/kg
- Salivary concentrations: levetiracetam is secreted into saliva and concentrations are similar to the unbound levels seen in plasma

Metabolism
- Levetiracetam undergoes minimal metabolism with ~30% of the dose metabolized by hydrolysis to a deaminated metabolite
- This metabolism is independent of the hepatic CYP system and is by means of a type B esterase enzyme located in whole blood
- The metabolites of levetiracetam are not pharmacologically active
- Autoinduction is not a feature of levetiracetam metabolism

Elimination
- The elimination half-life of levetiracetam is 6–8 hours in adults, 5–6 hours in children, and 10–11 hours in the elderly
- The renal clearance of levetiracetam is proportional to the CrCl
- Renal excretion: ~66% of an administered dose is excreted unchanged in urine

Drug Interaction Profile

Pharmacokinetic Drug Interactions
- Interactions between AEDs: effects on levetiracetam:
  - Carbamazepine, lamotrigine, methsuximide, oxcarbazepine, phenobarbital, and phenytoin can *increase* the clearance of levetiracetam and *decrease* levetiracetam plasma levels
- Interactions between AEDs: effects by levetiracetam:
  - To date, there have been no reports of levetiracetam affecting the clearance of other AEDs and affecting their plasma levels
- Interactions between AEDs and non-AED drugs: effects on levetiracetam:

    – Probenecid can *increase* ucbLO59 plasma levels, the non-pharmacologically active metabolite of levetiracetam
- Interactions between AEDs and non-AED drugs: effects by levetiracetam:
  – To date, there have been no reports of levetiracetam affecting the clearance of other non-AED drugs and affecting their plasma levels

Pharmacodynamic Drug Interactions
- An encephalopathic state induced by the addition of levetiracetam to valproate has been described
- Disabling symptoms compatible with carbamazepine toxicity were reported in patients in whom levetiracetam was added to carbamazepine
- Topiramate-related adverse effects were exacerbated in children co-prescribed with levetiracetam
- The efficacy of brivaracetam is decreased when co-administered with levetiracetam
- Perampanel in combination with levetiracetam is associated with an increased likelihood of developing fatigue
- Other central nervous depressants, such as alcohol, other AEDs, and MAOIs, may exacerbate the depressive effect of levetiracetam

Hormonal Contraception
- Levetiracetam does not enhance the metabolism of oral contraceptives and therefore does not compromise contraception control

Adverse Effects
How Drug Causes Adverse Effects
- Mechanism by which levetiracetam causes adverse effects has not been established
- CNS adverse effects may be due to excessive actions on SV2A synaptic vesicle proteins or to actions on various voltage-sensitive ion channels

Common Adverse Effects
- Somnolence, asthenia, ataxia, dizziness
- Behavioral symptoms (particularly common in children), including agitation, hostility, oppositional behavior, anxiety, aggression, emotional lability, depression

Life-threatening or Dangerous Adverse Effects
- Very rare liver failure
- Rare activation of suicidal ideation and acts

Rare and not Life-threatening Adverse Effects
- Psychosis

- Allergic reaction
- Bone marrow suppression

Weight Change
- Not common; weight gain reported but not expected

What to do About Adverse Effects
- Discuss common adverse effects with patients or parents before starting medication, including symptoms that should be reported to the physician
- Risk of adverse effects is greatest in the first few months of treatment
- Slower titration may decrease incidence or severity of some adverse effects
- Administration of pyridoxine (vitamin B$_6$) has been suggested to reduce behavioral adverse reactions in children and adult populations, but this has not yet been supported by controlled data
- Negative effect of levetiracetam on behavior and mood often persists and may require discontinuation of levetiracetam

Dosing and Use
Usual Dosage Range
- Adults: 1000–3000 mg/day
- Children: 30–40 mg/kg/day

Available Formulations
- Tablets: 250 mg, 500 mg, 750 mg, 1000 mg
- Oral solution: 100 mg/mL, 500 mg/5 mL
- Solution for iv injection: 100 mg/mL, 500 mg/5 mL
- Extended-release tablets: 500 mg, 750mg

How to Dose
- *For adults and children over 12 years of age*: start treatment with 250–500 mg twice daily; at intervals of 1–2 weeks increase as needed and as tolerated by 500 mg/day; maintenance dose is generally 2000–3000 mg/day; some patients may tolerate and respond to doses greater than 3000 mg/day
- *Children under 12 years of age*: start treatment with approximately 20 mg/kg/day, twice daily or three times daily; at intervals of 1–2 weeks increase as needed and as tolerated by approximately 10–20 mg/kg/day; maintenance dose generally 30–40 mg/kg/day; doses of up to 100 mg/kg/day may be necessary and well tolerated, especially in younger children

Dosing Tips
- Slower titration may decrease incidence or severity of some adverse effects

L

- In children, and at high doses, the daily dose may be preferably divided into three doses
- A dose for iv loading has not been determined, but 20–40 mg/kg has been administered safely to children with acute repetitive seizures or status epilepticus
- iv doses can be infused diluted in 100 mL of isotonic fluids (e.g., normal saline, lactated Ringer's, 5% dextrose) over 15 minutes
- For intolerable sedation, most of the dose can be given at night and less during the day

How to Withdraw Drug
- There is no need to adjust dosage of concurrent medications as levetiracetam is being discontinued, because plasma levels of other drugs do not change (see Pharmacokinetic Drug Interactions section)
- No data are available on potential for withdrawal seizures or symptoms upon rapid discontinuation
- Rapid discontinuation may increase the risk of seizures
- Taper dose over a period of several weeks

Overdose
- No fatalities have been reported: symptoms include sedation, agitation, aggression, respiratory depression, coma
- If indicated, the stomach should be emptied by lavage or by induction of emesis
- Hemodialysis removes levetiracetam from blood and, therefore, serves as a useful procedure in cases of overdose

Tests and Therapeutic Drug Monitoring
- Because levetiracetam may alter vitamin D metabolism and affect bone mineral density, 25-hydroxyvitamin D levels (and possibly bone mineral density) should be monitored, and vitamin D supplementation should be prescribed as needed
- There is no need to routinely monitor any other laboratory parameter during treatment with levetiracetam
- Therapeutic drug monitoring:
  - Optimum seizure control in patients on monotherapy is most likely to occur at levetiracetam plasma concentrations of 12–46 mg/L (70–270 μmol/L)
  - The conversion factor from mg/L to μmol/L is 5.88 (i.e., 1 mg/L = 5.88 μmol/L)
  - The reference range of levetiracetam in plasma is considered to be the same for children and adults, although no data are available to support this clinical practice
  - Levetiracetam can be monitored by use of saliva, which is a measure of the free non-protein-bound plasma concentration that is pharmacologically relevant

DOSING AND USE

Other Warnings / Precautions
• Patients should be monitored carefully for signs of depression or psychosis

Do not Use
• In patients with a history of allergic reaction to levetiracetam
• Because malitol is an excipient of levetiracetam, patients with rare hereditary problems of fructose intolerance should not take this medication

Special Populations
Renal Impairment
• Renal disease may decrease levetiracetam clearance by 35–60%
• Levetiracetam dosage should be individualized according to CrCl
  – Recommended dose for patients with mild impairment (CrCl 50–79 mL/min/1.73 m^2) is 500–1000 mg twice a day
  – Recommended dose for patients with moderate impairment (CrCl 30–49 mL/min/1.73 m^2) is 250–750 mg twice a day
  – Recommended dose for patients with severe impairment (CrCl <30 mL/min/1.73 m^2) is 250–500 mg twice a day
• Because levetiracetam can be removed by hemodialysis, patients receiving hemodialysis may require supplemental doses of levetiracetam; typically 500–1000 mg once a day will be required, followed by a supplemental dose of 250–500 mg following dialysis

Hepatic Impairment
• Levetiracetam is not metabolized in the liver and, therefore, no dosage adjustment is necessary

Children
• Children have an increased metabolic capacity and consequently higher doses in mg/kg/day are usually required to achieve the equivalent therapeutic plasma level

Elderly
• Elderly patients are more susceptible to adverse effects (especially somnolence) and therefore often do better at lower doses
• Because of an age-related reduction in renal function, lower levetiracetam doses are appropriate, and dosage may need to be guided by CrCl
• Elderly patients are often prescribed concurrent drug therapies for comorbidities and therefore may be at greater risk for pharmacokinetic and pharmacodynamic interactions; as the risk of pharmacokinetic interactions with levetiracetam is low or non-existent, levetiracetam may be advantageous for use in the elderly

- The safe profile of levetiracetam makes it a first-choice AED in the elderly

Pregnancy
- Specialist advice should be given to women who are of childbearing potential; they should be informed about the teratogenicity of all AEDs and the importance of avoiding an unplanned pregnancy; the AED treatment regimen should be reviewed when a woman is planning to become pregnant
- Rapid discontinuation of AEDs should be avoided as this may lead to breakthrough seizures, which could have serious consequences for the woman and the unborn child
- Levetiracetam was previously classified by the US FDA as risk category C (some animal studies show adverse effects); the current FDA Pregnancy and Lactation Rule has eliminated pregnancy risk category labels; in humans, levetiracetam has been found to be associated with a lower risk of major malformations compared to several other AEDs
- Use in women of childbearing potential requires weighing potential benefits to the mother against the risks to the fetus
- Use with other AEDs in combination may cause a higher risk for teratogenic effects than levetiracetam monotherapy
- Taper drug if discontinuing
- Seizures, even mild seizures, may cause harm to the embryo/fetus
- During pregnancy levetiracetam pharmacokinetics change significantly; levetiracetam plasma concentrations decrease by 40–60% due to increased clearance, so increases in levetiracetam dose are usually required. Blood levetiracetam levels are difficult to judge with confidence given its short half-life, but following trough concentrations may be useful at least once per trimester to guide further dose adjustment

Breast Feeding
- Breast milk: 80–130% of maternal plasma levels
- Breastfed infants: levetiracetam plasma levels are <20% of maternal plasma levels
- If drug is continued while breast feeding, infant should be monitored for possible adverse effects (irritability or sedation)
- If adverse effects are observed, recommend bottle feeding

The Overall Place of Levetiracetam in the Treatment of Epilepsy

Levetiracetam is a broad-spectrum AED and represents a first-line or second-line therapy in idiopathic generalized epilepsies (generalized and myoclonic seizures) and in partial/focal seizures with or without secondary generalization where it is one of the main alternatives to carbamazepine and oxcarbazepine. It is also a suitable alternative to the use of valproate in the treatment of juvenile myoclonic epilepsy and of idiopathic generalized epilepsies in general, especially in women (given the risk of teratogenesis and cognitive impairment in children exposed to valproate in utero). Because levetiracetam is associated with an excellent safety profile, does not cause significant idiosyncratic reactions, has simple pharmacokinetic characteristics, and has a low propensity to interact with other medications, its clinical use is straightforward and uncomplicated, making it a drug of choice for most epilepsies in adults, children, and adolescents.

Primary Seizure Types
• Partial (focal) seizures with or without secondary generalization
• Myoclonic seizures associated with juvenile myoclonic epilepsy
• Primary generalized tonic–clonic seizures associated with idiopathic generalized epilepsy

Secondary Seizure Types
• Absence seizures
• Progressive myoclonic epilepsy
• Severe myoclonic epilepsy of infancy (Dravet syndrome)
• Myoclonus

Potential Advantages
• Broad spectrum of seizure protection
• Has no organ toxicity (i.e., liver, kidneys, bone marrow, etc.) and has no dangerous or life-threatening adverse effects
• Simple straightforward pharmacokinetics
• Does not affect the pharmacokinetics of other drugs

Potential Disadvantages
• Behavioral and mood alterations are relatively common, especially in children, and may necessitate discontinuation
• Potential teratogen

Suggested Reading

Aiguabella M, Falip M, Villanueva V, de la Peña P, Molins A, Garcia-Morales I, Saiz RA, Pardo J, Tortosa D, Sansa G, Miró J. Efficacy of intravenous levetiracetam as an add-on treatment in status epilepticus: a multicentric observational study. *Seizure* 2011; **20**: 60–64.

Alsaadi T, El Hammasi K, Shahrour TM. Does pyridoxine control behavioral symptoms in adult patients treated with levetiracetam? Case series from UAE. *Epilepsy and Behavior Case Reports* 2015; **4**: 94–95.

Ben-Menachem E, Falter U; for the European Levetiracetam Study Group. Efficacy and tolerability of levetiracetam 3000 mg/d in patients with refractory partial seizures: a multicenter, double-blind, responder-selected study evaluating monotherapy. *Epilepsia* 2000; **41**: 1276–1283.

Beniczky SA, Viken J, Jensen LT, Andersen NB. Bone mineral density in adult patients treated with various antiepileptic drugs. *Seizure* 2012; **21**: 471–472.

Berkovic SF, Knowlton RC, Leroy RF, Schiemann J, Falter U; Levetiracetam N01057 Study Group. Placebo-controlled study of levetiracetam in idiopathic generalized epilepsy. *Neurology* 2007; **69**: 1751–1760.

Brodie MJ, Perucca E, Ryvlin P, Ben-Menachem E, Meencke HJ; Levetiracetam Monotherapy Study Group. Comparison of levetiracetam and controlled-release carbamazepine in newly diagnosed epilepsy. *Neurology* 2007; **68**: 402–408.

Crest C, Dupont S, Leguern E, Adam C, Baulac M. Levetiracetam in progressive myoclonic epilepsy: an exploratory study in 9 patients. *Neurology* 2004; **62**: 640–643.

Fattore C, Boniver C, Capovilla G, Cerminara C, Citterio A, Coppola G, Costa P, Darra F, Vecchi M, Perucca E. A multicenter, randomized, placebo-controlled trial of levetiracetam in children and adolescents with newly diagnosed absence epilepsy. *Epilepsia* 2011; **52**: 802–809.

Hernandez-Diaz S, Smith CR, Shen A, Mittendorf R, Hauser WA, Yerby M, Holmes LB. Comparative safety of antiepileptic drugs during pregnancy. *Neurology* 2012; **78**: 1692–1699.

Johannessen Landmark C, Patsalos PN. Drug interactions involving the new second- and third-generation antiepileptic drugs. *Expert Reviews in Neurotherapeutics* 2010; **10**: 119–140.

Kossoff EH, Bergey GK, Freeman JM, Vining EP. Levetiracetam psychosis in children with epilepsy. *Epilepsia* 2001; **42**: 1611–1613.

Krauss GL, Bergin MB, Kramer RE, Cho YW, Reich SG. Suppression of post-hypoxic and post-encephalitic myoclonus with levetiracetam. *Neurology* 2001; **56**: 411–412.

Major P, Greenberg E, Khan A, Thiele EA. Pyridoxine supplementation for the treatment of levetiracetam-induced behavior side effects in children: preliminary results. *Epilepsy and Behavior* 2008; **13**: 557–559.

Mawhinney E, Craig J, Morrow J, Russell A, Henry Smighson W, Parsons L, Morrison PJ, Liggan B, Irwin B, Delanty N, Hunt SJ. Levetiracetam in pregnancy. Result from the UK and Ireland epilepsy and pregnancy registers. *Neurology* 2013; **80**: 400–405.

Patsalos PN. *Antiepileptic drug interactions: a clinical guide*, 3rd edition. Springer, London, UK; 2016.

Patsalos PN. Levetiracetam: pharmacology and therapeutics in the treatment of epilepsy and other neurological conditions. *Reviews in Contemporary Pharmacotherapy* 2004; **13**: 1–168.

Pellock JM, Glauser TA, Bebin EM, Fountain NB, Ritter FJ, Coupez RM, Shileds WD. Pharmacokinetic study of levetiracetam in children. *Epilepsia* 2001; **42**: 1574–1579.

L

Rocamora R, Wagner K, Schulze-Bonhage A. Levetiracetam reduces frequency and duration of epileptic activity in patients with refractory primary generalized epilepsy. *Seizure* 2006; **15**: 428–433.

Shallcross R, Bromley RL, Irwin B, Bonnett LJ, Morrow J, Baker GA. Child development following in utero exposure. Levetiracetam vs sodium valproate. *Neurology* 2011; **76**: 383–389.

Shorvon SD, Lowenthal A, Janz D, Bielen E, Loiseau P; for the European Levetiracetam Study Group. Multicenter double-blind, randomized, placebo-controlled trial of levetiracetam as add-on therapy in patients with refractory partial seizures. *Epilepsia* 2000; **41**: 1179–1186.

Specchio LM, Gambardella A, Giallonardo AT, Michelucci R, Specchio N, Boero G, La Neve A. Open label, long-term, pragmatic study on levetiracetam in the treatment of juvenile myoclonic epilepsy. *Epilepsy Research* 2006; **71**: 32–39.

St. Louis EK, Gidal BE, Henry TR, Kaydanova Y, Krumholz A, McCabe PH, Montouris GD, Rosenfeld WE, Smith BJ, Stern JM, Waterhouse EJ, Schulz RM, Garnett WR, Bramley T. Conversions between monotherapies in epilepsy: expert consensus. *Epilepsy and Behavior* 2007; **11**: 222–234.

Striano P, Coppola A, Pezzella M, Ciampa C, Specchio N, Ragona F, Mancardi MM, Gennaro E, Beccaria F, Capovilla G, Rasmini P, Besana D, Coppola GG, Elia M, Granata T, Vecchi M, Vigevano F, Viri M, Gaggero R, Striano S, Zara F. An open-label trial of levetiracetam in severe myoclonic epilepsy of infancy. *Neurology* 2007; **69**: 250–254.

von Stülpnagel C, Kluger G, Leiz S, Holthausen H. Levetiracetam as add-on therapy in different subgroups of "benign" idiopathic focal epilepsies in childhood. *Epilepsy and Behavior* 2010; **17**: 193–198.

Westin AA, Reimers A, Helde G, Nakken KO, Brodtkorb E. Serum concentration/dose ratio of levetiracetam before, during and after pregnancy. *Seizure* 2008; **17**: 192–198.

LORAZEPAM

Therapeutics

Chemical Name and Structure

Lorazepam, 7-chloro-5-(2-chlorophenyl)-1,3-dihydro-3-dihydroxy-2H-1,4-benzodiazepine-2-one, is a nearly white crystalline substance, with a molecular weight of 321.16 and an empirical formula of $C_{15}H_{10}CI_2N_2O_2$.

Brand Names

- Abinol; Ansilor; Anxira; Anzepam; Aplacasse; Aripax; Ativan
- Bonatranquan
- Control
- Emoten; Emotival
- Larpose; Laubeel; Lauracalm; Lonza; Lopam; Lora; Lorabenz; Lorafen; Loram; Lorans; Lorapam; Lorax; Loraxepam-Efeka; Lorazene; Lorazep; Lorazepam-Eurogenerics; Lorazin; Lorazon; Lorenin; Loridem; Lorivan; Lorsilan; Lorzem
- Merlit; Merlopam
- Nervistop L; Neuropam; Novhepar; Nu-Loraz
- Orfidal
- Psicopax
- Renaquil
- Sedatival; Sidenar; Silence; Stapam
- Tavor; Temesta; Titus; Tranqipam; Trapax; Trapex
- Vigiten
- Zora

Generics Available

- Yes

Licensed Indications for Epilepsy

- Status epilepticus (UK SPC; FDA PI)

Licensed Indications for Non-epilepsy Conditions
• Acute excitement (UK SPC)
• Acute mania (UK SPC)
• Anxiety disorder (UK SPC; FDA PI)
• Anxiety associated with depressive symptoms (FDA PI)
• Insomnia (UK SPC)
• Sedation with amnesia (preoperative) (UK SPC)

Non-licensed Use for Epilepsy
• Acute repetitive seizures
• Myoclonic seizures
• Neonatal seizures

Non-licensed Use for Non-epilepsy Conditions
• Acute psychosis (adjunctive)
• Alcohol withdrawal psychosis
• Headache
• Muscle spasm
• Panic disorder
• Postanoxic myoclonus

Ineffective (Contraindicated)
• Lorazepam is potentially effective against all types of seizures and is not contraindicated for any form of epilepsy
• Lorazepam may cause tonic seizures in patients with epileptic encephalopathies being treated for atypical absence status epilepticus

Mechanism of Action
• Benzodiazepines bind to the neuronal $GABA_A$ receptor, a ligand-gated chloride channel
• Benzodiazepines do not act directly on the chloride channel, but enhance binding of GABA to the receptor
• When GABA binds to the $GABA_A$ receptor, it increases the frequency, but not the duration, of the opening of the chloride ion channel, which results in hyperpolarization of the membrane and reduction in neuronal firing
• Activation of the chloride channel enhances inhibitory neurotransmission
• Benzodiazepines also influence sodium channel function at high concentrations

Efficacy Profile
• The goal of treatment is complete remission of seizures
• The onset of action is very rapid, particularly after iv administration
• For the treatment of status epilepticus, the administration of lorazepam is usually followed by a bolus of phenytoin or fosphenytoin, particularly if there is no cessation of status after the lorazepam dose
• Like other benzodiazepines, lorazepam often loses its efficacy during chronic use

Pharmacokinetics

Absorption and Distribution

- First-pass hepatic transformation decreases the absolute systemic availability of oral lorazepam to 29% of that following iv administration
- When lorazepam is administered orally, peak plasma levels are achieved within 1.5–2 hours
- Lorazepam is absorbed more rapidly when administered sublingually than orally or intramuscularly and peak plasma levels are achieved within 1 hour
- Lorazepam entry into the brain is rapid, but probably slower than the brain penetration of diazepam
- Whereas iv bolus injection produces high brain levels rapidly, it is noteworthy that within 2 hours of administration, similar blood levels are produced by im injection or oral administration – thus any of these routes will suffice for non-urgent therapy (e.g., prevention of repetitive seizures)
- When lorazepam parenteral solution is administered rectally, absorption is slow; peak concentrations are lower than those achieved following iv administration, and may not be reached for 1–2 hours
- Pharmacokinetics: linear
- Volume of distribution: 1.0–2.0 L/kg
- Protein binding: 90%
- Salivary concentrations: it is not known whether lorazepam is secreted into saliva and whether such concentrations are similar to the unbound levels seen in plasma

Metabolism

- Lorazepam is metabolized rapidly in the liver by glucuronidation at the 3-hydroxy position
- Approximately 75% of the lorazepam dose is excreted by the kidneys as glucuronide
- The glucuronide metabolite is not pharmacologically active
- Autoinduction is not a feature of lorazepam metabolism

Elimination

- In adults the elimination half-life values for lorazepam are 8–24 hours
- In children the elimination half-life values for lorazepam are 7.6–13.4 hours
- In neonates half-life values are ~40 hours
- Renal excretion: <1% of an administered dose is excreted unchanged in urine

L

PHARMACOKINETICS

L

Drug Interaction Profile

Pharmacokinetic Drug Interactions

There have been no formal studies of interactions with lorazepam but there is a significant likelihood of interaction with some drugs (e.g., lamotrigine, oxcarbazepine, valproic acid) consequent to the mode of metabolism (glucuronidation) of lorazepam.

- Interactions between AEDs: effects on lorazepam:
  - Carbamazepine, phenobarbital, phenytoin, and primidone can *increase* the clearance of lorazepam and *decrease* lorazepam plasma levels
  - Valproate can *decrease* the clearance of lorazepam and *increase* lorazepam plasma levels
- Interactions between AEDs: effects by lorazepam:
  - To date, there have been no reports of lorazepam affecting the clearance of other AEDs and affecting their plasma levels
- Interactions between AEDs and non-AED drugs: effects on lorazepam:
  - Oral contraceptives may *increase* the clearance of lorazepam and *decrease* plasma lorazepam levels
  - Probenecid can *decrease* the clearance of lorazepam and *increase* lorazepam plasma levels
- Interactions between AEDs and non-AED drugs: effects by lorazepam:
  - To date, there have been no reports of lorazepam affecting the clearance of other non-AED drugs and affecting their plasma levels

Pharmacodynamic Drug Interactions

- Patients receiving long-term therapy with other benzodiazepines are less responsive to lorazepam in status epilepticus
- The cardiovascular and respiratory depression by lorazepam can be exacerbated by co-medication with phenobarbital
- Lorazepam potentiates the action of CNS-depressant drugs

Hormonal Contraception

- Lorazepam does not enhance the metabolism of oral contraceptives so as to decrease plasma levels of hormonal contraceptives and, therefore, does not compromise contraception control

Adverse Effects

How Drug Causes Adverse Effects

- Mechanism by which lorazepam causes adverse effects is probably the same as for seizure protection: enhancement of inhibitory neurotransmission through activation of the chloride ion channel
- Long-term adaptations in benzodiazepine receptors may explain the development of dependence, tolerance, and withdrawal
- Adverse effects are generally immediate, but often disappear in time

LORAZEPAM

L

Common Adverse Effects
• Sedation, drowsiness, fatigue
• Nausea
• Ataxia, dizziness, slurred speech, weakness
• Psychomotor slowing
• Cognitive dysfunction, forgetfulness, confusion
• Respiratory depression
• Hypotension
• Paradoxical reactions including agitation, restlessness, and hyperactivity
• Hypersecretion and drooling (hypersalivation), dry mouth
• Pain at injection site

Life-threatening or Dangerous Adverse Effects
• Other than respiratory depression, lorazepam has no life-threatening or dangerous adverse effects
• Hypersensitivity reactions are very rare
• Rare hepatic dysfunction, renal dysfunction, blood dyscrasias

Rare and not Life-threatening Adverse Effects
• Rare hallucinations
• Mania

Weight Change
• Not common; weight gain reported but not expected

What to do About Adverse Effects
• Because lorazepam is most commonly used in emergency situations, the only adverse effect that is of major relevance is respiratory depression
• All patients given more than 0.5–1.0 mg/kg of lorazepam should be monitored carefully for respiratory depression; adequate supportive equipment should be readily available
• Because of the development of tolerance associated with benzodiazepine therapy, starting at a low dose in non-urgent cases will usually decrease the incidence or severity of CNS adverse effects
• In patients treated with maintenance doses of lorazepam, some CNS-related adverse effects may be lessened by slow titration, but they may persist at low doses despite slow titration

Dosing and Use
Usual Dosage Range
• iv dose: 0.1 mg/kg, maintenance doses of 0.05–0.1 mg/kg (maximum dose 4 mg) every 6–8 hours
• Oral sublingual dose: 0.05–0.15 mg/kg, maintenance doses of 0.05–0.1 mg/kg (maximum dose 4 mg) every 6–8 hours

DOSING AND USE

L

Available Formulations
- Tablets: 0.5 mg, 1.0 mg, 2.0 mg, 2.5 mg
- Oral concentrate (Intensol) solution: 2 mg/mL
- Parenteral solution: 2 mg/mL (1 and 10 mL ampoule), 4 mg/mL (1 and 10 mL ampoule)

How to Dose
- The recommended iv dose of lorazepam is 0.1 mg/kg (maximum dose 4 mg); this dose may be repeated if necessary after 10 minutes and administration should not exceed 2 mg/min
- The recommended sublingual dose is 0.05–0.15 mg/kg (maximum 4 mg)
- Patients can be maintained on oral or iv maintenance doses of 0.05–0.1 mg/kg (maximum 4 mg) every 6–8 hours

Dosing Tips
- Slow dose titration may delay onset of therapeutic action but enhance tolerability to sedating effects
- Take liquid formulation with water, soda, apple sauce, or pudding
- Injectable lorazepam is intended for acute use; patients who require long-term treatment should be switched to the oral formulation
- Use lowest possible effective dose for the shortest possible period of time
- Assess need for continuous treatment regularly
- Risk of dependence may increase with dose and duration of treatment
- Frequency of dosing in practice is often greater than predicted from half-life, as duration of biological activity is often shorter than pharmacokinetic terminal half-life

How to Withdraw Drug
- There is no need to adjust dosage of concurrent medications as lorazepam is being discontinued, because plasma levels of other drugs do not change (see Pharmacokinetic Drug Interactions section)
- Abrupt discontinuation of lorazepam has been associated with withdrawal seizures, which may occur up to 60 hours following its discontinuation
- After acute or subacute treatment with repeated doses, the dose should be tapered down over 2–3 days
- In cases of chronic use, taper dose over a period of 1–2 months
- Taper by 0.5 mg every 3 days to reduce chances of withdrawal effects
- For difficult-to-taper cases, consider reducing dose much more slowly after reaching 3 mg/day, perhaps by as little as 0.25 mg per week or less
- For other patients with severe problems discontinuing a benzodiazepine, dosing may need to be tapered over many months (i.e., reduce dose by 1% every 3 days by crushing tablet and suspending or dissolving in 100 mL of fruit juice and then disposing of 1 mL while drinking the rest; 3–7 days later, dispose of 2 mL, and so on). This is

LORAZEPAM

both a form of very slow biological tapering and a form of behavioral desensitization

Overdose
- Fatalities can occur: symptoms include severe respiratory depression, hypotension, tiredness, ataxia, confusion, coma
- Lorazepam overdoses have also been found to cause specifically hallucinations, delirium, and transient global amnesia
- Treatment of overdoses consists of supportive care and the administration of the benzodiazepine receptor antagonist flumazenil. Aminophylline has also been used
- The stomach should be emptied immediately by lavage or by induction of emesis
- Hemodialysis does not remove lorazepam from blood and, therefore, does not serve as a useful procedure in cases of overdose

Tests and Therapeutic Drug Monitoring
- There is no need to monitor any laboratory parameter during treatment with lorazepam
- Therapeutic drug monitoring: uncommon
    - Optimum seizure control in patients on monotherapy is most likely to occur at plasma lorazepam concentrations of 20–30 μg/L (60–90 nmol/L)
    - The conversion factor from μg/L to nmol/L is 3.11 (i.e., 1 μg/L = 3.11 nmol/L)
    - The reference range of lorazepam in plasma is considered to be the same for children and adults, although no data are available to support this clinical practice

Other Warnings/Precautions
- Patients should be monitored carefully for evidence of respiratory depression, accumulation of secretions, and impairment of swallowing
- Lorazepam is a Schedule IV drug and the risk of dependence may increase with dose and duration of treatment
- Patients may develop dependence and/or tolerance with long-term use
- Use with caution in patients with pulmonary disease; there have been rare reports of death after initiation of benzodiazepines in patients with severe pulmonary impairment
- History of drug or alcohol abuse often creates greater risk for dependency
- Use oral formulation only with extreme caution if patient has obstructive sleep apnea; injection is contraindicated in patients with sleep apnea
- Some depressed patients may experience a worsening of suicidal ideation

DOSING AND USE

- Some patients may exhibit abnormal thinking or behavioral changes similar to those caused by other CNS depressants (i.e., either depressant actions or disinhibiting actions)
- Lorazepam must not be administered intra-arterially because it may cause arteriospasm and result in gangrene

Do not Use
- Use with caution in patients with a history of paradoxical or psychotic reaction to lorazepam, or to other benzodiazepines
- In patients who have narrow angle-closure glaucoma
- In patients who have untreated sleep apnea (injection)
- If there is a proven allergy to lorazepam or any other benzodiazepine

Special Populations
Renal Impairment
- Renal failure does not require a reduction in lorazepam dosage

Hepatic Impairment
- Severe hepatic failure may prolong the half-life of lorazepam and may lower protein binding
- Because of its short half-life and inactive metabolites, lorazepam may be a preferred benzodiazepine in some patients with liver disease

Children
- Children do not require additional precautions or monitoring

Elderly
- Elderly patients are more susceptible to adverse effects and, therefore, often do not tolerate higher doses
- Protein binding of lorazepam is slightly lower in the elderly
- A mean 20% reduction in total body clearance of lorazepam has been reported

Pregnancy
- Specialist advice should be given to women who are of childbearing potential; they should be informed about the teratogenicity of all AEDs and the importance of avoiding an unplanned pregnancy; the AED treatment regimen should be reviewed when a woman is planning to become pregnant
- Rapid discontinuation of AEDs should be avoided as this may lead to breakthrough seizures, which could have serious consequences for the woman and the unborn child
- Lorazepam is classified by the US FDA as risk category D (positive evidence of risk to human fetus; potential benefits may still justify its use during pregnancy, especially of seizure disorders); the current

FDA Pregnancy and Lactation Rule has eliminated pregnancy risk category labels
- Infants whose mothers received a benzodiazepine late in pregnancy may experience withdrawal effects
- Neonatal flaccidity has been reported in infants whose mothers took a benzodiazepine during pregnancy
- Use with other AEDs in combination may cause a higher risk for teratogenic effects than lorazepam monotherapy
- Taper drug if discontinuing
- Seizures, even mild seizures, may cause harm to the embryo/fetus
- It is not known whether during pregnancy lorazepam pharmacokinetics change, necessitating a dosage adjustment

Breast Feeding
- Breast milk: transfer of lorazepam into breast milk is minimal because of extensive binding to serum proteins
- Breastfed infants: it is not known what plasma lorazepam concentrations are achieved in breastfed infants compared with the levels of their mothers
- Lorazepam is virtually never used as an AED for long enough to have an impact on breast feeding
- If drug is continued while breast feeding, infant should be monitored for possible adverse effects (feeding difficulties, sedation, and weight loss)
- If adverse effects are observed, recommend bottle feeding

The Overall Place of Lorazepam in the Treatment of Epilepsy
As is the case with some other benzodiazepines, lorazepam use in the treatment of epilepsy is largely limited to acute and subacute situations and it is usually the drug of first choice in the treatment of status epilepticus. It has a high affinity for the benzodiazepine receptor so that its antiepileptic efficacy is similar to that of clonazepam. A very important potential advantage of lorazepam over diazepam is its longer duration of action, in both adults and children, and in neonates, where effects lasting 12 hours or more are usual.

Primary Seizure Types
- Emergency treatment of status epilepticus

Secondary Seizure Types
- Acute repetitive seizures
- Neonatal seizures
- Myoclonic seizures
- Postanoxic myoclonus

L

LORAZEPAM

Potential Advantages
- Rapid onset of action and availability in a variety of formulations (oral liquids as well as injectable formulations)
- Single injection produces a long-lasting effect
- iv lorazepam is as effective as iv diazepam in the treatment of status epilepticus
- Compared with diazepam, iv lorazepam has fewer adverse effects and a longer duration of action
- Sublingual lorazepam is a convenient and effective treatment of serial seizures in children
- Lorazepam has virtually no organ toxicity and has a low risk of hypotension
- Lorazepam may be preferred over other benzodiazepines for patients with liver or renal disease because its pharmacokinetics are unaffected in such patients

Potential Disadvantages
- The effectiveness of lorazepam in the chronic treatment of epilepsy is limited by its sedative and behavioral effects and by the development of tolerance to the protective effect against seizures
- Lorazepam may exacerbate or cause tonic seizures
- Abrupt discontinuation of lorazepam, and benzodiazepines in general, can lead to withdrawal seizures and withdrawal symptoms
- Potential teratogen

Suggested Reading

Appleton R, Sweeney A, Choonara I, Robson J, Molyneux E. Lorazepam versus diazepam in the acute treatment of epileptic seizures and status epilepticus. *Developmental Medicine and Child Neurology* 1995; **37**: 682–688.

Brigo F, Bragazzi NL, Bacigaluppi S, Nardone R, Trinka E. Is intravenous lorazepam realy more effective and safe than intravenous diazepam as first-line treatment for convulsive status epilepticus? A systematic review with meta-analysis of randomized control trials. *Epilepst & Behavor* 2016; **64**: 29–36.

DiMario FJ Jr, Clancy RR. Paradoxical precipitation of tonic seizures by lorazepam in a child with atypical absence seizures. *Pediatric Neurology* 1988; **4**: 249–251.

Greenblatt DJ, Ehrenberg BL, Gunderman J, Scavone JM, Tai NT, Harmatz JS, Shader RI. Kinetic and dynamic study of intravenous lorazepam: comparison with intravenous diazepam. *Journal of Pharmacology and Experimental Therapeutics* 1989; **250**: 134–140.

McDermott CA, Kowalczyk AL, Schnitzler ER, Mangurten HH, Rodvold KA, Metrick S. Pharmacokinetics of lorazepam in critically ill neonates with seizures. *Journal of Pediatrics* 1992; **120**: 479–483.

Prasad K, Al-Roomi K, Krishnan PR, Sequeira R. Anticonvulsant therapy for status epilepticus. *Cochrane Database Systematic Reviews* 2005; **4**: CD003723.

Relling MV, Mulhern RK, Dodge RK, Johnson D, Pieper JA, Rivera GK, Evans WE. Lorazepam pharmacodynamics and pharmacokinetics in children. *Journal of Pediatrics* 1989; **114**: 641–646.

Riviello JJ Jr, Holmes GL. The treatment of status epilepticus. *Seminars in Pediatric Neurology* 2004; **11**: 129–138.

L

SUGGESTED READING

METHSUXIMIDE

Therapeutics

Chemical Name and Structure

Methsuximide, *N*-2-dimethyl-2-phenyl-succinimide, is a white powder, with a molecular weight of 203.23 and an empirical formula of $C_{12}H_{13}NO_2$.

Brand Names
- Celontin
- Petinutin

Generics Available
- No

Licensed Indications for Epilepsy
- Absence seizures that are refractory to other AEDs (FDA PI)

Licensed Indications for Non-epilepsy Conditions
- There are none

Non-licensed Use for Epilepsy
- Partial seizures
- Myoclonic seizures
- Astatic seizures (drop attacks)

Non-licensed Use for Non-epilepsy Conditions
- There are none

Ineffective (Contraindicated)
- Generalized tonic–clonic seizures

Mechanism of Action
- Not established

Efficacy Profile
- The goals of treatment are to achieve complete seizure remission when possible, or at least improved frequency and severity of seizures, while also minimizing adverse effects and improving patient quality of life
- Onset of action may occur within the first few days

- Goal of therapy in typical absence seizures is not only full seizure control, but also normalization of EEG
- Once chronic therapy is initiated, it is usually continued for at least 2 years following the last seizure
- If partially effective, consider co-prescribing with lamotrigine or valproic acid, or switch to valproic acid, lamotrigine, levetiracetam, acetazolamide, topiramate, or zonisamide

M

Pharmacokinetics
Absorption and Distribution
- Oral bioavailability: not established
- Food co-ingestion: it is not known whether food co-ingestion affects the rate or extent of absorption
- Tmax: 1–4 hours (for pharmacologically active metabolite N-desmethylmethsuximide)
- Time to steady state: 8–16 days
- Pharmacokinetics: linear
- Protein binding: 45–60% (for N-desmethylmethsuximide)
- Volume of distribution: not established
- Salivary concentrations: it is not known whether methsuximide and N-desmethylmethsuximide are secreted into saliva and whether such concentrations are similar to the unbound levels seen in plasma

Metabolism
- Methsuximide is rapidly metabolized in the liver to its primary metabolite N-desmethylmethsuximide, which is then further hydroxylated before renal elimination
- The primary metabolite of methsuximide, N-desmethylmethsuximide, is pharmacologically active
- Autoinduction is not a feature of methsuximide metabolism

Elimination
- The elimination half-life of methsuximide is 1.0–2.6 hours
- The elimination half-life of N-desmethylmethsuximide is 34–80 hours in adults and 16–45 hours in children
- Renal excretion: <1% of an administered dose is excreted unchanged in urine

Drug Interaction Profile
Pharmacokinetic Drug Interactions
- Interactions between AEDs: effects on methsuximide:
  - Phenytoin and phenobarbital can *increase* the clearance of N-desmethylmethsuximide and *decrease* N-desmethylmethsuximide plasma levels

- Felbamate can *decrease* the clearance of N-desmethylmethsuximide and *increase* N-desmethylmethsuximide plasma levels
- Interactions between AEDs: effects by methsuximide:
  - Methsuximide can increase plasma levels of phenytoin and phenobarbital
  - Methsuximide can decrease plasma levels of carbamazepine, lamotrigine, levetiracetam, rufinamide, topiramate, and valproic acid
- Interactions between AEDs and non-AED drugs: effects on methsuximide:
  - To date, there have been no reports of other non-AED drugs affecting the clearance of methsuximide and affecting methsuximide plasma levels
- Interactions between AEDs and non-AED drugs: effects by methsuximide:
  - To date, there have been no reports of methsuximide affecting the clearance of other non-AED drugs and affecting their plasma levels

Pharmacodynamic Drug Interactions
- To date, none have been reported

Hormonal Contraception
- Methsuximide does not enhance the metabolism of oral contraceptives so as to decrease plasma levels of hormonal contraceptives and, therefore, does not compromise contraception control

Adverse Effects
The adverse effects of methsuximide are very similar to those caused by ethosuximide

How Drug Causes Adverse Effects
- Mechanism by which methsuximide causes adverse effects has not been determined

Common Adverse Effects
- Abdominal discomfort
- Vomiting
- Diarrhea
- Hiccups
- Headaches
- Sedation, drowsiness, fatigue

Life-threatening or Dangerous Adverse Effects
- Bone marrow reactions such as granulocytopenia, thrombocytopenia, or pancytopenia
- Systemic lupus erythematosus
- Stevens–Johnson syndrome

M

Rare and not Life-threatening Adverse Effects
• Behavioral disturbances: nervousness, irritability, depression, hallucinations, and even psychosis
• Attacks of hepatic porphyria may be precipitated by methsuximide
• Proteinuria
• Microscopic hematuria

Weight Change
• Weight gain is uncommon

What to do About Adverse Effects
• Discuss common and severe adverse effects with patients or parents before starting medication, including symptoms that should be reported to the physician
• Gastrointestinal adverse effects can improve when methsuximide is taken at the end of a meal

DOSING AND USE

Dosing and Use
Usual Dosage Range
• Adults: 600–1200 mg/day
• Children: 10–30 mg/kg/day (mean dose <30 kg body weight: 20 mg/kg/day; >30 kg body weight: 15 mg/kg/day)

Available Formulations
• Capsules: 150 mg, 300 mg

How to Dose
• *For adults:* start treatment with 300 mg/day; at intervals of 5–7 days increase by 300 mg/day as needed and tolerated; maintenance dose generally 600–1200 mg/day in two daily doses
• *Children:* start treatment with approximately 10 mg/kg/day, which is one-third of the initial target dose; there can be two or more subsequent increases by the same amount at intervals of 5–7 days; maintenance dose generally 10–30 mg/kg/day, in two daily doses

Dosing Tips
• Methsuximide should be given preferably after meals
• Because of the long half-life of N-desmethylmethsuximide, methsuximide can be taken twice daily

How to Withdraw Drug
• May need to adjust dosage of concurrent medications as methsuximide is being discontinued, because plasma levels of other drugs may change (see Pharmacokinetic Drug Interactions section)
• Rapid discontinuation may increase the risk of seizures

- Dose can be decreased linearly at weekly intervals over a period of 1–3 months
- Because recurrence of absence seizures may be subtle clinically, or because significant subclinical spike-and-wave discharges may require reintroduction of therapy, it is good practice to repeat an EEG 1–3 months after methsuximide has been discontinued

Overdose
- Usually not fatal and symptoms include: stupor, coma, respiratory depression, nausea, vomiting
- *N*-desmethylmethsuximide plasma levels above 40 mg/L cause toxicity, and levels above 150 mg/L have been associated with coma
- If indicated the stomach should be emptied by lavage or by induction of emesis
- Hemodialysis does not remove methsuximide or *N*-desmethylmethsuximide from blood and, therefore, is not a useful procedure in cases of overdose

Tests and Therapeutic Drug Monitoring
- There are no clear guidelines regarding the need to monitor blood counts for the rare occurrence of bone marrow suppression, and clinical education and observation are likely to provide the best probability of early detection; blood count can be determined after 2 months, then every 6 months
- Therapeutic drug monitoring:
  - Optimum seizure control in patients on monotherapy is most likely to occur at plasma *N*-desmethylmethsuximide levels of 10–40 mg/L (50–200 µmol/L)
  - The conversion factor from mg/mL to µmol/mL is 4.92 (i.e., 1 mg/L = 4.92 µmol/L)
  - Once the patient is doing well clinically, there is no need to determine blood levels routinely
  - The reference range of *N*-desmethylmethsuximide in plasma is considered to be the same for children and adults, although no data are available to support this clinical practice
  - There are no data indicating the usefulness of monitoring *N*-desmethylmethsuximide by use of saliva

Other Warnings/Precautions
- Patients should be instructed to promptly inform their physician if they develop a sore throat, fever, or other signs or symptoms suggestive of an infection
- Mental and/or physical abilities may be impaired

Do not Use
- In patients with generalized tonic–clonic seizures unless they also take a medication that is known to be effective against tonic–clonic seizures

Special Populations

Renal Impairment
• Renal impairment has little or no impact on methsuximide pharmacokinetics

Hepatic Impairment
• Liver failure may lower the clearance and decrease the dosage requirements of methsuximide

Children
• Children have an increased metabolic capacity and consequently higher doses on an mg/kg/day basis are usually required to achieve the equivalent therapeutic plasma levels
• Pharmacokinetic interactions in children are usually of a greater magnitude than that seen in adults

Elderly
• Methsuximide is used only very rarely in the elderly
• Elderly patients are more susceptible to adverse effects (especially somnolence) and, therefore, often do better at lower doses
• Because of an age-related reduction in renal and hepatic function, lower methsuximide doses are appropriate
• Elderly patients are often prescribed concurrent drug therapies for comorbidities and therefore may be at greater risk for pharmacokinetic and pharmacodynamic interactions; the risk of pharmacokinetic interactions with methsuximide is minimal

Pregnancy
• Specialist advice should be given to women who are of childbearing potential; they should be informed about the teratogenicity of all AEDs and the importance of avoiding an unplanned pregnancy; the AED treatment regimen should be reviewed when a woman is planning to become pregnant
• Rapid discontinuation of AEDs should be avoided as this may lead to breakthrough seizures, which could have serious consequences for the woman and the unborn child
• Methsuximide was previously classified by the US FDA as risk category C (some animal studies show adverse effects, no controlled studies in humans); the current FDA Pregnancy and Lactation Rule has eliminated pregnancy risk category labels
• Use with other AEDs in combination may cause a higher prevalence of teratogenic effects than methsuximide monotherapy
• Taper drug if discontinuing
• Seizures, even mild seizures, may cause harm to the embryo/fetus
• It is not known whether during pregnancy methsuximide pharmacokinetics change

Breast Feeding
- Breast milk: methsuximide: it is not known whether it is secreted into breast milk; *N*-desmethylmethsuximide: it is not known whether it is secreted into breast milk
- Breastfed infants: it is not known what plasma methsuximide and *N*-desmethylmethsuximide concentrations are achieved in breastfed infants compared with the levels of their mothers
- If drug is continued while breast feeding, infant should be monitored for possible adverse effects
- If adverse effects are observed, recommend bottle feeding

The Overall Place of Methsuximide in the Treatment of Epilepsy

The primary indication of methsuximide is in the treatment of childhood absence epilepsy. However, methsuximide appears to be less effective than ethosuximide. In contrast to ethosuximide, methsuximide has been reported to be effective as adjunctive therapy against partial seizures. Methsuximide has also been reported to be at times effective against myoclonic seizures, including juvenile myoclonic epilepsy and against astatic seizures (drop attacks)

Primary Seizure Types
- Childhood absence seizures

Secondary Seizure Types
- Partial (focal) seizures
- Myoclonic seizures, including juvenile myoclonic epilepsy
- Astatic seizures (drop attacks)

Potential Advantages
- Methsuximide has a mostly benign adverse effect profile and severe adverse reactions are extremely rare

Potential Disadvantages
- Narrow spectrum of seizure protection, limited mostly to absence seizures, with some efficacy against partial seizures
- Potential teratogen

Suggested Reading

Besag FM, Berry DJ, Pool F. Methsuximide lowers lamotrigine blood levels: a pharmacokinetic antiepileptic drug interaction. *Epilepsia* 2000; **41**: 624–627.

Browne TR, Feldman RG, Buchanan RA, Allan NC, Fawcett-Vickers L, Szako GK, Mattson GF, Norman SE, Greenblatt DJ. Methsuximide for complex partial seizures: efficacy, toxicity, clinical pharmacology, and drug interactions. *Neurology* 1983; **33**: 414–418.

Hurst DL. The use of methsuximide for juvenile myoclonic epilepsy. *Annals of Neurology* 1995; **38**: 517.

Strong JM, Abe T, Gibbs EL, Atkinson AJ. Plasma levels of methsuximide and N-desmethylmethsuximide during methsuximide therapy. *Neurology* 1974; **24**: 250–255.

Tennison MB, Greenwood RS, Miles MV. Methsuximide for intractable childhood seizures. *Pediatrics* 1991; **87**: 186–189.

Wilder BJ, Buchanan RA. Methsuximide for refractory complex partial seizures. *Neurology* 1981; **31**: 741–744.

M

SUGGESTED READING

MIDAZOLAM

Therapeutics

Chemical Name and Structure

Midazolam,8-chloro-6-(2-fluorophenyl)-1-methyl-4H-imidazol[1,5-a]
[1,4]benzodiazepine, is available as midazolam HCl and is a white to
light yellow crystalline compound, with a molecular weight of 362.25
and an empirical formula of $C_{18}H_{13}ClFN_3 \cdot HCl$.

Brand Names
- Benzosed
- Buccolam
- Dalam; Doricum; Dormicum; Dormonid
- Epistatus
- Flused; Fortanest; Fulsed
- Hypnovel
- Ipnovel
- Mezolam; Miben; Midacip; Midacum; Midanium; Midapic; Midaz;
  Midazo; Midazol; Midazolam Torrex; Midcalm; Midolam; Midosed;
  Midozor; Midzee; Midzol; Miloz; Mizolam
- Relacum
- Sedacum; Sedeven; Shortal; Sopodorm
- Uzolam
- Versed

Generics Available
- No

Licensed Indications for Epilepsy
- Buccolam is licensed for the treatment of prolonged, acute, convulsive
  seizures in infants, toddlers, children, and adolescents (from 3 months
  to <18 years) (UK SPC)

Licensed Indications for Non-epilepsy Conditions
- Anesthesia (UK SPC)
- Sedation (UK SPC; FDA PI)

- Preoperative induction of anesthesia (UK SPC; FDA PI)
- Drug-induced amnesia (UK SPC; FDA PI)

Non-licensed Use for Epilepsy
- Acute repetitive seizures
- Refractory neonatal seizures
- Refractory status epilepticus (convulsive and non-convulsive)
- Prehospital treatment of status epilepticus (im)

Non-licensed Use for Non-epilepsy Conditions
- There are none

Ineffective (Contraindicated)
- Midazolam is potentially effective against all types of seizures and is not contraindicated for any form of epilepsy

Mechanism of Action
- Benzodiazepines bind to the neuronal $GABA_A$ receptor, a ligand-gated chloride channel
- Benzodiazepines do not act directly on the chloride channel, but enhance binding of GABA to the receptor
- When GABA binds to the $GABA_A$ receptor, it increases the frequency, but not the duration, of the opening of the chloride ion channel, which results in hyperpolarization of the membrane and reduction in neuronal firing
- Activation of the chloride channel enhances inhibitory neurotransmission
- Benzodiazepines also influence sodium channel function at high concentrations

Efficacy Profile
- The goal of treatment is complete remission of seizures
- The onset of action is very rapid, particularly after iv administration
- Like other benzodiazepines, midazolam often loses its efficacy during chronic use
- Chronic use of midazolam in the treatment of epilepsy is unusual
- iv injection: onset 3–5 minutes
- im injection: onset 15 minutes, peak 20–30 minutes
- Patients generally recover 2–6 hours after awakening

Pharmacokinetics
Absorption and Distribution
- Oral bioavailability: first-pass hepatic transformation decreases the absolute systemic bioavailability of oral midazolam to 40–50% (27% in children) of that following iv administration
- After rectal administration (solution) absolute bioavailability is ~50%

175

- After oromucosal administration (solution) absolute bioavailability is ~75% (~87% in children with severe malaria and convulsions)
- Food co-ingestion: neither the rate of absorption nor the extent of absorption is affected by food co-ingestion
- Tmax: ~1 hour (oral), 20–30 minutes (im); ~30 minutes (rectal); ~30 minutes (oromucosal)
- Intranasal administration of midazolam is followed by very rapid absorption, and a time to seizure control of 2.5–5 minutes has been reported
- After iv administration, there is rapid distribution, with a distribution half-life of 6–15 minutes
- Time to steady state: not appropriate
- Pharmacokinetics: linear
- Protein binding: 96–98% (midazolam); 89% (1-hydroxymidazolam)
- Volume of distribution: 1.0–2.5 L/kg
- Salivary concentrations: it is not known whether midazolam or 1-hydroxymidazolam is secreted into saliva and whether such concentrations are similar to the unbound levels seen in plasma

Metabolism
- Midazolam is rapidly metabolized in the liver, primarily by CYP3A4, to 1-hydroxymidazolam (~63–80% of an administered dose) and to two minor metabolites (a 4-hydroxy metabolite (~3% of the dose) and a 1,4-dihydroxy metabolite (~1% of the dose)
- 1-hydroxymidazolam and its two minor metabolites are subsequently glucuronidated and eliminated predominantly through the kidneys
- 1-hydroxymidazolam has weak pharmacological activity (approximately 10% of the pharmacological activity of midazolam after iv administration)
- Autoinduction is not a feature of midazolam metabolism

Elimination
- The elimination half-life of midazolam is 1.5–4 hours in adults
- The elimination half-life of midazolam is 1–3 hours in children and can be as long as 6.5–12 hours in sick neonates
- Renal excretion: <1% of the midazolam dose is excreted unchanged in the urine

Drug Interaction Profile
Pharmacokinetic Drug Interactions
- Interactions between AEDs: effects on midazolam:
  - Carbamazepine, perampanel, and phenytoin can *increase* the clearance of midazolam and can *decrease* midazolam plasma levels
- Interactions between AEDs: effects by midazolam:
  - To date, there have been no reports of midazolam affecting the clearance of other AEDs and affecting their plasma levels

MIDAZOLAM

- Interactions between AEDs and non-AED drugs: effects on midazolam:
  - Atorvastatin, cimetidine, clarithromycin, diltiazem, erythromycin, fluconazole, grapefruit juice, itraconazole, ketoconazole, omeprazole, posaconazole, ranitidine, ritonavir-boosted lopinavir, verapamil, and voriconazole can *decrease* the clearance of midazolam and *increase* midazolam plasma levels
  - Rifampin and St. John's wort can *increase* the clearance of midazolam and *decrease* midazolam plasma levels
- Interactions between AEDs and non-AED drugs: effects by midazolam:
  - To date, there have been no reports of midazolam affecting the clearance of other non-AED drugs and affecting their plasma levels

Pharmacodynamic Drug Interactions
- Patients receiving long-term therapy with other benzodiazepines may be less responsive to midazolam in status epilepticus
- The cardiovascular and respiratory depression by midazolam can be exacerbated by co-medication with phenobarbital
- Midazolam may potentiate the action of CNS-depressant drugs
- Midazolam decreases the minimum alveolar concentration of halothane needed for general anesthesia
- Hypotension has occurred in neonates given midazolam and fentanyl

Hormonal Contraception
- Midazolam does not enhance the metabolism of oral contraceptives so as to decrease plasma levels of hormonal contraceptives and, therefore, does not compromise contraception control

Adverse Effects
How Drug Causes Adverse Effects
- Mechanism by which midazolam causes adverse effects is probably the same as for seizure protection: enhancement of inhibitory neurotransmission through activation of the chloride ion channel
- Actions at benzodiazepine receptors that carry over to the next day can cause daytime sedation, amnesia, and ataxia

Common Adverse Effects
- Oversedation: impaired recall, agitation, involuntary movements, headache
- Drowsiness, fatigue
- Ataxia
- Psychomotor slowing
- Cognitive dysfunction
- Respiratory depression
- Hypotension

M

ADVERSE EFFECTS

- Paradoxical reactions, including agitation, restlessness, and hyperactivity
- Nausea, vomiting
- Irritation/pain at site of injection

Life-threatening or Dangerous Adverse Effects
- Other than respiratory depression, midazolam has no life-threatening or dangerous adverse effects
- Hypersensitivity reactions are very rare
- Respiratory depression, apnea, respiratory arrest
- Cardiac arrest

Rare and not Life-threatening Adverse Effects
- Skin rash, urticarial reaction, pruritus at site of injection
- Euphoria, hallucinations
- Anterograde amnesia

Weight Change
- Not common; weight gain reported but not expected

What to do About Adverse Effects
- Because midazolam is most commonly used in emergency situations, the only adverse effect that is of major relevance is respiratory depression
- All patients given midazolam for repetitive seizures or status epilepticus should be monitored carefully for respiratory depression; adequate supportive equipment should be readily available

Dosing and Use
Usual Dosage Range
- The recommended initial iv bolus dose of midazolam is 0.15 mg/kg, administered over 2–5 minutes (no more than 2 mg/min)
- If necessary, the initial iv bolus may be followed by continuous iv infusion at an initial rate of 1 µg/kg/min

Available Formulations
- Tablets: 15 mg
- Syrup: 2 mg/mL (2.5 mL bottle or 118 mL bottle)
- Ampoules for iv, im, and rectal administration: 1 mg/mL, 2 mg/mL, 5 mg/mL, 10 mg/2 mL, 10 mg/5 mL
- Ampoules for injection: 5 mg/mL, 10 mg/2 mL, 15 mg/3 mL
- Prefilled syringes with oromucosal solution: 2.5 mg in 0.5 mL; 5 mg in 1 mL; 7.5 mg in 1.5 mL; 10 mg in 2 mL

MIDAZOLAM

How to Dose
- In most instances, midazolam is administered acutely or subacutely as described above
- The iv loading dose of midazolam should be administered over 2–5 minutes or no more than 2 mg/min
- The infusion rate maybe increased by 1 µg/kg/min every 15 minutes until seizure control is achieved
- Seizure control is often achieved at infusion rates of <3 µg/kg/min
- The use of rates up to 18 µg/kg/min has been reported
- The recommended im dose is 5–10 mg in adults (0.2 mg/kg in children); this dose can be repeated once
- The recommended intranasal and buccal dose is also 5–10 mg in adults (0.2 mg/kg in children)

Dosing Tips
- Better to underdose, observe for effects, and then prudently raise dose while monitoring carefully
- Although bioavailability after im administration is good (~80%), there is considerable interpatient variability
- The full syringe amount of oromucosal solution should be inserted slowly into the space between the gum and the cheek
- Care should be exercised to avoid excessive swallowing of midazolam during oromucosal administration; this can be achieved by administering half of the dose into one side of the mouth, then the other half slowly into the other side

How to Withdraw Drug
- There is no need to adjust dosage of concurrent medications as midazolam is being discontinued, because plasma levels of other drugs do not change (see Pharmacokinetic Drug Interactions section)
- Abrupt discontinuation of midazolam may be associated with withdrawal seizures
- After acute or subacute treatment with repeated doses or iv infusion, the dose should be tapered down over 2–3 days
- Chronic use of midazolam for the treatment of epilepsy is exceedingly rare

Overdose
- Overdose with a benzodiazepine can cause all of the adverse effects listed above and can lead to severe respiratory depression, hypotension, coma, and death
- Treatment of overdose consists of supportive care and the administration of the benzodiazepine receptor antagonist flumazenil
- The stomach should be emptied immediately by lavage or by induction of emesis
- It is not known whether hemodialysis removes midazolam from blood and, therefore, could serve as a useful procedure in case of overdose

M

DOSING AND USE

M

Tests and Therapeutic Drug Monitoring
- There is no need to monitor any laboratory parameter during treatment with midazolam
- Therapeutic drug monitoring: uncommon
  - Subjective CNS effects have been reported at threshold plasma levels of 30–100 µg/L (82.8–276 nmol/L), and mean peak plasma level after 1 mg/kg orally in patients 2–12 years old was approximately 200 µg/L (552 nmol/L). A therapeutic range is not used clinically
  - The conversion factor from mg/mL to µmol/L, or µg/mL to nmol/L, is 2.76 (i.e., 1 µg/L = 2.76 nmol/L)
  - There are no data indicating the usefulness of monitoring midazolam by use of saliva

Other Warnings / Precautions
- Patients should be monitored carefully for evidence of respiratory depression, accumulation of secretions, and impairment of swallowing
- Patients with chronic obstructive pulmonary disease should receive lower doses
- Use with caution in patients with impaired respiratory function

Do not Use
- Use with caution in patients with a history of paradoxical reaction to midazolam, or to other benzodiazepines
- If patient has narrow angle-closure glaucoma

MIDAZOLAM

Special Populations
Renal Impairment
- Renal failure may prolong the half-life of midazolam

Hepatic Impairment
- Severe hepatic failure may prolong the half-life of midazolam

Children
- Children do not require additional precautions or monitoring
- In sick neonates, clearance is reduced and the elimination half-life of midazolam is longer (6.5–12 hours)
- Seriously ill neonates have reduced clearance and longer elimination half-life values
- The effect of inhibitors of midazolam metabolism may be larger in infants administered oromucosal midazolam because of the likelihood that more of the dose will be swallowed, compared to adults, and absorbed in the gastrointestinal tract

Elderly
- Elderly patients are more susceptible to adverse effects and, therefore, often do better at lower doses
- The elimination half-life of midazolam may be prolonged in the elderly

Pregnancy
- Specialist advice should be given to women who are of childbearing potential; they should be informed about the teratogenicity of all AEDs and the importance of avoiding an unplanned pregnancy; the AED treatment regimen should be reviewed when a woman is planning to become pregnant
- Midazolam was previously classified by the US FDA as risk category D (positive evidence of risk to human fetus; potential benefits may still justify its use during pregnancy, especially of seizure disorders); the current FDA Pregnancy and Lactation Rule has eliminated pregnancy risk category labels
- Possible increased risk of birth defects when benzodiazepines are taken during pregnancy
- Infants whose mothers received a benzodiazepine late in pregnancy may experience withdrawal effects
- Neonatal flaccidity has been reported in infants whose mothers took a benzodiazepine during pregnancy
- Midazolam is virtually never used as an AED for long enough to have an impact on the pregnancy or the fetus

Breast Feeding
- Breast milk: transfer into breast milk is minimal (0.6% of that attained in the mother's circulation) because of extensive binding to plasma proteins (albumin)
- Midazolam is virtually never used as an AED for long enough to have an impact on breast feeding
- Breastfed infants: it is not known what plasma midazolam concentrations are achieved in breastfed infants compared with the levels of their mothers
- Effects on infants have been observed and include feeding difficulties, sedation, and weight loss
- If drug is continued while breast feeding, infant should be monitored for possible adverse effects
- If adverse effects are observed, recommend bottle feeding

The Overall Place of Midazolam in the Treatment of Epilepsy

As is the case with some other benzodiazepines, midazolam use in the treatment of epilepsy is largely limited to acute and subacute management of convulsive and non-convulsive seizures. Midazolam is the only drug used in the management of status epilepticus which can be given by rectal administration, by im or iv injection, or oromucosal administration. Its im use in premonitory status is a great advantage, and midazolam has an important clinical role at this stage in status as an alternative to iv or rectal diazepam, or iv lorazepam.

Primary Seizure Types
• Status epilepticus

Secondary Seizure Types
• None

Potential Advantages
• Midazolam is very rapidly absorbed following im and intranasal administration
• Midazolam has a relatively short half-life and is well suited for continuous iv infusion
• Midazolam has virtually no organ toxicity
• It has less tendency to accumulate than diazepam
• The use of the oromucosal formulation avoids the awkward and embarrassing use of rectal formulations

Potential Disadvantages
• The effectiveness of midazolam in the chronic treatment of epilepsy is limited by its sedative and behavioral effects, by its short elimination half-life, and by the development of tolerance to the protective effect against seizures
• Abrupt discontinuation of midazolam, and benzodiazepines in general, can lead to withdrawal seizures and withdrawal symptoms
• Short-acting with tendency to relapse following a single injection
• The lipid solubility of midazolam and hence its cerebral action are reduced as blood and cerebral pH fall
• Elimination dependent on blood flow
• Potential teratogen

Suggested Reading

Bell DM, Richards G, Dhillon S, Oxley JR, Cromarty J, Sander JW, Patsalos PN. A comparative pharmacokinetic study of intravenous and intramuscular midazolam in patients with epilepsy. *Epilepsy Research* 1991; **10**: 183–190.

Chamberlain JM, Altieri MA, Futterman C, Young GM, Ochsenschlager DW, Waisman Y. A prospective, randomized study comparing intramuscular midazolam with intravenous diazepam for the treatment of seizures in children. *Pediatric Emergency Care* 1997; **13**: 92–94.

Claassen J, Hirsch LJ, Emerson RG, Bates JE, Thompson TB, Mayer SA. Continuous EEG monitoring and midazolam infusion for refractory nonconvulsive status epilepticus. *Neurology* 2001; **57**: 1036–1042.

MIDAZOLAM

Garnock-Jones KP. Oromucosal midazolam. A review of its use in pediatric patients with prolonged acute convulsive seizures. *Pediatric Drugs* 2012; **14**: 251–261.

Holmes GL, Riviello JJ Jr. Midazolam and pentobarbital for refractory status epilepticus. *Pediatric Neurology* 1999; **20**: 259–264.

Koul RL, Aithala GR, Chacko A, Joshi R, Elbualy MS. Continuous midazolam as treatment of status epilepticus. *Archives of Diseases of Childhood* 1997; **76**: 445–448.

Lahat E, Goldman M, Barr J, Eshel G, Berkovitch M. Intranasal midazolam for childhood seizures. *Lancet* 1998; **352**: 620.

Moretti R, Julliand S, Rinaldi VE, Titomanlio L. Buccal midazolam compared with rectal diazepam reduces seizure duration in children in the outpatient setting. *Pediatric Emergency Care* 2017 Mar 27. doi: 10.1097/PEC.0000000000001114.

Prasad K, Al-Roomi K, Krishnan PR, Sequeira R. Anticonvulsant therapy for status epilepticus. *Cochrane Database of Systematic Reviews* 2005; **4**: CD003723.

Riviello JJ Jr, Holmes GL. The treatment of status epilepticus. *Seminars in Pediatric Neurolology* 2004; **11**: 129–138.

Sheth RD, Buckley DJ, Gutierrez AR, Gingold M, Bodensteiner JB, Penney S. Midazolam in the treatment of refractory neonatal seizures. *Clinical Neuropharmacology* 1996; **19**: 165–170.

Silbergleit R, Durkalski V, Conwit R, Pancioli A, Palesch Y, Barsan W. Intramuscular versus intravenous therapy for prehospital status epilepticus. *New England Journal of Medicine* 2012; **366**: 591–600.

Singhi S, Murthy A, Singhi P, Jayashree M. Continuous midazolam versus diazepam infusion for refractory convulsive status epilepticus. *Journal of Child Neurology* 2002; **17**: 106–110.

M

SUGGESTED READING

OXCARBAZEPINE

Therapeutics

Chemical Name and Structure

Oxcarbazepine, 10,11-dihydro-10-oxo-5H-dibenz(b,f)azepine-4-carboxamide, is a white to faintly orange crystalline powder, with a molecular weight of 254.29 and an empirical formula of $C_{15}H_{12}N_2O_2$.

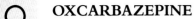

Brand Names
- Actinium; Apydan extent
- Carbamac; Carbox
- Deprectal
- Epex
- Lonazet
- Mezalog
- Neurtrol
- Oleptal; Oscar; Oxana; Oxcarb; Oxcazo; Oxemazetol; Oxep; Oxepin; Oxeptal; Oxetol; Oxital; Oxpine; Oxrate; Oxtellar XR; Oxycarb; Oxzey
- Prolepsi
- Seizurone; Selzic
- Timox; Trexapin; Trileptal; Trileptin
- Zenoxa; Zepox

Generics Available
- Yes

Licensed Indications for Epilepsy
- Monotherapy or adjunctive treatment of partial (focal) seizures with or without secondary generalization in patients ≥ 4 years (FDA PI)
- Monotherapy or adjunctive treatment of partial (focal) seizures with or without secondary generalization in patients ≥ 6 years of age (UK SPC)
- Adjunctive treatment of partial (focal) seizures with or without secondary generalization in patients ≥ 2 years of age (FDA PI)

Licensed Indications for Non-epilepsy Conditions
• There are none

Non-licensed Use for Epilepsy
• There are none

Non-licensed Use for Non-epilepsy Conditions
• Bipolar disorder
• Trigeminal neuralgia

Ineffective (Contraindicated)
• Oxcarbazepine is contraindicated for primary generalized seizures such as absence or myoclonic seizures in idiopathic generalized epilepsies; this may be the result of oxcarbazepine per se and not of its pharmacologically active metabolite 10-hydroxycarbazepine
• Efficacy is as yet unproven in neonates and children <2 years of age

Mechanism of Action
• The pharmacological activity of oxcarbazepine is primarily exerted through its 10-monohydroxy metabolite (hydroxy-10,11-dihydro-5H-dibenzapine-5-carboxamide)
• Acts as a use-dependent blocker of voltage-sensitive sodium channels
• This results in stabilization of hyperexcited neural membranes, inhibition of repetitive neuronal firing, and diminution of propagation of synaptic impulses so that seizure spread is prevented
• Increases potassium conductance
• Modulates high-voltage-activated calcium channels, and reduces the release of glutamate

Efficacy Profile
• The goals of treatment are to achieve complete seizure remission when possible, or at least improved frequency and severity of seizures, while also minimizing adverse effects and improving patient quality of life
• Efficacy should be apparent within 2 weeks of treatment initiation
• If it is not producing clinical benefits within 6–8 weeks, it may require a dosage increase or it may not work at all
• If oxcarbazepine is ineffective or only partially effective, it can be replaced by or combined with another AED that is appropriate for the patient's seizure type or epilepsy syndrome

Pharmacokinetics
Absorption and Distribution
• Oral bioavailability: 100% (oxcarbazepine)
• Food co-ingestion: neither delays the rate of absorption nor decreases the extent of absorption (oxcarbazepine)

PHARMACOKINETICS

- Tmax: 3–6 hours (oxcarbazepine)
- Time to steady state: 2–3 days (10-hydroxycarbazepine)
- Pharmacokinetics: linear
- Protein binding: 40% (10-hydroxycarbazepine); 60% (oxcarbazepine)
- Volume of distribution: 0.75 L/kg (10-hydroxycarbazepine)
- Salivary concentrations: 10-hydroxycarbazepine is secreted into saliva and concentrations are similar to the unbound levels seen in plasma

Metabolism
- Oxcarbazepine is rapidly metabolized in the liver to its pharmacologically active metabolite, 10-hydroxycarbazepine (also known as S-licarbazepine and eslicarbazepine), by stereoselective biotransformation mediated by cytosolic arylketone reductase
- 10-hydroxycarbazepine comprises a racemic mixture of 80% S and 20% R
- 10-hydroxycarbazepine is subsequently primarily metabolized by conjugation with glucuronic acid
- Minor amounts (4% of dose) of 10-hydroxycarbazepine are oxidized to an inactive 10,11-dihydroxy metabolite
- Metabolites (other than 10-hydroxycarbazepine) are not pharmacologically active
- Autoinduction is not a feature of oxcarbazepine metabolism

Elimination
- Half-life of oxcarbazepine is ~2 hours; thus oxcarbazepine is essentially a prodrug rapidly converted to its 10-hydroxycarbazepine metabolite
- In the absence of enzyme-inducing co-medication, half-life values for 10-hydroxycarbazepine are 8–15 hours
- In the presence of enzyme-inducing co-medication, half-life values for 10-hydroxycarbazepine are 7–12 hours
- Renal excretion: >95% of an administered dose is excreted as metabolites in urine; 49% as glucuronides of 10-hydroxycarbazepine and 27% as unchanged 10-hydroxycarbazepine
- Renal excretion: <1% of an administered dose is excreted unchanged as oxcarbazepine in urine

Drug Interaction Profile
Pharmacokinetic Drug Interactions
- Interactions between AEDs: effects on 10-hydroxycarbazepine:
  - Carbamazepine, lacosamide, perampanel, phenobarbital, and phenytoin can *increase* the clearance of 10-hydroxycarbazepine and *decrease* 10-hydroxycarbazepine plasma levels
  - Valproic acid can displace 10-hydroxycarbazepine from its plasma protein-binding sites

• Interactions between AEDs: effects by 10-hydroxycarbazepine:
  – 10-hydroxycarbazepine can *decrease* plasma levels of carbamazepine, lamotrigine, levetiracetam, perampanel, rufinamide, and topiramate
  – 10-hydroxycarbazepine can *increase* plasma levels of phenobarbital and phenytoin
• Interactions between AEDs and non-AED drugs: effects on 10-hydroxycarbazepine:
  – Viloxazine can *increase* 10-hydroxycarbazepine plasma levels
  – Atkins diet (modified), rifampicin and verapamil can *decrease* 10-hydroxycarbazepine plasma levels
  – Oral contraceptives can *increase* the clearance and *decrease* plasma levels of 10-hydroxycarbazepine
• Interactions between AEDs and non-AED drugs: effects by 10-hydroxycarbazepine:
  – 10-hydroxycarbazepine can decrease plasma levels of cyclosporine, felodipine, glufosfamide, and imatinib

Pharmacodynamic Drug Interactions
• Concomitant administration with lamotrigine has been associated with an increased risk of adverse effects (nausea, somnolence, dizziness, and headache)
• Concomitant administration with lithium has been associated with enhanced neurotoxicity
• Concomitant administration with amisulpride has been associated with a neuroleptic malignant syndrome
• Concomitant administration with diuretics such as furosemide or hydrochlorothiazide may increase the risk of hyponatremia

Hormonal Contraception
• Oxcarbazepine enhances the metabolism of oral contraceptives and decreases plasma levels of hormonal contraceptives, potentially reducing effectiveness and leading to breakthrough bleeding and contraceptive failure; medium- or high-dose oral contraceptive preparations are indicated in patients taking oxcarbazepine; in addition to recommendations for additional barrier contraceptives and folic acid 1,000 mg daily in all women of childbearing potential

Adverse Effects
How Drug Causes Adverse Effects
• CNS adverse effects may be due to actions at voltage-sensitive sodium channels

Common Adverse Effects
• Somnolence, dizziness, headache
• Depression, apathy, agitation, confusional state
• Diplopia, blurred vision, vertigo
• Nausea, vomiting

ADVERSE EFFECTS

187

- Hyponatremia
- Rash, alopecia, acne
- Fatigue, asthenia

Life-threatening or Dangerous Adverse Effects
- Rare serious rash, including Stevens–Johnson syndrome, toxic epidermal necrolysis (Lyell syndrome), and erythema multiforme; median time of onset is 19 days; these have been shown to be strongly associated with the HLA-B*1502 allele in Southeast Asian populations treated with carbamazepine, and possibly also with oxcarbazepine
- Skin rash rate is 5% with oxcarbazepine, which is lower than the approximate 10–15% rash rate with carbamazepine; however, there is substantial cross-reactivity, as approximately 25–33% of patients who experience skin rash with carbamazepine will also develop rash with oxcarbazepine, whereas up to 71.4% of those who develop rash with oxcarbazepine will also develop rash with carbamazepine
- Hypersensitivity reactions, including multiorgan hypersensitivity reactions, may occur: oxcarbazepine should be withdrawn immediately if these symptoms present
- Hyponatremia (sodium levels <130 mmol/L) is seen in up to 46%, which is generally asymptomatic and thought to be mediated by an oxcarbazepine-induced SIADH mechanism; hyponatremia may be dose-related, and generally occurs within the first weeks after initiation of therapy; risk for hyponatremia is higher in the elderly and in those receiving diuretic co-medications
- Very rare hematologic dyscrasias, including agranulocytosis, aplastic anemia, pancytopenia, and thrombocytopenia
- Rare arrhythmia and atrioventricular block
- Very rare angioedema, including laryngeal edema

Rare and not Life-threatening Adverse Effects
- Hepatitis
- Pancreatitis

Weight Change
- Not common; weight gain reported but not expected

What to do About Adverse Effects
- Discuss common and severe adverse effects with patients or parents before starting medication, including symptoms that should be reported to the physician
- Sedation is dose-related and can subside with time
- Lower the dose
- If hyponatremia is symptomatic, or serum sodium is below 130 mmol/L, consider dose reduction, fluid restriction, or switching to another drug

Dosing and Use

Usual Dosage Range
- Adults: 600–2400 mg/day
- Children:
  - 600–900 mg/day – for body weight of <20 kg
  - 900–1200 mg/day – for body weight of 20–29 kg
  - 900–1500 mg/day – for body weight of 30–39 kg
  - 1500–1800 mg/day – for body weight 40–59 kg

Available Formulations
- Tablets: 150 mg, 300 mg, 600 mg
- Oral suspension: 300 mg/5 mL

How to Dose
- When initiating oxcarbazepine treatment, start with a low dose and titrate slowly so as to minimize adverse effects.
  - *For adults:* start treatment with 300 mg/day in two divided doses; subsequently in 2-day intervals increase in steps of 150 mg daily; maintenance dose generally up to 2400 mg/day given in two equally divided doses
  - *Children 2–16 years old:* start treatment with 10 mg/kg/day in two divided doses; subsequently increase in steps of 10 mg/kg/day at weekly intervals to a maximum of 30–45 mg/kg/day; maintenance dose generally up to 1800 mg/day (depending on body weight) given in two equally divided doses

Dosing Tips
- Titration of dose should be undertaken based on individual tolerability and response to the drug
- Slow dose titration may delay onset of therapeutic action but enhance tolerability to sedating adverse effects
- Should titrate slowly in the presence of other sedating agents, such as other AEDs to best tolerate additive sedative adverse effects
- Doses of oxcarbazepine need to be approximately one-third higher than those of carbamazepine for similar results
- Suspension formulation, which is useful for patients with difficulties swallowing, can be administered mixed in a glass of water or directly from the oral dosing syringe supplied
- Patients who have exhibited a rash with carbamazepine should be informed of the risk of cross-reactivity with oxcarbazepine use, which occurs in ~25–33%

How to Withdraw Drug
- May need to adjust dosage of concurrent medications as oxcarbazepine is being discontinued, because plasma levels of other drugs may change (see Pharmacokinetic Drug Interactions section)

DOSING AND USE

- Taper: a gradual dose reduction over several weeks should be undertaken
- Rapid discontinuation may induce withdrawal seizures

Overdose
- In overdoses up to 24 g, no serious adverse effects were observed
- The most common adverse effects observed with oxcarbazepine overdose include somnolence, dizziness, nausea, vomiting, hyperkinesia, hyponatremia, ataxia, and nystagmus
- If indicated, the stomach should be emptied by lavage or by induction of emesis
- It is not known whether hemodialysis removes oxcarbazepine and 10-hydroxycarbazepine from blood, so the value of hemodialysis in cases of oxcarbazepine overdose remains unknown

Tests and Therapeutic Drug Monitoring
- Before starting: check serum sodium levels and CBC
- Because severe dermatologic reactions (Stevens–Johnson syndrome) to carbamazepine and oxcarbazepine have been shown to be associated with the HLA-B★1502 allele in Southeast Asian populations, testing for this allele should be considered before starting oxcarbazepine in patients of Southeast Asian descent
- During treatment: recheck sodium level in 1–2 months after initiating therapy (or sooner if symptoms of hyponatremia evolve), and sporadically thereafter (i.e., approximately every 12 months)
- Because oxcarbazepine can alter vitamin D metabolism and affect bone mass, 25-hydroxyvitamin D levels should be monitored in all patients, and vitamin D supplementation should be prescribed as needed; consider also dual-energy X-ray absorptiometry (DEXA) bone scan in patients at risk for osteopenia
- Therapeutic drug monitoring:
  - Optimum seizure control in patients on monotherapy is most likely to occur at plasma 10-hydroxycarbazepine concentrations of 3–35 mg/L (12–137 µmol/L)
  - The conversion factor from mg/L to µmol/L is 3.96 (i.e., 1 mg/L = 3.96 µmol/L)
  - The reference range of 10-hydroxycarbazepine in plasma is considered to be the same for children and adults, although no data are available to support this clinical practice
  - 10-hydroxycarbazepine can be monitored by use of saliva, which is a measure of the free non-protein-bound plasma concentration and is pharmacologically relevant

Other Warnings/Precautions
- Use cautiously in patients who have demonstrated hypersensitivity to carbamazepine
- Because oxcarbazepine has a tricyclic chemical structure, it is not recommended to be taken with MAOIs, including 14 days after

MAOIs are stopped; do not start an MAOI until 2 weeks after discontinuing oxcarbazepine
- May exacerbate narrow angle-closure glaucoma
- In patients with pre-existing renal conditions associated with low sodium, or in patients treated with sodium-lowering medications (e.g., diuretics, desmopressin, non-steroidal anti-inflammatory drugs (e.g., indometacin)), sodium levels should be measured before initiating treatment with oxcarbazepine; thereafter, sodium levels should be measured after ~1–2 months, and thereafter approximately annually or according to clinical need
- Usually hyponatremia (sodium levels <130 mmol/L) is asymptomatic and dose adjustment is not necessary; clinically significant hyponatremia is seen in 2–3% and generally occurs within 3 months of treatment initiation, and can be reversed by restricting fluid intake and reduction in oxcarbazepine dose
- Patients with cardiac insufficiency and heart failure should be weighed regularly as an index of fluid retention; if worsening of the cardiac condition or fluid retention is observed, water restriction is indicated
- Rarely oxcarbazepine may lead to impairment of cardiac conductance and patients with pre-existing conduction disturbances (e.g., atrioventricular block, arrhythmia) should be followed carefully
- Some patients may experience dizziness and somnolence, and thus caution needs to be exercised if patient intends to drive or use machinery

Do not Use
- If patient has a proven allergy to oxcarbazepine or to any of the excipients
- Because oxcarbazepine has a tricyclic chemical structure, it is not recommended to be taken with MAOIs
- If patient has hypersensitivity to other carboxamide derivatives (e.g., carbamazepine and eslicarbazepine acetate)

Special Populations
Renal Impairment
- Oxcarbazepine is renally excreted, so the dose needs to be adjusted according to CrCl as follows:
  - CrCl of <30 mL/min – starting dose: 300 mg/day taken twice a day; increase dose, in at least weekly intervals, to achieve desired clinical response

Hepatic Impairment
- Oxcarbazepine is extensively metabolized in the liver to 10-hydroxycarbazepine which is in turn substantially metabolized; consequently lower doses may be required in patients with hepatic impairment

Children
- Children have an increased metabolic capacity and consequently higher mg/kg doses are usually required to achieve the equivalent therapeutic plasma levels seen in adults
- Pharmacokinetic interactions in children are usually of a greater magnitude than that seen in adults

Elderly
- Elderly patients are generally more susceptible to adverse effects and therefore may not tolerate higher doses
- Because of an age-related reduction in renal function, lower oxcarbazepine target doses are appropriate and should be based on CrCl values
- Because oxcarbazepine is associated with dizziness and somnolence, the elderly may be at increased risk of falls
- Elderly have an increased risk of developing hyponatremia with oxcarbazepine use
- Elderly patients are often prescribed concurrent drug therapies for comorbidities and therefore may be at greater risk for pharmacokinetic and pharmacodynamic interactions; the risk of pharmacokinetic interactions with oxcarbazepine is moderate

Pregnancy
- Specialist advice should be given to women who are of childbearing potential; they should be informed about the teratogenicity of all AEDs and the importance of avoiding an unplanned pregnancy; the AED treatment regimen should be reviewed when a woman is planning to become pregnant
- Rapid discontinuation of AEDs should be avoided, as this may lead to breakthrough seizures which could have serious consequences for the woman and the unborn child
- Oxcarbazepine was previously classified by the US FDA as risk category C (some animal studies show adverse effects, no controlled studies in humans); the current FDA Pregnancy and Lactation Rule has eliminated pregnancy risk category labels
- Oxcarbazepine is structurally similar to carbamazepine, which has been shown to be teratogenic in humans
- Use in women of childbearing potential requires weighing potential benefits to the mother against the risks to the fetus
- Use with other AEDs in combination may cause a higher prevalence of teratogenic effects than oxcarbazepine monotherapy
- Taper drug if discontinuing
- Seizures, even mild seizures, may cause harm to the embryo/fetus
- During pregnancy, oxcarbazepine pharmacokinetics change significantly so that 10-hydroxycarbazepine concentrations decrease by 30–38% due to increased clearance consequent to enhanced glucuronidation; an increase in oxcarbazepine dose is usually required, and regular monitoring of 10-hydroxycarbazepine levels is indicated

to ensure stability through pregnancy, monitoring at least once per trimester; in the postpartum state, as glucuronidation returns to normal, oxcarbazepine dose reduction is usually also necessary to avoid toxicity

Breast Feeding
- Breast milk: 10-hydroxycarbazepine: 50–80% of maternal plasma levels
- Breastfed infants: 10-hydroxycarbazepine plasma levels are 7–12% of maternal plasma levels
- If drug is continued while breast feeding, the infant should be monitored for possible adverse effects
- If adverse effects are observed, recommend bottle feeding

The Overall Place of Oxcarbazepine in the Treatment of Epilepsy

Oxcarbazepine is similar to carbamazepine in its antiepileptic efficacy and is an effective drug of first choice both as monotherapy and as adjunctive therapy for all types of partial (focal) seizures with or without secondary generalization. It may be particularly useful in patients who responded to carbamazepine, but were unable to tolerate full dosage titration with that drug.

Primary Seizure Types
- Partial (focal) seizures with or without secondary generalization

Secondary Seizure Types
- None

Potential Advantages
- Oxcarbazepine is better tolerated than carbamazepine, probably because it is not metabolized to the pharmacologically active metabolite carbamazepine-epoxide
- Oxcarbazepine has much less prominent actions on CYP enzyme systems than carbamazepine, and thus fewer pharmacokinetic interactions

Potential Disadvantages
- Patients are at greater risk of hyponatremia than with carbamazepine
- May need to restrict fluid and/or monitor sodium because of risk of hyponatremia
- Potential teratogen
- There is cross-reactivity for rash between carbamazepine and oxcarbazepine; approximately 25–33% of patients who develop rash with carbamazepine also develop rash with oxcarbazepine

Suggested Reading

Bang LM, Goa KL. Spotlight on oxcarbazepine in epilepsy. *CNS Drugs* 2004; **18**: 57–61.

Beniczky SA, Viken J, Jensen LT, Andersen NB. Bone mineral density in adult patients treated with various antiepileptic drugs. *Seizure* 2012; **21**: 471–472.

Berghuis B, van der Palen J, de Haan GJ, Lindhout D, Koeleman BPC, Sander JW; EpiPGX Consortium. Carbamazepine- and oxcarbazepine-induced hyponatremia in people with epilepsy. *Epilepsia* 2017; **58**: 1227–1233.

Borusiak P, Langer T, Heruth M, Karenfort M, Bettendorf U, Jenke AC. Antiepileptic drugs and bone metabolism in children: data from 128 patients. *Journal of Child Neurology* 2013; **28**: 176–183.

Chen YC, Chu CY, Hsiao CH. Oxcarbazepine-induced Stevens–Johnson syndrome in a patient with HLA-B★1502 genotype. *Journal of the European Academy of Dermatology and Venereology* 2009; **23**: 702–703.

Christensen J, Sabers A, Sidenius P. Oxcarbazepine concentrations during pregnancy: a retrospective study in patients with epilepsy. *Neurology* 2006; **67**: 1497–1499.

French JA, Kanner AM, Bautista J, et al. Therapeutics and Technology Assessment Subcommittee of the American Academy of Neurology; Quality Standards Subcommittee of the American Academy of Neurology; American Epilepsy Society. Efficacy and tolerability of the new antiepileptic drugs I: treatment of new onset epilepsy: report of the Therapeutics and Technology Assessment Subcommittee and Quality Standards Subcommittee of the American Academy of Neurology and the American Epilepsy Society. *Neurology* 2004; **62**: 1252–1260.

French JA, Kanner AM, Bautista J, et al. Therapeutics and Technology Assessment Subcommittee of the American Academy of Neurology; Quality Standards Subcommittee of the American Academy of Neurology; American Epilepsy Society. Efficacy and tolerability of the new antiepileptic drugs II: treatment of refractory epilepsy: Efficacy and tolerability of the new antiepileptic drugs II: treatment of refractory epilepsy: report of the Therapeutics and Technology Assessment Subcommittee and Quality Standards Subcommittee of the American Academy of Neurology and the American Epilepsy Society. *Neurology* 2004; **62**: 1261–1273.

Gelisse P, Genton P, Kuate D, Pesenti A, Baldy-Moulinier M, Crespel A. Worsening of seizures by oxcarbazepine in juvenile idiopathic generalized epilepsies. *Epilepsia* 2004; **45**: 1282–1288.

Harden CL, Pennell PB, Koppel BS, et al. American Academy of Neurology; American Epilepsy Society. Practice parameter update: management issues for women with epilepsy-focus on pregnancy (an evidence-based review): vitamin K, folic acid, blood levels, and breastfeeding: report of the Quality Standards Subcommittee and Therapeutics and Technology Assessment Subcommittee of the

OXCARBAZEPINE

American Academy of Neurology and American Epilepsy Society. *Neurology* 2009; **73**:142–149.

Hirsch LJ, Arif H, Nahm EA, Buchsbaum R, Resor SR Jr, Bazil CW. Cross-sensitivity of skin rashes with antiepileptic drug use. *Neurology* 2008; **71**: 1527–1534.

Hu FY, Wu XT, An DM, Yan B, Stefan H, Zhou D. Pilot association study of oxcarbazepine-induced mild cutaneous adverse reactions with HLA-B*1502 allele in Chinese Han population. *Seizure* 2011; **20**: 160–162.

Johannessen Landmark C, Patsalos PN. Drug interactions involving the new second- and third-generation antiepileptic drugs. *Expert Reviews in Neurotherapeutics* 2010; **10**: 119–140.

Marson AG, Al-Kharusi AM, Alwaidh M, et al. SANAD Study group. The SANAD study of effectiveness of carbamazepine, gabapentin, lamotrigine, oxcarbazepine, or topiramate for treatment of partial epilepsy: an unblinded randomised controlled trial. *Lancet* 2007; **369**: 1000–1015.

Patsalos PN. *Antiepileptic drug interactions: a clinical guide*, 3rd edition. Springer, London, UK; 2016.

Patsalos PN, Berry DJ. Therapeutic drug monitoring of antiepileptic drugs by use of saliva. *Therapeutic Drug Monitoring* 2013; **35**: 4–29.

Reisinger TL, Newman M, Loring DW, Pennell PB, Meador MD. Antiepileptic drug clearance and seizure frequency during pregnancy in women with epilepsy. *Epilepsy and Behavior* 2013; **29**: 13–18.

Rouan MC, Lecaillon JB, Godbillon J, Menard F, Darragon T, Meyer P, Kourilsky O, Hillion D, Aldigier JC, Jungers P. The effect of renal impairment on the pharmacokinetics ofoxcarbazepine and its metabolites. *European Journal of Clinical Pharmacology* 1994; **47**: 161–167.

Schmidt D, Elger CE. What is the evidence that oxcarbazepine and carbamazepine are distinctly different antiepileptic drugs? *Epilepsy and Behavior* 2004; **5**: 627–635.

Shellhaas RA, Barks AK, Joshi SM. Prevalence and risk factors for vitamin D insufficiency among children with epilepsy. *Pediatric Neurology* 2010; **42**: 422–426.

St. Louis EK. The art of managing conversions between antiepileptic drugs; maximizing patient tolerability and quality of life. *Pharmaceuticals* 2010; **3**: 2956–2969.

St. Louis EK, Gidal BE, Henry TR, Kaydanova Y, Krumholz A, McCabe PH, Montouris GD, Rosenfeld WE, Smith BJ, Stern JM, Waterhouse EJ, Schulz RM, Garnett WR, Bramley T. Conversions between monotherapies in epilepsy: expert consensus. *Epilepsy and Behavior* 2007; **11**: 222–234.

Vestergaard P, Rejnmark L, Mosekilde L. Fracture risk associated with use of antiepileptic drugs. *Epilepsia* 2004; **45**: 1330–1337.

Zheng T, Clarke AL, Morris MJ, Reid CA, Petrou S, O'Brien TJ. Oxcarbazepine, not its active metabolite, potentiates GABA A activation and aggravates absence seizures. *Epilepsia* 2009; **50**: 83–87.

SUGGESTED READING

P PARALDEHYDE

Therapeutics

Chemical Name and Structure
Paraldehyde, a cyclic polymer of acetaldehyde (2,4,6-trimethyl-1,3,5-trioxane), is a colorless liquid, with a molecular weight of 132.2 and an empirical formula of $C_6H_{12}O_3$. It crystallizes at and below 12°C.

Brand Names
• There are none

Generics Available
• Yes

Licensed Indications for Epilepsy
• There are none

Licensed Indications for Non-epilepsy Conditions
• There are none

Non-licensed Use for Epilepsy
• Acute repetitive convulsive seizures refractory to traditional AED therapy

Non-licensed Use for Non-epilepsy Conditions
• There are none

Ineffective (Contraindicated)
• Paraldehyde should not be used chronically in the treatment of epileptic seizures

Mechanism of Action
• The mechanism by which paraldehyde exerts its anticonvulsant activity has not been established

Efficacy Profile
• It is for the treatment of status epilepticus, particularly when other drugs are inappropriate or ineffective
• The onset of action is very rapid, particularly after iv administration

Pharmacokinetics
Absorption and Distribution
- Oral bioavailability: 90–100%
- Rectal bioavailability: 75–90%
- Food co-ingestion: it is not known whether the rate of absorption or the extent of absorption is affected by food co-ingestion
- Tmax: ~0.5 hours (oral ingestion); ~1.5–2 hours (rectal administration); ~20–60 minutes (im administration)
- Time to steady state: not applicable (paraldehyde is practically never used chronically in the treatment of epileptic seizures)
- Pharmacokinetics: linear
- Protein binding: not known
- Volume of distribution: 0.89 L/kg (adults); 3.18 L/kg (infants)
- Salivary concentrations: it is not known whether paraldehyde is secreted into saliva and whether such concentrations are similar to the unbound levels seen in plasma

Metabolism
- 70–90% of the dose is metabolized in the liver to acetaldehyde, which is then oxidized to acetic acid by the enzyme aldehyde dehydrogenase
- Acetic acid is then metabolized further into CO_2 and water
- Some of the drug (11–28%) is excreted unchanged through the lungs, which gives a characteristic unpleasant odor to the breath

Elimination
- The elimination half-life of paraldehyde in neonates is 10.2–23.6 hours
- The elimination half-life of paraldehyde in children and adults is 3.5–9.5 hours
- Renal excretion: <1% of an administered dose is excreted unchanged as paraldehyde in urine

Drug Interaction Profile
Pharmacokinetic Drug Interactions
- Interactions between AEDs: effects on paraldehyde:
  - To date, there have been no reports of AEDs affecting the clearance of paraldehyde and affecting plasma levels
- Interactions between AEDs: effects by paraldehyde:
  - To date, there have been no reports of paraldehyde affecting the clearance of other AEDs and affecting their plasma levels
- Interactions between AEDs and non-AED drugs: effects on paraldehyde:
  - Disulfiram, which inhibits acetaldehyde dehydrogenase, can *decrease* the clearance of paraldehyde and *increase* paraldehyde (and acetaldehyde) plasma levels

P

PARALDEHYDE

- Interactions between AEDs and non–AED drugs: effects by paraldehyde:
  - To date, there have been no reports of paraldehyde affecting the clearance of other non-AED drugs and affecting their plasma levels

Pharmacodynamic Drug Interactions
- Paraldehyde may potentiate the effect of other CNS depressants such as barbiturates and alcohol
- Disulfiram may enhance the toxicity of paraldehyde

Hormonal Contraception
- Because paraldehyde is only used for the acute treatment of seizures, its potential effect on hormonal contraception is of limited relevance

Adverse Effects
How Drug Causes Adverse Effects
- Mechanism by which paraldehyde causes adverse effects has not been established

Common Adverse Effects
- Drowsiness, lethargy
- Nausea, vomiting, or abdominal pain, when administered orally
- Muscle cramps
- Unusual sweating
- Unpleasant odor of breath
- Allergic skin rash
- Paraldehyde can be irritating to the eyes and to the skin
- Yellow discoloration of the skin and eyes with long-term use

Life-threatening or Dangerous Adverse Effects
- Metabolic acidosis, especially after administration of partly decomposed paraldehyde
- iv administration may cause pulmonary edema and hemorrhage, cardiac dilatation, and cardiovascular shock, and this route of administration should be discouraged
- Hepatitis and nephrosis have been observed after prolonged use of paraldehyde
- Deaths have been reported due to corrosive poisoning by decomposed paraldehyde
- When a higher than 5% concentration is used for iv infusion, droplets of pure paraldehyde may form and act as emboli

Rare and not Life-threatening Adverse Effects
- Impaired coordination and ataxia
- May aggravate colitis when given rectally
- May aggravate gastric ulcer when given orally

P

- May cause severe pain, redness, swelling, or sterile abscess at im injection site, as well as thrombophlebitis when administered iv
- im injection close to nerve trunks may cause severe and permanent nerve damage
- im injection may cause severe causalgia if the injection is too close to the sciatic nerve

Weight Change
- Not common; paraldehyde is practically never used chronically in the treatment of epileptic seizures

What to do About Adverse Effects
- Heart rate, respiration, and blood pressure must be monitored closely during paraldehyde administration

Dosing and Use
Usual Dosage Range
- Rectal: 1:1 paraldehyde: vegetable oil solution, 0.3 mL/kg per dose (300 mg/kg of paraldehyde); may repeat every 2–4 hours
- im: adults 5–10 mL/dose, children 0.1–0.15 mL/kg/dose, every 4–8 hours
- iv: 100–150 mg/kg (0.1–0.15 mL/kg) over 10–15 minutes, followed by a drip of 20 mg/kg/hour (0.4 mL/kg/hour of a 5% solution)
- Maintenance: paraldehyde is virtually never administered chronically for the treatment of epileptic seizures

Available Formulations
- Ampoules (darkened glass): 5 mL/ampoule for im, rectal, or iv administration (contains hydroquinone 100 µg/mL as an antioxidant)

How to Dose
- For iv administration, paraldehyde should be diluted into a 5% solution by adding normal saline (20 mL of normal saline for each 1 mL of paraldehyde)
- Dosages are commonly cited in volume units (e.g., mL) as well as mass units (e.g., g) which for practical purposes can be considered equivalent (strictly speaking, 1 mL weighs 1.006 g); 1 mL of paraldehyde is 1 g or 1000 mg of paraldehyde

Dosing Tips
- Never use any plastic containers, spoons, or syringes to administer paraldehyde, because of its solvent effect on plastic; use only glass or metal, unless the 5% solution is used
- Paraldehyde should be diluted with normal saline before iv administration

DOSING AND USE

- Before rectal administration, the paraldehyde solution should be mixed 1:1 with an equal volume of olive oil, peanut oil, or other vegetable oil to reduce mucosal irritation
- When taken orally, paraldehyde can be mixed with milk or fruit juice to reduce the unpleasant taste
- Breakdown of paraldehyde, consequent to exposure to light, leads to a brownish discoloration and an acetic acid odor of the solution, indicating that it should no longer be used
- Paraldehyde has a short shelf-life and decomposes after the container has been opened
- Administration of partly decomposed paraldehyde is highly toxic and may cause: metabolic acidosis or death if administered by injection; severe proctitis and excoriating anal rash or even large-bowel perforation if administered by means of the rectal route

How to Withdraw Drug
- Because paraldehyde is used only for the acute treatment of seizures, gradual withdrawal is not necessary

Overdose
- Can be fatal: symptoms include confusion, nausea, vomiting, severe abdominal pain, weakness, oliguria, cloudy urine, metabolic acidosis, hyperventilation, respiratory depression, pulmonary edema, bradycardia, hypotension, cardiac failure, renal failure, toxic hepatitis, coma
- Fatalities are uncommon and usually secondary to respiratory failure, heart failure, or metabolic acidosis
- The main aspect of treatment is respiratory support
- Bicarbonate for metabolic acidosis and vasopressors for hypotension may be considered
- The stomach should be emptied immediately by lavage or by induction of emesis
- It is not known whether hemodialysis removes paraldehyde from blood and, therefore, could serve as a useful procedure in cases of overdose

Tests and Therapeutic Drug Monitoring
- Electrolytes and blood gases may be obtained when metabolic acidosis is suspected
- Therapeutic drug monitoring: because paraldehyde is not administered chronically, plasma level monitoring is not necessary or helpful
- The minimum therapeutic plasma concentration for the control of status epilepticus is considered to be ~300 ng/mL

Other Warnings/Precautions
- Patients should be monitored carefully for signs of unusual bleeding or bruising
- Heart rate, respiration, and blood pressure must be monitored closely during administration

P

Do not Use
- Rectally in patients with colitis
- Orally in patients with gastric ulcer
- In patients with chronic lung disease, such as emphysema, asthma, or bronchitis
- In patients with severe hepatic failure
- In patients with a history of hypersensitivity to paraldehyde

Special Populations
Renal Impairment
- Renal impairment has little or no impact on paraldehyde pharmacokinetics and elimination

Hepatic Impairment
- Hepatic impairment may lead to decreased clearance of paraldehyde
- Paraldehyde is contraindicated in patients with severe hepatic failure

Children
- No specific or different information is available on children

Elderly
- No information is available

Pregnancy
- Paraldehyde should not be administered chronically for the treatment of epileptic seizures, nor should it be given acutely to pregnant women
- Paraldehyde was previously classified by the US FDA as risk category D (positive evidence of risk to human fetus; potential benefits may still justify its use during pregnancy); the current FDA Pregnancy and Lactation Rule has eliminated pregnancy risk category labels
- Paraldehyde should not be used during labor, because it diffuses across the placenta and has been shown to cause respiratory depression in newborns

Breast Feeding
- Breast milk: paraldehyde is secreted into breast milk
- Breastfed infants: it is not known what plasma paraldehyde concentrations are achieved in breastfed infants compared with the levels of their mothers

The Overall Place of Paraldehyde in the Treatment of Epilepsy
Although paraldehyde is an old-fashioned medication (first introduced into clinical practice in 1882), it may have a place in the treatment of super refractory status epilepticus. In current practice, given the wide availability of several other better-established parenteral therapies, it

P

should be reserved for cases of refractory established status epilepticus that have failed most other agents. Paraldehyde may be particularly useful where iv administration is difficult, or where conventional AEDs have proved ineffective and all other good options have been exhausted. The drug is usually given rectally or intramuscularly and absorption is fast and complete.

Primary Seizure Types
• The use of paraldehyde in the treatment of epilepsy is limited solely to the treatment of super refractory convulsive status epilepticus

Secondary Seizure Types
• None

Potential Advantages
• Paraldehyde can be administered rectally or intramuscularly when no venous access is available
• Seizures do not often recur after seizure control has been established
• Longer duration of action compared with other benzodiazepines

Potential Disadvantages
• Paraldehyde has a slower onset of action and less efficacy compared with the current traditional therapies of status epilepticus
• Decomposed or inadequately diluted solutions are highly toxic
• iv administration carries the risk of potentially serious toxic effects and careful monitoring is essential

Suggested Reading

Ahmad S, Ellis JC, Amend H, Molyneux E. Efficacy and safety of intranasal lorazepam versus intramuscular paraldehyde for protracted convulsions in children: an open randomized trial. *Lancet* 2006; **367**: 1555–1556.

Appleton R, Macleod S, Maryland T. Drug management for acute tonic-clonic convulsions including convulsive status epilepticus in children. *Cochrane Database of Systematic Reviews* 2008; **3**: CD001905.

Armstrong DL, Battin MR. Pervasive seizures caused by hypoxic-ischemic encephalopathy: treatment with intravenous paraldehyde. *Journal of Child Neurology* 2001; **16**: 915–917.

Bostrom B. Paraldehyde toxicity during treatment of status epilepticus. *American Journal of Diseases in Children* 1982; **136**: 414–415.

Chin RF, Neville BG, Packham C, Wade A, Bedford H, Scott RC. Treatment of community-onset, childhood convulsive status epilepticus: a prospective, population-based study. *Lancet Neurology* 2008; **7**: 696–703.

Curless RG, Holzman BH, Ramsay RE. Paraldehyde therapy in childhood status epilepticus. *Archives of Neurology* 1983; **40**: 477–480.

Jain P, Sharma S, Dua T, Barbui S, Das RR, Aneja S. Efficacy and safety of anti-epileptic drugs in patients with active convulsive seizures when no IV access is available: systematic review. *Epilepsy Research* 2016; **122**: 47–55.

Johnson CE, Vigoreaux JA. Compatibility of paraldehyde with plastic syringes and needle hubs. *American Journal of Hospital Pharmacy* 1984; **41**: 306–308.

Ramsay RE. Pharmacokinetics and parenteral use of phenytoin, phenobarbital, and paraldehyde. *Epilepsia* 1989; **30** (Suppl 2): S1–S3.

Welty TE, Cloyd JC, Abdel-Monem MM. Delivery of paraldehyde in 5% dextrose and 0.9% sodium chloride injections through polyvinyl chloride IV sets and burettes. *American Journal of Hospital Pharmacy* 1988; **45**: 131–135.

P

SUGGESTED READING

PERAMPANEL

Therapeutics

Chemical Name and Structure

Perampanel, 2-(2-oxo-1-phenyl-5-pyridin-2-yl-1,2-dihydropyridin-3-yl)-benzonitrile, is a white to yellowish-white powder, with a molecular weight of 349.4 and an empirical formula of $C_{23}H_{15}N_3O$.

Brand Names
• Fycompa

Generics Available
• No

Licensed Indications for Epilepsy
• Adjunctive treatment of partial-onset seizures with or without secondary generalization in patients aged 12 years and older (UK SPC; FDA PI)
• Adjunctive treatment of primary generalized tonic–clonic seizures in adults and adolescents from 12 years of age with idiopathic generalized epilepsy (UK SPC; FDA PI)

Licensed Indications for Non-epilepsy Conditions
• There are none

Non-licensed Use for Epilepsy
• Lafora disease
• Lance–Adams syndrome (posthypoxic non-epileptic myoclonus)
• Lennox–Gastaut syndrome
• Posthypoxic myoclonus
• Status epilepticus
• Unverricht–Lundborg disease

Non-licensed Use for Non-epilepsy Conditions
- There are none

Ineffective (Contraindicated)
- There is no contraindication for perampanel
- There is no published experience in neonatal seizures
- There is no information regarding its effectiveness for prophylaxis of febrile seizures

Mechanism of Action
- Perampanel is a non-competitive antagonist of the AMPA-type glutamate receptor, thereby inhibiting AMPA-induced increases in intracellular calcium and reducing neuronal excitability. Because the AMPA receptor is involved in the generation and propagation of seizures, perampanel may prove to have antiepileptogenic properties.

Efficacy Profile
- The goals of treatment are to achieve complete seizure remission when possible, or at least improved frequency and severity of seizures, while also minimizing adverse effects and improving patient quality of life
- Once chronic therapy is initiated, it is usually continued for at least 2 years following the last seizure
- If perampanel is ineffective or only partially effective, it can be replaced by or combined with another AED that is appropriate for the patient's seizure type or epilepsy syndrome

Pharmacokinetics
Absorption and Distribution
- Oral bioavailability: 100%
- Food co-ingestion: decreases the rate by 2 hours but not the extent of absorption
- Tmax: 0.25–2.0 hours
- Time to steady state: 14 days
- Pharmacokinetics: linear
- Protein binding: 95%
- Volume of distribution: 1.1 L/kg
- Saliva concentrations: it is not known whether perampanel is secreted into saliva and whether such concentrations are similar to the unbound levels seen in plasma

Metabolism
- Perampanel undergoes substantial metabolism (98%) in the liver primarily by oxidation followed by glucuronidation; the major metabolites are hydroxylated perampanel and various glucuronide conjugates

P

PHARMACOKINETICS

P

- The isoenzyme CYP3A4 is considered to be principally responsible for the hydroxylation of perampanel, although CYP3A5 may also be involved
- The metabolites of perampanel are not pharmacologically active
- Autoinduction is not a feature of perampanel metabolism

Elimination
- The plasma half-life of perampanel in adult healthy volunteers is 51–129 hours (mean, 105 hours) after single-dose and 66–90 hours after multiple-dose administration
- In the presence of enzyme-inducing co-medication, half-life values for perampanel are 25 hours
- Renal excretion: approximately 2% of an administered dose is excreted as unchanged perampanel in urine

Drug Interaction Profile
Pharmacokinetic Drug Interactions
- Interactions between AEDs: effects on perampanel:
  – Carbamazepine, oxcarbazepine, phenytoin, and topiramate can *increase* the clearance of perampanel and *decrease* perampanel plasma levels
- Interactions between AEDs: effects by perampanel:
  – Perampanel can *decrease* plasma levels of carbamazepine, clobazam, lamotrigine, midazolam, and valproic acid
  – Perampanel can *increase* plasma levels of oxcarbazepine
- Interactions between AEDs and non-AED drugs: effects on perampanel:
  – Ketoconazole can *increase* perampanel plasma levels
- Interactions between AEDs and non-AED drugs: effects by perampanel:
  – To date, there have been no reports of perampanel affecting the clearance of other non-AED drugs and affecting their plasma levels

Pharmacodynamic Drug Interactions
- Perampanel has an additive or superadditive effect on the effects of alcohol with increased levels of anger, confusion, and depression consequent to a pharmacodynamic interaction
- Carbamazepine in combination with perampanel is associated with increased sedation. This effect may be the consequence of a pharmacodynamic interaction
- Levetiracetam in combination with perampanel is associated with increased likelihood of developing fatigue. This effect may be the consequence of a pharmacodynamic interaction
- Oxcarbazepine in combination with perampanel is associated with increased risk of decreased appetite. This effect may be the consequence of a pharmacodynamic interaction

P

ADVERSE EFFECTS

- Phenobarbital in combination with perampanel is associated with increased irritability. This effect may be the consequence of a pharmacodynamic interaction
- Primidone in combination with perampanel is associated with increased risk of decreased appetite. This effect may be the consequence of a pharmacodynamic interaction

Hormonal Contraception
- Perampanel does not enhance the metabolism of the estrogen (ethinylestrodiol) component of hormonal contraceptives, and, therefore, does not compromise contraception control
- Perampanel can, however, enhance the metabolism of the progesterone (levonogestrel) component of hormonal contraceptives and potentially lead to contraceptive failure when progesterone-only contraceptive formulations are used: medium- or high-dose progesterone preparations are advisable in patients taking perampanel, with additional recommendations for use of barrier methods and supplemental folic acid 1000 mg in all women of childbearing potential

Adverse Effects
How Drug Causes Adverse Effects
- The mechanism by which perampanel causes adverse effects has not been established

Common Adverse Effects
- Somnolence, dizziness
- Ataxia, dysarthria, balance disorder, irritability
- Aggression, anger, anxiety, confusional state
- Diplopia, blurred vision
- Vertigo, nausea, gait disturbance, fatigue

Life-threatening or Dangerous Adverse Effects
- As with other AEDs, there can be depression and activation of suicidal ideation and acts

Rare and not Life-threatening Adverse Effects
- To date, none have been reported

Weight Change
- Weight gain is common

What to do About Adverse Effects
- Discuss common adverse effects with patients or parents before starting medication, including symptoms that should be reported to the physician
- Risk of adverse effects is greatest in the first few months of treatment

- Slower titration may decrease incidence or severity of some adverse effects
- Patients treated with any AED should be monitored for depression, worsening of depression, suicidal thoughts or behaviors, as well as changes in mood that are not usual for the patient
- When treating patients with psychiatric comorbidities, caution should be exercised and they should be monitored carefully for neuropsychiatric adverse effects

Dosing and Use
Usual Dosage Range
- Partial-onset seizures: 4–12 mg/day
- Primary generalized tonic–clonic seizures: up to 8 mg/day

Available Formulations
- Tablets: 2 mg, 4 mg, 6 mg, 8 mg, 10 mg, 12 mg

How to Dose
- *For adults and children over 12 years of age:* start treatment with 2 mg once a day; at intervals of 2 weeks, increase by 2 mg daily; maintenance dose generally 4–8 mg daily, as needed and as tolerated; for patients co-prescribed AEDs that enhance the clearance of perampanel, dose increments can be undertaken at intervals of 1 week; in the clinical trials of perampanel, patients treated with 10–12 mg/day experienced limited improvement in seizure control but more adverse events
- *Children under 12 years of age:* the safety, effectiveness, and dosage requirements of perampanel in patients younger than 12 years have not been established
- *For patients over 65 years of age:* start treatment with 2 mg once a day; at intervals of 2 weeks, increase by 2 mg daily; maintenance dose generally 4–8 mg daily, as needed and as tolerated

Dosing Tips
- Tablets should be swallowed whole, with water and without food
- Take once daily before bedtime so as to mitigate somnolence and dizziness

How to Withdraw Drug
- May need to adjust dosage of concurrent medications as perampanel is discontinued, because plasma levels of other drugs may change (see Pharmacokinetic Drug Interactions section)
- No data are available on potential for withdrawal seizures or symptoms upon rapid discontinuation
- Rapid discontinuation may increase the risk of seizures; however, because of its long half-life and subsequent slow decline in plasma

P

concentrations, perampanel can be abruptly discontinued if absolutely necessary

Overdose
- No fatalities have been reported
- Symptoms in a patient who may have ingested up to 264 mg of perampanel included altered mental status, agitation, and aggressive behavior and irritability; the patient fully recovered without any sequelae
- If indicated, the stomach should be emptied by lavage or by induction of emesis
- Standard medical practice for the management of any overdose should be applied
- It is not known whether hemodialysis removes perampanel from blood and, therefore, serves as a useful procedure in cases of overdose

Tests and Therapeutic Drug Monitoring
- There is no need to monitor any laboratory parameter during treatment with perampanel
- Therapeutic drug monitoring:
  - Optimum seizure control in patients on monotherapy is most likely to occur at perampanel plasma concentrations of 200–1000 μg/L (572–2860 nmol/L)
  - The conversion factor from μg/L to nmol/L is 2.86 (i.e., 1 μg/L = 2.86 nmol/L)
  - There are no data indicating the usefulness of monitoring perampanel in saliva

Other Warnings / Precautions
- There appears to be an increased risk of falls, particularly in the elderly; the underlying reason is unknown

Do not Use
- If patient is hypersensitive to perampanel or its excipients, which include lactose
- Because formulations contains lactose, patients with rare hereditary problems of galactose intolerance, Lapp lactose deficiency, or glucose-galactose malabsorption should not take this medicine

Special Populations
Renal Impairment
- Perampanel is renally secreted, thus, the dose may need to be lowered in renally impaired patients
- Perampanel clearance is not influenced by CrCl

SPECIAL POPULATIONS

- Dose adjustment is not necessary in patients with mild renal impairment
- Use in patients with moderate or severe renal impairment or patients undergoing hemodialysis is not recommended

Hepatic Impairment
- Perampanel is extensively metabolized in the liver and consequently lower doses are required
  - With mild hepatic impairment (Child–Pugh A score 5–6), perampanel plasma clearance was decreased by 44%, whereas for moderate hepatic impairment (Child–Pugh B score 7–9), clearance was decreased by 69%
  - Perampanel half-life values are prolonged in subjects with mild hepatic impairment (306 vs. 125 hours) and in subjects with moderate impairment (295 vs. 139 hours)
  - Perampanel free (non-protein-bound) AUC values are 1.8-fold and 3.3-fold greater in mild and moderate hepatic impairment respectively compared to matched healthy individuals

Children
- Based on limited data of perampanel in patients under 12 years it appears that efficacy and tolerability are similar to that seen in adolescents, adults, and the elderly
- The pharmacokinetics of perampanel in children have yet to be reported

Elderly
- The efficacy and safety of perampanel in this population appear to be similar to that observed in adults and adolescents
- Elderly patients are more susceptible to adverse effects (especially somnolence, dizziness, and falls) and, therefore, often do better at lower doses
- Because of an age-related reduction in hepatic and renal function, lower perampanel doses are appropriate (see How to Dose section)
- Elderly patients are often prescribed concurrent drug therapies for comorbidities and therefore may be at greater risk for pharmacokinetic and pharmacodynamic interactions; the risk of pharmacokinetic interactions with perampanel is substantial

Pregnancy
- Specialist advice should be given to women who are of childbearing potential; they should be informed about the teratogenicity of all AEDs and the importance of avoiding an unplanned pregnancy; the AED treatment regimen should be reviewed when a woman is planning to become pregnant
- Rapid discontinuation of AEDs should be avoided as this may lead to breakthrough seizures, which could have serious consequences for the woman and the unborn child

P

- Perampanel was previously classified by the US FDA as risk category C (some animal studies show adverse effects, no controlled studies in humans); the current FDA Pregnancy and Lactation Rule has eliminated pregnancy risk category labels
- Use in women of childbearing potential requires weighing potential benefits to the mother against the risks to the fetus
- Use with other AEDs in combination may cause a higher prevalence of teratogenic effects than perampanel monotherapy
- Taper drug if discontinuing
- Seizures, even mild seizures, may cause harm to the embryo/fetus
- There are no available data on whether the pharmacokinetics of perampanel change during pregnancy

Breast Feeding
- Breast milk: it is not known whether perampanel is excreted in breast milk
- Breastfed infants: it is not known what plasma perampanel concentrations are achieved in breastfed infants compared with the levels of their mothers
- If drug is continued while breast feeding, infant should be monitored for possible adverse effects (irritability or sedation)
- If adverse effects are observed, recommend bottle feeding

The Overall Place of Perampanel in the Treatment of Epilepsy
Perampanel is a first-in-class selective non-competitive antagonist of the postsynaptic AMPA glutamate receptor. It was initially licensed as add-on therapy for partial/focal-onset seizures, but has recently been licensed for the management of primary generalized tonic–clonic seizures in drug-resistant patients; however, additional indications may be identified once trials are carried out in patients with other types of seizures or epilepsies. Because of its relatively recent introduction, it is too early to ascertain the place of perampanel in the treatment of patients with epilepsy.

Primary Seizure Types
- Partial/focal-onset seizures with or without secondary generalization
- Primary generalized tonic–clonic seizures

Secondary Seizure Types
- None

Potential Advantages
- Has no known organ toxicity (i.e., liver, kidneys, bone marrow, etc.)
- Novel mechanism of action that is not shared with any of the other available AEDs
- Dosing schedule is once per day

P

Potential Disadvantages
- Associated with significant pharmacokinetic interactions whereby its metabolism is readily inducible (and possibly readily inhibitable)
- Somnolence is a common adverse effect
- Potential teratogen

Suggested Reading

Auvin S, Dozieres B, Ilea A, Delanoë C. Use of perampanel in children and adolescents with Lennox–Gastaut syndrome. *Epilepsy and Behavior* 2017; **74**: 59–63.

Besag FMC, Patsalos PN. Clinical efficacy of perampanel for partial-onset and primary generalized tonic-clonic seizures. *Neuropsychiatric Decease and Treatment* 2016; **12**: 1215–1220.

Crespel A, Gelisse P, Tang NPL, Genton P. Perampanel in 12 patients with Unverricht–Lundborg disease. *Epilepsia* 2017; **58**: 543–547.

French JA, Krauss GL, Biton V, Squillacote D, Yang H, Laurenza A, Kumar D, Rogawski MA. Adjunctive perampanel for refractory partial-onset seizures. Randomized phase III study 304. *Neurology* 2011; **79**: 589–596.

French JA, Krauss GL, Wechsler RT, Wang XF, DiVentura B, Brandt C, Trinke E, O'Brien TJ, Laurenza A, Patten A, Bibbiani F. Perampanel for tonic-clonic seizures in idiopathic generalized epilepsy. A randomized trial. *Neurology* 2015; **85**: 950–957.

Goldsmith D, Minassian BA. Efficacy and tolerability of perampanel in ten patients with Lafora disease. *Epilepsy and Behavior* 2016; **62**: 132–135.

Hanada T, Hashizume Y, Tokuhara N, Takenaka O, Kohmura N, Ogasawara A, Hatekeyama S, Ohgoh M, Ueno M, Nishizawa Y. Perampanel: a novel, orally active, noncompetitive AMPA-receptotr antagonist that reduces seizure activity in rodent models of epilepsy. *Epilepsia* 2011; **52**: 1331–1340.

Heyman E, Lahat E, Levin N, Epstein O, Lazinger M, Berkovitch M Gandelman-Marton R. Tolerability and efficacy of perampanel in children with refractory epilepsy. *Developmental Medicine and Child Neurology* 2017; **59**: 441–444.

Krauss GL, Bar M, Biton V, Klapper JA, Rektor I, Vaiciene-Magistris N, Squillacote D, Kumar D. Tolerability and safety of perampanel: two randomized dose-escalation studies. *Acta Neurologica Scandinavica* 2012; **125**: 8–15.

Krauss GL, Serratosa JM, Villanueva V, Endziniene E, Hong Z, French J, Yang H, Squillacote D, Edwards HB, Zhu J, Laurenza A. Randomized phase III study 306. Adjunctive perampanel for refractory partial-onset seizures. *Neurology* 2012; **78**: 1408–1415.

Ledingham DRM, Patsalos PN. Perampanel: what is its place in the management of partial epilepsy? *Neurology and Therapy* 2013; **2**: 13–24.

PERAMPANEL

Leppik IE, Wechsler RT, Williams B, Yang H, Zhou S, Laurenza A. Efficacy and safety of perampanel in the subgroup of elderly patients included in the phase III epilepsy clinical trials. *Epilepsy Research* 2015; **110**: 216–220.

Patsalos PN. The clinical pharmacology profile of the new antiepileptic drug perampanel: a novel noncompetitive AMPA receptor antagonist. *Epilepsia* 2015; **56**: 12–27.

Patsalos PN. Gougoulaki N, Sander JW. Perampanel serum concentrations in adults with epilepsy: effect of dose, age, sex and concomitant anti-epileptic drugs. *Therapeutic Drug Monitoring* 2016; **38**: 358–364.

Patsalos PN, Zugman M, Lake C, James A, Ratnaraj N, Sander JW. Serum protein binding of 25 antiepileptic drugs in a routine clinical setting: a comparison of free non-protein-bound concentrations. *Epilepsia*, 2017; **58**: 1234–1243.

Redecker J, Wittstock M, Benecke R, Rosche J. Efficacy of perampanel in refractory nonconvulsive stutas epilepticus and simple partial status epilepticus. *Epilepsy and Behavior* 2015; **45**: 176–179.

P

SUGGESTED READING

P PHENOBARBITAL

Therapeutics

Chemical Name and Structure
Phenobarbital, 5-ethyl-5-phenylbarbituric acid, is a white powder, with a molecular weight of 232.23 and an empirical formula of $C_{12}H_{12}N_2O_3$.

Brand Names
- Alepsal; Ancalixir; Andral; Aphenylbarbit; Atrofen
- Barbee; Barbilettae; Barbilixir; Barbinol; Barbiphenyl; Bialminal
- Comizial
- Dormital
- Edhanol; Emgard; Epigard; Epikon; Epinil; Epitan
- Fenemal; Fenobarb; Fenobarbital; Fenobarbitale; Fenobarbitale Sodico; Fenton
- G-30; G-60; Gardenal; Gardenal Sodium; Gardenale; Gee; Gratusminal
- Lepinal natrium; Lethyl; Lumcalcio; Luminal; Luminale; Luminaletas; Luminalette; Luminaletten; Luminalum
- Menobarb
- Neurobiol
- Pevalon; Phenaemal; Phenobarbital SOD; Phenobarbiton; Phenobarbiton-natrium; Phenobarbitone; Phenobarbitone Sodium; Phenotal
- Sevenal; Shenobar; Shinosun; Solfoton
- Tridezibarbitur
- Uni-Feno

Generics Available
- Yes

Licensed Indications for Epilepsy
- Generalized tonic–clonic and partial seizures in patients of any age (FDA PI)
- All forms of epilepsy, except absence seizures, in patients of any age (UK SPC)

Licensed Indications for Non-epilepsy Conditions
- Sedative/hypnotic (FDA PI)

P

Non-licensed Use for Epilepsy
- Acute convulsive episodes and status epilepticus
- Lennox–Gastaut syndrome
- Myoclonic seizures
- Neonatal seizures
- Prophylaxis of febrile seizures

Non-licensed Use for Non-epilepsy Conditions
- Treatment of sedative or hypnotic drug withdrawal

Ineffective (Contraindicated)
- Absence seizures

Mechanism of Action
- Enhancement of GABA inhibition
- Enhances postsynaptic $GABA_A$ receptor-mediated chloride currents by prolonging the opening of the chloride ionophore
- Concentration-dependent reduction of calcium-dependent action potentials

Efficacy Profile
- The goals of treatment are to achieve complete seizure remission when possible, or at least improved frequency and severity of seizures, while also minimizing adverse effects and improving patient quality of life
- Onset of action is rapid following iv administration
- In the absence of a loading dose, maintenance doses do not achieve a steady-state level until approximately 2–3 weeks, because of the long elimination half-life; accordingly, the onset of action may be delayed
- Once chronic therapy is initiated, it is usually continued for at least 2 years following the last seizure
- Phenobarbital is a drug of first choice only in neonates with seizures
- Phenobarbital is a drug of third choice for the iv treatment of status epilepticus, after a benzodiazepine and phenytoin
- If phenobarbital is ineffective or only partially effective, it can be replaced by or combined with another AED that is appropriate for the patient's seizure type or epilepsy syndrome

Pharmacokinetics
Absorption and Distribution
- Oral bioavailability: >90% (tablets)
- Bioavailability: >90% after im administration (parenteral solution); 90% after rectal administration (parenteral solution)
- Food co-ingestion: causes a slight delay in the rate of absorption but the extent of absorption is unaffected
- Tmax: 2–4 hours (oral ingestion); <4 hours (im administration)

PHARMACOKINETICS

P

- Time to steady state: 15–29 days (adults)
- Pharmacokinetics: linear
- Protein binding: 55%
- Volume of distribution: 0.54 L/kg (adult volunteers); 0.61 L/kg (adult patients with epilepsy); ~1.0 L/kg (newborns)
- Salivary concentrations: phenobarbital is secreted into saliva, and concentrations are similar to the unbound levels seen in plasma

Metabolism
- Phenobarbital undergoes significant metabolism in the liver to two major metabolites, *p*-hydroxyphenobarbital (~20–30% of administered dose) which partially (50%) undergoes sequential metabolism to a glucuronic acid conjugate, and 9-D-glucopyran-osylphenobarbital (~25–30% of administered dose), a nitrogen glucosidation conjugate
- CYP2C9 plays a major role in the metabolism of phenobarbital to *p*-hydroxyphenobarbital with minor metabolism by CYP2C19 and CYP2E1
- The identity of the UGT enzyme responsible for the formation of 9-D-glucopyranosylphenobarbital is unknown
- The metabolites of phenobarbital are not pharmacologically active
- Phenobarbital undergoes autoinduction so that its clearance can increase and this may require an upward dosage adjustment when prescribed as monotherapy

Elimination
- The elimination half-life is 70–140 hours (adults); 100–200 hours (newborn)
- During the neonatal period, phenobarbital elimination accelerates markedly; thereafter, half-lives are very short, with average values of 63 hours during the first year of life and 69 hours between ages 1 and 5 years
- Renal excretion: ~20–25% of an administered dose is excreted unchanged in urine in adults, with large interindividual variability

Drug Interaction Profile
Pharmacokinetic Drug Interactions
- Interactions between AEDs: effects on phenobarbital:
  - Felbamate, oxcarbazepine, phenytoin, rufinamide, stiripentol, and valproic acid can *decrease* the clearance of phenobarbital and *increase* phenobarbital plasma levels
- Interactions between AEDs: effects by phenobarbital:
  - Phenobarbital can *increase* the clearance and *decrease* the levels of brivaracetam, carbamazepine, clobazam, clonazepam, diazepam, ethosuximide, felbamate, lacosamide, lamotrigine, levetiracetam, midazolam, oxcarbazepine, phenytoin, rufinamide, stiripentol, tiagabine, topiramate, valproic acid, and zonisamide

PHENOBARBITAL

P

- Interactions between AEDs and non-AED drugs: effects on phenobarbital:
  - Chloramphenicol and propoxyphene can *increase* phenobarbital plasma levels
  - Dicoumarol, thioridazine, tipranavir (in combination with ritonavir), and troleandomycin can *decrease* phenobarbital plasma levels
- Interactions between AEDs and non-AED drugs: effects by phenobarbital:
  - Phenobarbital can *increase* the clearance and *decrease* the plasma levels of acetaminophen (paracetamol), albendazole, 9-aminocampthothecin, atenolol, cimetidine, chloramphenicol, chlorpromazine, clozapine, cortisol, cyclosporin, delavirdine, desipramine, dexamethasone, doxycycline, etoposide, felodipine, fentanyl, glufosfamide, griseofulvin, haloperidol, imipramine, irinotecan, itraconazole, lidocaine, meperidine, methadone, methotrexate, methylprednisolone, metronidazole, mianserin, nifedipine, nimodipine, nortriptyline, paclitaxel, paroxetine, prednisolone, procarbazine, propranolol, quinidine, rifampicin, tacrolimus, teniposide, theophylline, thioridazine, tirilazad, verapamil, and warfarin

Pharmacodynamic Drug Interactions
- Phenobarbital can exacerbate the effects of alcohol and other CNS depressants
- Phenobarbital in combination with perampanel is associated with increased irritability. This effect may be the consequence of a pharmacodynamic interaction
- A pharmacodynamic interaction between phenobarbital and ifosfamide, resulting in encephalopathy, can occur

Hormonal Contraception
- Phenobarbital enhances the metabolism of oral contraceptives so as to decrease plasma levels of hormonal contraceptives and to reduce their effectiveness, leading to breakthrough bleeding and contraceptive failure; medium- or high-dose oral contraceptive preparations are indicated in patients taking phenobarbital, with additional recommendations for use of barrier methods and supplemental folic acid 1000 mg in all women of childbearing potential

Adverse Effects
How Drug Causes Adverse Effects
- Mechanism by which phenobarbital causes adverse effects has not been established and is presumed to be the same as the mechanism invoked for efficacy

ADVERSE EFFECTS

P

Common Adverse Effects
• Sedation and drowsiness
• Hyperactivity and irritability (especially in children)
• Dysarthria, ataxia, incoordination, nystagmus
• Depression
• Cognitive impairment
• Decreased bone mineral density

Life-threatening or Dangerous Adverse Effects
• Very rare: Stevens–Johnson syndrome, erythema multiforme, toxic epidermal necrolysis
• Hypersensitivity reactions, may lead to hepatic failure

Rare and not Life-threatening Adverse Effects
• Movement disorders, such as dyskinesia
• Seizure exacerbation or de novo seizures
• Hematologic toxicity, mainly megaloblastic anemia
• Exacerbation of acute intermittent porphyria
• Vitamin K-deficient hemorrhagic disease in newborns of mothers treated with phenobarbital; can be prevented by administration of vitamin K to the mother before delivery
• Connective tissue disorders associated with long-term phenobarbital therapy (unusual in children), such as Dupuytren contractures, plantar fibromatosis, heel and knuckle pads, frozen shoulder, Peyronie disease, and diffuse joint pain
• Loss of libido and erectile dysfunction

Weight Change
• Not common

What to do About Adverse Effects
• Discuss common and severe adverse effects with patients or parents before starting medication, including symptoms that should be reported to the physician
• Dosage reduction in case of presumably dose-related adverse effects
• CNS-related adverse effects are usually dose-dependent and are reversible
• Many adverse effects disappear over time (usually within a few weeks) and include dizziness, sleepiness, drowsiness, tiredness, loss of appetite, nausea, and vomiting
• Consider calcium and vitamin D supplements in cases of low 25-hydroxyvitamin D levels and/or decreased bone mineral density

Dosing and Use

Usual Dosage Range
- Adults and children over 12 years of age: 1.5–4 mg/kg/day
- Children:
  - Children (2 months to 1 year): 4–11 mg/kg per day
  - Children (1–3 years): 3–7 mg/kg per day
  - Children (3–6 years): 2–5 mg/kg per day
- The initial loading dose of 15–20 mg/kg in newborns is similar to the dose in children and adults and will achieve a plasma level of approximately 20 mg/L (86.2 µmol/L); this level can usually be maintained in newborns with a maintenance dose of 3–4 mg/kg per day

Available Formulations
- Tablets: 15 mg, 30 mg, 32 mg, 32.4 mg, 60 mg, 64.8 mg, 65 mg, 97.2 mg, 100 mg
- Solution: 20 mg/5 mL
- Solution for iv injection: 15 mg/mL, 30 mg/mL, 60 mg/mL, 65 mg/mL, 130 mg/mL, 200 mg/mL
- Elixir: 15 mg/5 mL; 20 mg/5 mL

How to Dose
- *For adults and children over 12 years of age:* start treatment with 1.5–4 mg/kg/day
- *Children:* start treatment with 2–11 mg/kg/day (2 months to 1 year: 4–11 mg/kg per day; 1–3 years: 3–7 mg/kg per day; 3–6 years: 2–5 mg/kg per day); doses above 11 mg/kg may be necessary in some infants to achieve high therapeutic levels
- Because of the long elimination half-life and slow accumulation of phenobarbital, the full maintenance dose can be given on the first day; steady-state plasma levels will be reached only after 2–3 weeks
- The iv loading dose of phenobarbital in the treatment of status epilepticus varies between 10 and 30 mg/kg; 15–20 mg/kg is most common. The rate of administration should not exceed 100 mg/min (2 mg/kg/min in children weighing <40 kg)

Dosing Tips
- Given its long half-life, dividing the daily dose of phenobarbital into two or more doses, even in children, appears unnecessary
- Salt formulations are more rapidly absorbed than are the acid formulations
- The rate of absorption is increased if the sodium salt is ingested as a dilute solution or taken on an empty stomach

How to Withdraw Drug
- May need to adjust dosage of concurrent medications as phenobarbital is being discontinued, because plasma levels of other drugs may change (see Pharmacokinetic Drug Interactions section)

- After long-term administration, phenobarbital should always be discontinued gradually over several weeks
- Barbiturates and benzodiazepines are the AEDs most commonly associated with withdrawal seizures upon rapid discontinuation
- Unless there is a specific reason to proceed faster, it is appropriate to taper the phenobarbital dose linearly over 3–6 months, with reductions every 2–4 weeks

Overdose
- The toxic dose of phenobarbital varies considerably; in general 1 g produces serious adverse effects and 2–10 g commonly results in death and is mostly secondary to cardiorespiratory failure
- In individuals who have not been previously exposed to phenobarbital, plasma levels at or above 80 mg/L (345 μmol/L) are considered lethal; higher plasma levels may be tolerated by patients on chronic phenobarbital therapy
- Symptoms include: constricted pupils, nystagmus, ataxia, somnolence, stupor or coma, pulmonary edema, and respiratory failure
- Treatment consists mainly of cardiorespiratory support
- Alkalinization with sodium bicarbonate, iv hydration, and forced diuresis accelerate the elimination of phenobarbital through the kidneys
- The stomach should be emptied immediately by lavage or by induction of emesis
- Hemodialysis removes phenobarbital from blood and, therefore, serves as a useful procedure in cases of overdose

Tests and Therapeutic Drug Monitoring
- Monitoring of blood count and liver function tests usually not necessary
- Because phenobarbital can alter vitamin D metabolism and affect bone mineral density, 25-hydroxyvitamin D levels should be monitored in all patients, and vitamin D supplementation should be prescribed as needed; consider also DEXA bone scan in patients at risk for osteopenia
- Therapeutic drug monitoring:
  - Optimum seizure control in patients on monotherapy is most likely to occur at phenobarbital plasma concentrations of 10–40 mg/L (43–172 μmol/L)
  - The conversion factor from mg/L to μmol/L is 4.31 (i.e., 1 mg/L = 4.31 μmol/L)
  - The reference range of phenobarbital in plasma is considered to be the same for children and adults, although no data are available to support this clinical practice
  - Phenobarbital can be monitored by use of saliva which is a measure of the free non-protein-bound plasma concentration and is pharmacologically relevant

P

Other Warnings / Precaution
- Phenobarbital may be habit forming
- Tolerance and psychological and physical dependence may occur with long-term use
- Should be prescribed with caution to patients with a history of mental depression, or suicidal tendencies, or a history of drug abuse

Do not Use
- In patients with known history of allergic reaction to barbiturates
- In patients with known history of intermittent acute porphyria
- Because the tablet formulation contains lactose, patients with rare hereditary problems of galactose intolerance, Lapp lactose deficiency, or glucose–galactose malabsorption should not take this formulation
- If patient has a proven allergy to phenobarbital or to any of the excipients

Special Populations
Renal Impairment
- Phenobarbital is renally secreted and thus the dose may need to be lowered in renally impaired patients
- Because phenobarbital can be removed by hemodialysis, patients receiving hemodialysis may require supplemental doses of phenobarbital

Hepatic Impairment
- Phenobarbital is extensively metabolized in the liver and consequently lower doses may be required

Children
- Children have an increased metabolic capacity and consequently higher doses on a mg/kg/day basis are usually required to achieve the equivalent therapeutic plasma levels seen in adults
- Pharmacokinetic interactions in children are usually of a greater magnitude than that seen in adults

Elderly
- Elderly patients are more susceptible to adverse effects of phenobarbital (especially somnolence) and may be unable to tolerate higher doses; slower titration to a lower initial target dosage should be considered
- Because of an age-related reduction in renal and hepatic function, lower phenobarbital doses are appropriate
- Elderly patients are often prescribed concurrent drug therapies for comorbidities and therefore may be at greater risk for pharmacokinetic and pharmacodynamic interactions; the risk of pharmacokinetic interactions with phenobarbital is substantial

P

PHENOBARBITAL

Pregnancy

- Specialist advice should be given to women who are of childbearing potential; they should be informed about the teratogenicity of all AEDs and the importance of avoiding an unplanned pregnancy; the AED treatment regimen should be reviewed when a woman is planning to become pregnant
- Rapid discontinuation of AEDs should be avoided as this may lead to breakthrough seizures, which could have serious consequences for the woman and the unborn child
- Phenobarbital was previously classified by the US FDA as risk category D (positive evidence of risk to human fetus; potential benefits may still justify its use during pregnancy); the current FDA Pregnancy and Lactation Rule has eliminated pregnancy risk category labels
- Analysis of a recent pregnancy registry revealed that phenobarbital was associated with a higher risk of congenital malformations than most other AEDs, in particular, cardiac defects and oral clefts
- Use in women of childbearing potential requires weighing potential benefits to the mother against the risks to the fetus
- Supplementation with folic acid may reduce the risk of congenital abnormalities
- Seizures, even mild seizures, may cause harm to the embryo/fetus
- Use with other AEDs in combination may cause a higher prevalence of teratogenic effects than phenobarbital monotherapy
- Taper drug if discontinuing
- Vitamin K-deficient hemorrhagic disease in newborns of mothers treated with phenobarbital can be prevented by administration of vitamin K to the mother before delivery
- During pregnancy phenobarbital pharmacokinetics change significantly so that in the first trimester total and free phenobarbital plasma concentrations decrease by 50–55% due to increased clearance and reduction in albumin concentrations; an increase in phenobarbital dose may be required in some patients

Breast Feeding

- Breast milk: 30–50% of maternal plasma levels
- Breastfed infants: phenobarbital plasma levels may reach 50–100% of maternal plasma levels
- If drug is continued while breast feeding, infant should be monitored for possible adverse effects, including sedation, poor sucking and weight gain, and vomiting
- If adverse effects are observed, recommend bottle feeding

The Overall Place of Phenobarbital in the Treatment of Epilepsy

Phenobarbital is a highly effective broad-spectrum AED, being effective in all seizure types with the exception of absences. It is associated with rapid onset and prolonged action, and there is extensive experience of its use in adults and children and also in neonates for neonatal or febrile seizures. Phenobarbital has a significant role in the management of established status epilepticus, although it is usually the drug of third choice after a benzodiazepine and phenytoin. Because of its sedative and cognitive effects, it is never a drug of first choice, except for the treatment of neonatal seizures.

Primary Seizure Types
• Partial (focal) and secondary generalized seizures
• Acute convulsive episodes and status epilepticus

Secondary Seizure Types
• Prophylaxis of febrile seizures
• Myoclonic seizures
• Primarily generalized tonic–clonic seizures
• Lennox–Gastaut syndrome

Potential Advantages
• Broad spectrum of activity
• Low systemic toxicity
• Long half-life enabling once-daily dosing
• Can be administered intravenously and intramuscularly
• Tolerance does not occur
• Is effective in status epilepticus
• Inexpensive

Potential Disadvantages
• Phenobarbital produces more sedative and behavioral adverse effects than most other AEDs
• Requires frequent blood testing and close monitoring
• Associated with significant pharmacokinetic interactions and usually acts as an inducer of hepatic metabolism
• Potential teratogen

Suggested Reading
Boreus LO, Jalling B, Kallberg N. Phenobarbital metabolism in adults and in newborn infants. *Acta Paediatrica Scandinavica* 1978; **67**: 193–200.

Hernandez-Diaz S, Smith CR, Shen A, Mittendorf R, Hauser WA, Yerby M, Holmes LB. Comparative safety of antiepileptic drugs during pregnancy. *Neurology* 2012; **78**: 1692–1699.

Hirtz DG, Sulzbacher SI, Ellenberg JH, Nelson KB. Phenobarbital for febrile seizures – effects on intelligence and on seizure recurrence. *New England Journal of Medicine* 1990; **322**: 364–369.

Kjaer D, Horvath-Puho E, Christensen J, Vestergaard M, Czeizel AE, Sorensen HT, Olsen J. Antiepileptic drug use, folic acid supplementation, and congenital abnormalities: a population-based

P

case-control study. *British Journal of Obstetrics and Gynaecology* 2008; **115**: 98–103.

Mattson RH, Cramer JA, Collins JF, Smith DB, Delgado-Escueta AV, Browne TR, Williamson PD, Treiman DM, McNamara JO, McCutchen CB. Comparison of carbamazepine, phenobarbital, phenytoin, and primidone in partial and secondarily generalized tonic-clonic seizures. *New England Journal of Medicine* 1985; **313**: 145–151.

Painter MJ, Scher MS, Stein AD, Armatti S, Wang Z, Gardiner JC, Paneth N, Minnigh B, Alvin J. Phenobarbital compared with phenytoin for the treatment of neonatal seizures. *New England Journal of Medicine* 1999; **341**: 485–489.

Patsalos PN. *Antiepileptic drug interactions: a clinical guide*, 3rd edition. Springer, London, UK; 2016.

Patsalos PN, Berry DJ. Therapeutic drug monitoring of antiepileptic drugs by use of saliva. *Therapeutic Drug Monitoring* 2013; **35**: 4–29.

Patsalos PN, Berry DJ, Bourgeois BFD, Cloyd JC, Glauser TA, Johannessen SI, Leppik IE, Tomson T, Perucca E. Antiepileptic drugs – best practice guidelines for therapeutic drug monitoring: a position paper by the Subcommission on Therapeutic Drug Monitoring, ILAE Commission on Therapeutic Strategies. *Epilepsia* 2008; **49**: 1239–1276.

Shellhaas RA, Barks AK, Joshi SM. Prevalence and risk factors for vitamin D insufficiency among children with epilepsy. *Pediatric Neurology* 2010; **42**: 422–426.

Vestergaard P, Rejnmark L, Mosekilde L. Fracture risk associated with use of antiepileptic drugs. *Epilepsia* 2004; **45**: 1330–1337.

Vining EP, Mellitis ED, Dorsen MM, Cataldo MF, Quaskey SA, Spielberg SP, Freeman JM. Psychologic and behavioral effects of antiepileptic drugs in children: a double-blind comparison between phenobarbital and valproic acid. *Pediatrics* 1987; **80**: 165–174.

Wilensky AJ, Friel PN, Levy RH, Comfort CF, Kaluzny SP. Kinetics of phenobarbital in normal subjects and epileptic patients. *European Journal of Clinical Pharmacology* 1982; **23**: 87–92.

Wolf S, Forsythe A. Behavior disturbance, phenobarbital and febrile seizures. *Pediatrics* 1978; **61**: 729–731.

PHENYTOIN

Therapeutics

Chemical Name and Structure

Phenytoin, 5,5-diphenyl-2,4-imidazolidinedione, is a white powder, with a molecular weight of 252.26 for the free acid and a molecular weight of 274.25 for the sodium salt, which is equivalent to an acid content of 91.98%. It has an empirical formula of $C_{15}H_{12}N_2O_2$.

Brand Names
- Aleviatin; Antisacer; Aurantin
- Clerin; Cumatil
- Difetoin; Di-Hydan; Dilantin; Dintoina; Diphantoine; Diphantoine Z; Diphedan; Ditoin; Ditomed
- Epamin; Epanutin; Epilan-D; Epilantin; Epileptin; Epinat; Eptoin
- Felantin; Fenatoin; Fenidantoin S; Fenitoina; Fenitoina Rubio; Fenitoina Sodica; Fenitron; Fenytoin; Fomiken
- Hidanil; Hidantoína; Hydantin; Hydantol
- Ikaphen
- Kutoin
- Lantidin; Lehydan
- Movileps
- Neosidantoina
- Pepsytoin-100; Phenhydan; Phenilep; Phenytoin KP; Phenytoinum; Pyoredol
- Sinergina
- Utoin

Generics Available
- Yes

Licensed Indications for Epilepsy
- Monotherapy or adjunctive therapy for patients of any age for the treatment of tonic–clonic seizures, focal seizures, or a combination of these, and for the treatment of seizures occurring during or following neurosurgery and/or severe head injury (UK SPC)
- iv administration for the management of status epilepticus (UK SPC)
- Monotherapy or adjunctive therapy in adults and children (lower age not defined) with generalized tonic–clonic seizures and complex focal

P

PHENYTOIN

(psychomotor, temporal lobe) seizures, and prevention and treatment of seizures occurring during or following neurosurgery (FDA PI)

Licensed Indications for Non-epilepsy Conditions
- Monotherapy for the treatment of trigeminal neuralgia in patients who have not responded to carbamazepine or in patients who are intolerant to carbamazepine (UK SPC)

Non-licensed Use for Epilepsy
- There are none

Non-licensed Use for Non-epilepsy Conditions
- Arrhythmias

Ineffective (Contraindicated)
- Phenytoin is contraindicated for absence seizures, myoclonic jerks, progressive myoclonic epilepsies such as Unverricht syndrome and probably in Lennox–Gastaut syndrome, and other childhood epileptic encephalopathies (although it may be effective in tonic seizures)

Mechanism of Action
- Acts as a use-dependent blocker of voltage-sensitive sodium channels
- Interacts with the open-channel conformation of voltage-sensitive sodium channels
- Modulates sustained repetitive firing
- Regulates calmodulin and second messenger systems
- Inhibits calcium channels and calcium sequestration

Efficacy Profile
- The goals of treatment are to achieve complete seizure remission when possible, or at least improved frequency and severity of seizures, while also minimizing adverse effects and improving patient quality of life
- Efficacy should be apparent within 4 weeks of treatment initiation
- If it is not producing clinical benefits within 6–8 weeks, it may require a dosage increase or it may not work at all
- If phenytoin is ineffective or only partially effective, it can be replaced by or combined with another AED that is appropriate for the patient's seizure type or epilepsy syndrome

Pharmacokinetics
Absorption and Distribution
- Oral bioavailability: ≥ 80% (bioavailability is formulation-dependent)
- Food co-ingestion: nasogastric feeding and co-ingestion of certain foods can reduce phenytoin absorption from the gastrointestinal tract

- Tmax: 1–12 hours (rate of absorption is formulation-dependent)
- Time to steady state: 6–21 days
- Pharmacokinetics: non-linear due to saturable metabolism so that clearance decreases with increasing dose
- Protein binding: 90%
- Volume of distribution: 0.5–0.8 L/kg
- Salivary concentrations: phenytoin is secreted into saliva and concentrations are similar to the unbound levels seen in plasma

Metabolism
- Phenytoin undergoes extensive metabolism in the liver by hydroxylation to various metabolites, the principal metabolites being 5-(p-hydroxyphenyl)-5-phenylhydantoin (pHPPH; 67–88%) and a dihydrodiol derivative (7–11%)
- The isoenzymes responsible for the hydroxylation of phenytoin are CYP2C9 (~80%) and CYP2C19 (~20%)
- In excess of 60% of pHPPH is subsequently glucuronidated and excreted in urine
- The metabolites of phenytoin are not pharmacologically active
- Phenytoin undergoes autoinduction, primarily by means of CYP2C19, so that its clearance can increase, and this may require an upward dosage adjustment when prescribed as monotherapy

Elimination
- In the absence of enzyme-inducing AEDs, half-life values for phenytoin are 30–100 hours
- In the presence of enzyme-inducing co-medication, half-life values for phenytoin are 30–100 hours
- Phenytoin elimination is not first-order and, therefore, half-life values increase with increasing plasma concentrations
- Renal excretion: ~5% of an administered dose is excreted as unchanged phenytoin in urine

Drug Interaction Profile
Pharmacokinetic Drug Interactions
- Interactions between AEDs: effects on phenytoin:
  - Carbamazepine, clonazepam, and phenobarbital can *increase* the clearance of phenytoin and *decrease* phenytoin plasma levels
  - Acetazolamide, brivaracetam, carbamazepine, clobazam, clonazepam, eslicarbazepine acetate, felbamate, methsuximide, oxcarbazepine, phenobarbital, rufinamide, stiripentol, sulthiame, and topiramate can *decrease* the clearance of phenytoin and *increase* phenytoin plasma levels
  - Vigabatrin can *decrease* phenytoin plasma levels by means of an unknown mechanism

DRUG INTERACTION PROFILE

- Valproic acid can *increase* the free fraction of phenytoin by displacing phenytoin from its plasma protein (albumin) binding site and a concurrent inhibition of phenytoin clearance
- Interactions between AEDs: effects by phenytoin:
  - Phenytoin can *decrease* plasma levels of brivaracetam, carbamazepine, clobazam, clonazepam, eslicarbazepine, ethosuximide, felbamate, lacosamide, lamotrigine, levetiracetam, methsuximide, oxcarbazepine, perampanel, pregabalin, primidone, rufinamide, stiripentol, tiagabine, topiramate, valproic acid, and zonisamide
  - Phenytoin can *increase* plasma levels of phenobarbital
- Interactions between AEDs and non-AED drugs: effects on phenytoin:
  - Allopurinol, amiodarone, azapropazone, capecitabine, chloramphenicol, chlorphenamine, cimetidine, clarithromycin, clinafloxacin, co-trimoxazole, danazole, dexamethasone, disulfiram, dextropropoxyphene (propoxyphene), dicoumarol, diltiazem, doxifluridine, efavirenz, fenyramidol, fluconazole, 5-fluorouracil, fluoxetine, fluvoxamine, imipramine, isoniazid, itraconazole, methaqualone, methylphenidate, metronidazole, miconazole, nifedipine, Noni juice, nortriptyline, omeprazole, piperine, posaconazole, risperidone, ritonavir, sertraline, sulfadiazine, sulfamethizole, sulfamethoxazole, sulfaphenazole, sulfinpyrazone, tacrolimus, tamoxifen, ticlopidine, trazodone, trimethoprim, UFT, verapamil, viloxazine, and voriconazole can *increase* phenytoin plasma levels
  - Antacids, acyclovir, bleomycin, carboplatin, cisplatin, danazol, dexamethasone, diazoxide, lopinavir/ritonavir, loxapine, methotrexate, nelfinavir, nevirapine, POMP-24, rifampicin, shankhapushpi, sucralfate, theophylline, and vinblastine can *decrease* phenytoin plasma levels
  - Phenylbutazole, salicylates, and tolbutamide can *increase* the free fraction of phenytoin by displacing phenytoin from its plasma protein (albumin) binding site and a concurrent inhibition of phenytoin clearance
- Interactions between AEDs and non-AED drugs: effects by phenytoin:
  - Phenytoin can *decrease* plasma levels of acetaminophen (paracetamol), albendazole, 9-aminocamptothecin, amiodarone, atorvastatin, atracurium, busulphan, CCNU, cisatracurium, clozapine, cortisol, cyclophosphamide, cyclosporin, delavirdine, desipramine, dexamethasone, diazepam, diazoxide, dicoumarol, digoxin, disopyramide, doxacurium, doxycycline, efavirenz, etoposide, felodipine, fentanyl, gefitinib, glufosfamide, haloperidol, ifosfamide, imatinib, irinotecan, isoxicam, itraconazole, ivabradine, ketoconazole, lidocaine, lopinavir, mebendazole, meperidine, methadone, methotrexate, methylprednisolone, metyrapone, mexiletine, mianserin, midazolam, mirtazapine, nevirapine, nimodipine, nisoldipine, nortriptyline, paclitaxel, pancuronium, paroxetine, posaconazole, praziquantel, prednisolone, procarbazine, propranolol, quetiapine, quinidine, rapacuronium, ritonavir,

rocuronium, sertraline, simvastatin, sirolimus, tacrolimus, temozolomide, temsirolimus, teniposide, theophylline, thiorida-zine, thiotepa, tirilazad, topotecan, vecuronium, verapamil, vincris-tine, and voriconazole
- Phenytoin can *increase* plasma levels of chloramphenicol, losartan, and risperidone

Pharmacodynamic Drug Interactions
- The diuretic effect of furosemide is substantially reduced by con-comitant administration with phenytoin
- Neurotoxicity may occur in combination with lacosamide conse-quent to a pharmacodynamic interaction
- In combination with lamotrigine, a drug-induced chorea can occur consequent to a pharmacodynamic interaction

Hormonal Contraception
- Phenytoin enhances the metabolism of oral contraceptives so as to decrease plasma levels of hormonal contraceptives and to reduce their effectiveness, leading to breakthrough bleeding and contraceptive failure; medium- or high-dose oral contraceptive preparations are indicated in patients taking phenytoin; in addition to recommendations for additional barrier contraceptives and folic acid 1,000 mg daily in all women of childbearing potential

Adverse Effects
How Drug Causes Adverse Effects
- CNS adverse effects theoretically due to excessive actions at voltage-sensitive sodium channels
- Rash hypothetically an allergic reaction

Common Adverse Effects
- Ataxia, nystagmus, slurred speech, decreased coordination, mental confusion
- Paresthesia, drowsiness, vertigo, dizziness, insomnia, headache
- Nausea, vomiting, constipation
- Toxic hepatitis, liver damage
- Gingival hyperplasia, hirsutism, dysmorphism, hypertrichosis
- Decreased bone mineral density

Life-threatening or Dangerous Adverse Effects
- Rare serious rash, including Stevens–Johnson syndrome and toxic epidermal necrolysis (Lyell syndrome), can occur
- Lymphadenopathy, including benign lymph node hyperplasia, pseudolymphoma, lymphoma, and Hodgkin disease
- Rare hematological abnormalities, some fatal, have been associated with phenytoin and these include leukopenia, anemia,

thrombocytopenia, agranulocytosis, pancytopenia, with and without bone marrow suppression, and aplastic anemia
* Occasionally macrocytosis and megaloblastic anemia have occurred but these usually respond to folic acid therapy
* Phenytoin may be associated with an increased risk of suicidal ideation and patients should be monitored for such behavior
* Vitamin K-deficient hemorrhagic disease in newborns of mothers treated with phenytoin can be prevented by administration of vitamin K to the mother before delivery

Rare and not Life-threatening Adverse Effects
* Cerebellar dysfunction (irreversible)
* Peripheral neuropathy (irreversible)
* Movement disorders such as chorea, dystonia, tremor, and asterixis
* Hypoglycemia
* Confusional states such as delirium, psychosis, or encephalopathy

Weight Change
* Not common, reported but not expected

What to do About Adverse Effects
* Discuss common and severe adverse effects with patients or parents before starting medication, including symptoms that should be reported to the physician
* Dosage reduction in case of presumably dose-related adverse effects
* Risk of serious adverse effects is greatest in the first few months of treatment
* If patient develops signs of a rash, phenytoin should be discontinued and patient should be monitored and investigated for organ involvement (hepatic, renal, hematological)
* If the rash is of the severe type (Stevens–Johnson syndrome or Lyell syndrome) the drug should not be resumed; if the rash is of the milder type (measles type or scarlatiniform), phenytoin may be resumed after the rash has completely disappeared; if the rash recurs upon reinstituting phenytoin, further phenytoin medication is contraindicated
* Consider calcium and vitamin D supplements in case of low 25-hydroxyvitamin D levels and/or decreased bone mineral density

Dosing and Use
Usual Dosage Range
* Adults: 200–400 mg/day
* Children: 5–10 mg/kg/day

Available Formulations
* Capsules: 25 mg, 50 mg, 100 mg, 300 mg
* Tablets: 50 mg, 100 mg

P

- Infatabs chewable tablets: 50 mg
- Oral suspension: 30 mg/5 mL
- Parenteral solution: 250 mg/5 mL

How to Dose
- When initiating phenytoin treatment start with a low dose and titrate slowly so as to minimize adverse effects
  - *For adults:* start treatment with 150–300 mg/day either as a single dose (nocte) or in two equally divided doses; every 3–4 weeks increase by up to 50 mg/day in divided doses; maintenance dose generally 200–400 mg/day; some patients may require up to 500 mg/day
  - *Children:* start treatment with 5 mg/kg/day either as a single dose (nocte) or in two equally divided doses; every 3–4 weeks increase by up to 5 mg/kg/day in divided doses; maintenance dose generally 5–10 mg/kg/day; some patients may require up to 300 mg/day
  - *Neonates:* because phenytoin absorption is unreliable after oral ingestion, a loading dose of 15–20 mg/kg of the parenteral solution will usually produce plasma levels within the generally accepted therapeutic range; maintenance dose may be >10 mg/kg/day
  - *For status epilepticus:* current practice favors the preferential use of the fosphenytoin parenteral formulation (see fosphenytoin chapter). For conventional parenteral phenytoin, the usual preparation for emergency treatment is a 5-mL ampoule containing 250 mg phenytoin. For the treatment of established status epilepticus, the rate of infusion should not exceed 50 mg/min (to avoid hypotension) and it is prudent to reduce this to 20–30 mg/min in the elderly and to <25 mg/min in children – the usual dose for adults is approximately 1000 mg, therefore, taking approximately 20 minutes to administer; phenytoin is constituted in propylene glycol (40%), ethanol (10%), and water (250 mg in 5 mL), and thus is highly basic and potentially toxic to soft tissue with extravasation

Dosing Tips
- Because of the non-linear pharmacokinetics of phenytoin, and the fact that non-linearity occurs at different doses for different patients, there is wide interpatient variability in phenytoin plasma levels with equivalent doses and, therefore, dosing should be accompanied by regular checks on phenytoin plasma levels
- Dosage changes should not be undertaken at intervals shorter than 7–10 days; typically the interval should be 3–4 weeks
- Epanutin capsules contain phenytoin sodium whereas Epanutin suspension and Epanutin infatabs contain phenytoin; although 100 mg of phenytoin sodium is equivalent to 92 mg of phenytoin on a molecular basis, these molecular equivalents are not necessarily biologically equivalent and care needs to be exercised where it is necessary to change the dosage form and plasma level monitoring is recommended

DOSING AND USE

- Epanutin infatabs may be chewed
- Parenteral infusion solution should not be added to drip bottles or mixed with other drugs because of serious risk of precipitation; administration by means of a side arm or directly using an infusion pump is preferable, and infusion through a large-bore peripheral iv or central venous access line should be considered (with caveat that some fear potential for cardiac arrhythmia with central venous infusion, although to date no cases of acute phenytoin-related cardiac toxicity due to central venous administration have been reported, to our knowledge)
- im administration should not be used in the treatment of status epilepticus because the attainment of peak phenytoin plasma levels may require up to 24 hours, and because tissue toxicity of highly basic, insoluble parenteral phenytoin could cause serious tissue reactions; for im administration, conventional parenteral phenytoin is contraindicated, and only fosphenytoin formulation should instead be considered for use in this setting (see instead fosphenytoin)

How to Withdraw Drug
- May need to adjust dosage of concurrent medications as phenytoin is being discontinued, because plasma levels of other drugs may change (see Pharmacokinetic Drug Interactions section)
- Taper: a gradual dose reduction over a period of many weeks should be undertaken
- Rapid discontinuation may induce withdrawal seizures and should only be undertaken if there are safety concerns (e.g., a rash with serious characteristics)

Overdose
- The mean lethal dose for adults is considered to be 2–5 g; the lethal dose in children is unknown
- Initial symptoms include ataxia, nystagmus, and dysarthria; subsequently the patient becomes comatose, the pupils are unresponsive, and hypotension occurs followed by respiratory depression and apnea; death is the consequence of respiratory and circulatory depression
- If indicated the stomach should be emptied by lavage or by induction of emesis
- Hemodialysis removes phenytoin from blood and, therefore, serves as a useful procedure in cases of overdose

Tests and Therapeutic Drug Monitoring
- Before starting: liver and kidney function tests
- During treatment: liver and kidney function tests every 12 months; folate levels should be monitored every 6 months
- Because phenytoin can alter vitamin D metabolism and affect bone mineral density, 25-hydroxyvitamin D levels should be monitored in all patients, and vitamin D supplementation should be prescribed

P

as needed; consider also DEXA bone scan in patients at risk for osteopenia
- Therapeutic drug monitoring:
  - Optimum seizure control in patients on monotherapy is most likely to occur at plasma phenytoin concentrations of 10–20 mg/L (40–80 µmol/L)
  - The conversion factor from mg/L to µmol/L is 3.96 (i.e., 1 mg/L = 3.96 µmol/L)
  - In clinical settings whereby the phenytoin free fraction is changed (e.g., by drugs (valproic acid, phenylbutazole, salicylates, and tolbutamide) that act as protein-binding displacers or by physiologies/pathologies associated with reduced albumin concentrations (children, elderly, pregnancy, renal and hepatic disease, malnutrition, and after surgery)), patient management is best guided by use of phenytoin free non-protein-bound plasma concentrations
  - The reference range of phenytoin in plasma is considered to be the same for children and adults, although no data are available to support this clinical practice
  - Phenytoin can be monitored by use of saliva, which is a measure of the free non-protein-bound plasma concentration and is pharmacologically relevant

Other Warnings/Precautions
- Life-threatening rashes have developed in association with phenytoin use; phenytoin should generally be discontinued at the first sign of serious rash
- Caution is required when treating patients with a history of allergy or rash to other AEDs
- Because phenytoin exacerbates porphyria, caution should be exercised in patients suffering from this disorder
- An effect on glucose metabolism, inhibition of insulin release, and hyperglycemia may occur, particularly at high phenytoin levels
- Lowers calcium and folic acid blood levels: folic acid supplementation may be necessary
- Plasma levels of phenytoin sustained above the optimum range may result in confusional states referred to as "delirium," "psychosis," or "encephalopathy," or rarely, irreversible cerebellar dysfunction
- Parenteral phenytoin should not be administered by im injection because the medication will crystallize within muscles and cause significant pain
- Whenever possible, parenteral phenytoin preparations should be avoided, with preferential use instead of fosphenytoin formulations for iv or im administration (see fosphenytoin chapter); if parenteral phenytoin must be used, infuse through a large-bore peripheral iv in a limb preferentially, monitoring regularly for signs of extravasation with termination of infusion if this occurs to avoid the potentially catastrophic tissue reaction of purple glove syndrome (severe

DOSING AND USE

P

purplish-black skin discoloration, edema, and pain that may be complicated by compartment syndrome that rarely requires limb amputation)
• iv administration should be accompanied by continuous monitoring of the ECG and of blood pressure and respiratory depression; cardiac resuscitation equipment should be available

Do not Use
• If patient has a proven allergy to phenytoin or to any of the excipients
• Because formulations contain lactose, patients with rare hereditary problems of galactose intolerance, Lapp lactose deficiency, or glucose–galactose malabsorption should not take this medicine

Special Populations
Renal Impairment
• Phenytoin is renally secreted and thus the dose may need to be lowered in renally impaired patients
• Because phenytoin can be removed by hemodialysis, patients receiving hemodialysis may require supplemental doses of phenytoin

Hepatic Impairment
• Phenytoin is extensively metabolized and consequently lower doses will be required in patients with hepatic impairment

Children
• Children have an increased metabolic capacity and consequently higher doses on a mg/kg basis are usually required to achieve the equivalent therapeutic plasma levels seen in adults
• Pharmacokinetic interactions in children are usually of a greater magnitude than that seen in adults
• The absorption of phenytoin following oral absorption in neonates is unpredictable and phenytoin metabolism is depressed; it is particularly important to monitor plasma levels in neonates

Elderly
• Elderly patients are more susceptible to adverse effects and may be unable to tolerate higher doses; slower titration to a lower initial target dosage should be considered
• Because of an age-related reduction in hepatic and renal function, lower initial and target phenytoin doses are appropriate
• Elderly patients are often prescribed concurrent drug therapies for comorbidities and therefore may be at greater risk for pharmacokinetic and pharmacodynamic interactions; the risk of pharmacokinetic interactions with phenytoin is substantial
• Because of a tendency for lower serum albumin values, elderly patients may have a higher free (unbound) fraction of phenytoin

- Given frequent gastric achlorydia in elderly nursing home residents, absorption of oral phenytoin in elderly is highly variable, so consequently plasma phenytoin levels may vary; regular plasma phenytoin level monitoring to ensure adequate and consistent absorption, without overreaction and dose adjustments to single measurements, needs to be considered, and dose adjustments should be considered only when phenytoin levels show consistently low or high values over serial measurement

Pregnancy
- Specialist advice should be given to women who are of childbearing potential; they should be informed about the teratogenicity of all AEDs and the importance of avoiding an unplanned pregnancy; the AED treatment regimen should be reviewed when a woman is planning to become pregnant
- Rapid discontinuation of AEDs should be avoided as this may lead to breakthrough seizures, which could have serious consequences for the woman and the unborn child
- Phenytoin is classified by the US FDA as risk category D (positive evidence of risk to human fetus; potential benefits may still justify its use during pregnancy); the current FDA Pregnancy and Lactation Rule has eliminated pregnancy risk category labels
- Supplementation with folic acid may reduce the risk of congenital abnormalities
- Use in women of childbearing potential requires weighing potential benefits to the mother against the risks to the fetus
- Use with other AEDs in combination may cause a higher prevalence of teratogenic effects than phenytoin monotherapy
- Taper drug if discontinuing
- Vitamin K-deficient hemorrhagic disease in newborns of mothers treated with phenytoin can be prevented by administration of vitamin K to the mother before delivery
- Seizures, even mild seizures, may cause harm to the embryo/fetus
- During pregnancy phenytoin pharmacokinetics change significantly so that phenytoin plasma concentrations decrease by 39–56% and free phenytoin plasma concentrations decrease by 31–82% due to increased clearance consequent to enhanced hydroxylation and also due to reduced gastrointestinal absorption; an increase in phenytoin dose may be required in some patients

Breast Feeding
- Breast milk: 10–60% of maternal plasma levels
- Breastfed infants: phenytoin plasma levels are <10% of maternal plasma levels
- If drug is continued while breast feeding, infant should be monitored for possible adverse effects (irritability or sedation)
- If adverse effects are observed, recommend bottle feeding

P

The Overall Place of Phenytoin in the Treatment of Epilepsy

Phenytoin is highly effective in partial (focal) seizures and generalized tonic–clonic seizures, and to date no other AED has been shown to be more effective in this regard. However, its adverse effects and its complicated pharmacokinetic characteristics hinder its use. If phenobarbital fails, phenytoin is very useful in neonatal seizures. Phenytoin is often considered the drug of choice for the management of established status epilepticus, following initial therapy with iv lorazepam. However, it should be noted that given risk for serious soft-tissue reactions (i.e., purple glove syndrome) with parenteral phenytoin which is highly basic and insoluble, current practice now instead favors preferential use instead of fosphenytoin formulation for parenteral administration.

Primary Seizure Types
- Partial (focal) seizures
- Generalized tonic–clonic seizures

Secondary Seizure Types
- None

Potential Advantages
- No other AED has been shown to have superior efficacy in partial (focal) and generalized tonic–clonic seizures in randomized controlled trials
- Inexpensive

Potential Disadvantages
- Associated with non-linear pharmacokinetics so that plasma levels increase disproportionately to dose and dosing can only be undertaken with guidance of therapeutic drug monitoring (measurement of blood levels)
- Associated with more pharmacokinetic interactions than any other AED, and usually acts as an inducer of hepatic metabolism
- Long-term use of phenytoin in women is unsuitable because of aesthetic adverse effects
- Potential teratogen

Suggested Reading

Birnbaum A, Hardie NA, Leppik IE, Conway JM, Bowers SE, Lackner T, Graves NM. Variability of total phenytoin serum concentrations within elderly nursing home residents. *Neurology* 2003; **60**: 555–559.

de Silva M, MacArdle B, McGowan M, Hughes E, Stewart J, Neville BG, Johnson AL, Reynolds EH. Randomized comparative monotherapy trial of phenobarbitone, phenytoin, carbamazepine or sodium valproate for newly diagnosed childhood epilepsy. *Lancet* 1996; **347**: 709–713.

Heller AJ, Chesterman P, Elwes RD, Crawford P, Chadwick D, Johnson AL, Reynolds EH. Phenobarbitone, phenytoin, carbamazepine, or sodium valproate for newly diagnosed epilepsy: a randomised comparative monotherapy trial. *Journal of Neurology Neurosurgery and Psychiatry* 1995; **58**: 44–50.

Kjaer D, Horvath-Puho E, Christensen J, Vestergaard M, Czeizel AE, Sorensen HT, Olsen J. Antiepileptic drug use, folic acid supplementation, and congenital abnormalities: a population-based case-control study. *British Journal of Obstetrics and Gynaecology* 2008; **115**: 98–103.

Mattson RH, Cramer JA, Collins JF, Smith DB, Delgado-Escueta AV, Browne TR, Williamson PD, Treiman DM, McNamara JO, McCutchen CB. Comparison of carbamazepine, phenobarbital, phenytoin and primidone in partial and secondarily generalized tonic-clonic seizures. *New England Journal of Medicine* 1985; **313**: 145–151.

Pack AM, Morrell MJ, Randall A, McMahon DJ, Shane E. Bone health in young women with epilepsy after one year of antiepileptic drug monotherapy. *Neurology* 2008; **70**: 1586–1593.

Patsalos PN, Berry DJ, Bourgeois BF, Cloyd JC, Glauser TA, Johannessen SI, Leppik IE, Tomson T, Perucca E. Antiepileptic drugs – best practice guidelines for therapeutic drug monitoring: a position paper by the Subcommission on Therapeutic Drug Monitoring, ILAE Commission on Therapeutic Strategies. *Epilepsia* 2008; **49**: 1239–1276.

Patsalos PN, Froscher W, Pisani F, van Rijn CM. The importance of drug interactions in epilepsy therapy. *Epilepsia* 2002; **43**: 365–385.

Patsalos PN, Perucca E. Clinically important interactions in epilepsy: general features and interactions between antiepileptic drugs. *Lancet Neurology* 2003; **2**: 347–356.

Patsalos PN, Perucca E. Clinically important interactions in epilepsy: interactions between antiepileptic drugs and other drugs. *Lancet Neurology* 2003; **2**: 473–481.

Reynolds EH. Chronic antiepileptic drug toxicity: a review. *Epilepsia* 1975; **16**: 319–352.

Shellhaas RA, Barks AK, Joshi SM. Prevalence and risk factors for vitamin D insufficiency among children with epilepsy. *Pediatric Neurology* 2010; **42**: 422–426.

P

SUGGESTED READING

P

PIRACETAM

Therapeutics

Chemical Name and Structure

Piracetam, 2-oxo-1-pyrrolidine acetamide, is a white powder, with a molecular weight of 142.2 and an empirical formula of $C_6H_{10}N_2O_2$.

Brand Names

- Acetar; Avigilen; Axonyl
- Braintop
- Cerebroforte; Cerebropan; Cerebrosteril; Cerebryl; Cerepar N; Cetam; Ciclofalina; Cintilan; Cleveral; Cuxabrain
- Dinagen; Docpirace
- Encefalux; Encetrop
- Flavis
- Gabacet; Genogris; Geram; Geratam
- Huberdasen
- Kalicor
- Lucetam; Lytenur
- Merapiran; Myocalm
- Neuronova; Noodis; Noostan; Nootron; Nootrop; Nootropicon; Nootropil; Nootropyl; Normabrain; Norzetam; Novocephal
- Oikamid
- Pirabene; Piracebral; Piracemed; Piracetam AbZ; Piracetam AL; Piracetam EG; Piracetam Elbe-Med; Piracetam-Farmatrading; Piracetam Faro; Piracetam Heumann; Piracetam Interpharm; Piracetam-neuraxpharm; Piracetam Prodes; Piracetam-ratiopharm; Piracetam-RPh; Piracetam Stada; Piracetam Verla; Piracetam von ct; Piracetop; Piracetrop; Pirax; Pirazetam-Eurogenerics; Psycoton; Pyramen
- Qropi
- Sinapsan; Stimubral; Synaptine

Generics Available
- Yes

Licensed Indications for Epilepsy
- Adjunctive treatment of myoclonus of cortical origin irrespective of etiology (UK SPC)

Licensed Indications for Non-epilepsy Conditions
- There are none

Non-licensed Use for Epilepsy
- There are none

Non-licensed Use for Non-epilepsy Conditions
- Antiaging agent
- Clotting, coagulation, and vasospastic disorders
- Cognitive enhancer: particularly after stroke and in chronic ischemia
- Treatment of alcoholism
- Verbal memory enhancer

Ineffective (Contraindicated)
- There is some evidence to suggest that piracetam may aggravate seizures in some patients

Mechanism of Action
- Although disturbances of serotonergic and GABAergic function are implicated in cortical myoclonus, piracetam does not seem to modify these systems and, therefore, its mechanism of action is unknown
- Actions associated with piracetam include: enhancement of oxidative glycolysis, anticholinergic effects, increases cerebral blood flow, reduces platelet aggregation, and improves erythrocyte function; however, how these properties contribute to the suppression of myoclonus is unclear

Efficacy Profile
- The goals of treatment are to achieve complete seizure remission when possible, or at least improved frequency and severity of seizures, while also minimizing adverse effects and improving patient quality of life
- Often the effects of piracetam are immediate, profound, and long-term in that tolerance does not develop
- Discontinuation should occur in the absence of definitive, meaningful seizure reduction

P

PIRACETAM

Pharmacokinetics

Absorption and Distribution
- Oral bioavailability: ~100%
- Food co-ingestion: neither delays the rate of absorption nor decreases the extent of absorption
- Tmax: 0.5–1.5 hours
- Time to steady state: 1–2 days
- Pharmacokinetics: linear
- Protein binding: 0%
- Volume of distribution: 0.6 L/kg
- Salivary concentrations: it is not known whether piracetam is secreted into saliva and whether such concentrations are similar to the unbound levels seen in plasma

Metabolism
- Piracetam is not metabolized

Elimination
- Following a single dose, half-life values in young men are 4–6 hours
- Renal excretion: ~100% of an administered dose is excreted unchanged in urine

Drug Interaction Profile

Pharmacokinetic Drug Interactions
- Interactions between AEDs: effects on piracetam:
  - To date, there have been no reports of AEDs affecting the clearance of piracetam and affecting piracetam plasma levels
- Interactions between AEDs: effects by piracetam:
  - To date, there have been no reports of piracetam affecting the clearance of other AEDs and affecting their plasma levels
- Interactions between AEDs and non-AED drugs: effects on piracetam:
  - To date, there have been no reports of other non-AED drugs affecting the clearance of piracetam and affecting piracetam plasma levels
- Interactions between AEDs and non-AED drugs: effects by piracetam:
  - To date, there have been no reports of piracetam affecting the clearance of other non-AED drugs and affecting their plasma levels

Pharmacodynamic Drug Interactions
- In combination with clonazepam, piracetam may be particularly efficacious in suppressing myoclonic seizures
- In combination with acenocoumarol, piracetam can significantly decrease platelet aggregation, β-thromboglobulin release, levels of fibrinogen, and von Willebrand factors, and whole blood and plasma viscosity
- Confusion, irritability, and sleep disorders have been reported in a patient administered with thyroid extract (triiodothyronine + thyroxine) and piracetam

P

Hormonal Contraception
- Piracetam is not expected to affect the metabolism of oral contraceptives so as to decrease plasma levels of hormonal contraceptives and, therefore, should not compromise contraception control

Adverse Effects
How Drug Causes Adverse Effects
- Unknown

Common Adverse Effects
- Dizziness, insomnia
- Nausea, gastrointestinal discomfort
- Agitation, anxiety, confusion, hallucination

Life-threatening or Dangerous Adverse Effects
- Anaphylactic reaction, hypersensitivity
- Rare rash may occur

Rare and not Life-threatening Adverse Effects
- Asthenia
- Depression
- Somnolence

Weight Change
- Weight gain is common

What to do About Adverse Effects
- Discuss common and severe adverse effects with patients or parents before starting medication, including symptoms that should be reported to the physician
- Typically adverse effects are mild and transient
- If necessary reduce piracetam dose

Dosing and Use
Usual Dosage Range
- Adults: up to 20 g/day
- Children <16 years of age: not recommended

Available Formulations
- Tablets: 800 mg, 1200 mg
- Solution (300 mL): 333.3 mg/mL

How to Dose
- When initiating piracetam treatment start with a low dose and titrate slowly so as to minimize adverse effects

- *For adults:* start treatment with 7.2 g/day in two or three divided doses; each 3–4 days increase by 4.8 g daily; maintenance dose generally <20 g/day given in two or three equally divided doses

Dosing Tips
- The solution formulation can be used in patients who have difficulty swallowing and after ingestion should be followed by water or a soft drink to reduce the bitter taste of piracetam solution
- At the higher doses the major drawback is the number of tablets that need to be taken and their bulk, although drowsiness is occasionally dose-limiting at the high dose range

How to Withdraw Drug
- There is no need to adjust dosage of concurrent medications as piracetam is being discontinued, because plasma levels of other drugs do not change (see Pharmacokinetic Drug Interactions section)
- Taper: a gradual dose reduction over a 1–3-week period should be undertaken
- Rapid discontinuation may induce myoclonic or generalized seizures

Overdose
- No specific measures are indicated; to date, no fatalities have been reported
- If indicated the stomach should be emptied by lavage or by induction of emesis
- Hemodialysis removes 50–60% of piracetam from blood and, therefore, may be a useful procedure in cases of overdose

Tests and Therapeutic Drug Monitoring
- Before starting: coagulation tests, liver and kidney function tests
- During treatment: coagulation tests, liver and kidney function tests every 6–12 months
- Therapeutic drug monitoring:
  - There are no data relating the plasma concentration of piracetam with that of seizure suppression
  - Thus, although routine monitoring of piracetam is not recommended, measurement of plasma piracetam concentrations may be useful as a check on compliance
  - There are no data indicating the usefulness of monitoring piracetam by use of saliva

Other Warnings/Precautions
- Due to the effect of piracetam on platelet aggregation, caution is recommended in patients with underlying disorders of hemostasis, major surgery, or severe hemorrhage
- Some patients may experience hyperkinesia, somnolence, nervousness, and depression and thus caution needs to be exercised if patient intends to drive or use machinery

P

Do not Use
- If patient has severe renal (CrCl <20 mL/min) or hepatic impairment
- If patient has a cerebral hemorrhage
- If patient has a proven allergy to piracetam, other pyrrolidone derivatives, or to any of the excipients

Special Populations
Renal Impairment
- Piracetam is renally excreted, so the dose needs to be lowered: recommended adjustments are:
  - Mild renal impairment (CrCl 50–79 mL/min) – 2/3 usual daily dose
  - Moderate impairment (CrCl 30–49 mL/min) – 1/3 usual daily dose
  - Severe impairment (CrCl 20–30 mL/min) – 1/6 usual daily dose
- Because piracetam can be removed by hemodialysis, patients receiving hemodialysis may require supplemental doses of piracetam

Hepatic Impairment
- Even though piracetam is not metabolized, its use is contraindicated in hepatically impaired patients

Children
- Piracetam is not licensed for use in children

Elderly
- Elderly patients are generally more susceptible to adverse effects and therefore may not tolerate higher doses
- Because of an age-related reduction in renal function, lower piracetam doses are appropriate and should be based on CrCl values
- Elderly patients are often prescribed concurrent drug therapies for comorbidities and therefore may be at greater risk for pharmacokinetic and pharmacodynamic interactions; as the risk of pharmacokinetic interactions with piracetam is low or non-existent, piracetam may be advantageous for use in the elderly

Pregnancy
- Specialist advice should be given to women who are of childbearing potential; they should be informed about the teratogenicity of all AEDs and the importance of avoiding an unplanned pregnancy; the AED treatment regimen should be reviewed when a woman is planning to become pregnant
- Rapid discontinuation of AEDs should be avoided as this may lead to breakthrough seizures, which could have serious consequences for the woman and the unborn child

- Piracetam was previously classified by the US FDA as risk category C (some animal studies show adverse effects, no controlled studies in humans); the current FDA Pregnancy and Lactation Rule has eliminated pregnancy risk category labels
- Use in women of childbearing potential requires weighing potential benefits to the mother against the risks to the fetus
- Use with other AEDs in combination may cause a higher prevalence of teratogenic effects than piracetam monotherapy
- Taper drug if discontinuing
- Seizures, even mild seizures, may cause harm to the embryo/fetus
- There are no available data on the pharmacokinetic changes of piracetam during pregnancy

Breast Feeding
- Breast milk: piracetam is excreted in breast milk
- Breastfed infants: it is not known what plasma piracetam concentrations are achieved in breastfed infants compared with the levels of their mothers
- If drug is continued while breast feeding, infant should be monitored for possible adverse effects
- If adverse effects are observed, recommend bottle feeding

The Overall Place of Piracetam in the Treatment of Epilepsy

Cortical myoclonus, with or without epilepsy, can result in profound disability. The jerks are often exacerbated by action, and the patient may be bed-bound and immobile, unable to move without severe myoclonic jerking disrupting all motor activity. Piracetam is particularly effective for the treatment of myoclonic seizures and often its effects are immediate, profound, and long-term in that tolerance does not develop. Furthermore, in some cases, piracetam can have a truly remarkable effect, suppressing the myoclonus and reversing completely even severe disability. Piracetam is the only drug that improves the myoclonus in some patients with progressive myoclonic epilepsy syndromes.

Primary Seizure Types
- Myoclonic seizures

Secondary Seizure Types
- None

Potential Advantages
- Piracetam is an efficacious AED for the treatment of cortical myoclonus and its associated profound disability
- It is well tolerated and is associated with very few adverse effects, which are typically mild and transient

- Because it is excreted exclusively by renal elimination, piracetam is not associated with any significant pharmacokinetic interactions

Potential Disadvantages
- Not effective in many cases of cortical myoclonus
- Bulky tablets which have to be ingested in large numbers (particularly at the higher doses)
- Potential teratogen

Suggested Reading

Brown P, Steiger MJ, Thompson PD, Rothwell JC, Day BL, Salama M, Waegemans T, Marsden CD. Effectiveness of piracetam in cortical myoclonus. *Movement Disorders* 1993; **8**: 63–68.

Koskiniemi M, van Vleyman B, Hakamies L, Lamusuo S, Taalas J. Piracetam relieves symptoms in progressive myoclonic epilepsy: a multicentre, randomised, double-blind, crossover study comparing the efficacy and safety of three dosages of oral piracetam with placebo. *Journal of Neurology, Neurosurgery, and Psychiatry* 1998; **64**: 344–348.

Obeso JA, Artieda J, Quinn N, Rothwell JC, Luquin MR, Vaamonde J, Marsden CD. Piracetam in the treatment of different types of myoclonus. *Clinical Neuropharmacology* 1988; **11**: 529–536.

Shorvon SD. Pyrrolidine derivatives. *Lancet* 2001; **358**: 1885–1892.

P # PREGABALIN

Therapeutics

Chemical Name and Structure

Pregabalin, S-3-(aminomethyl)-5-methylhexanoic acid, is a white powder, with a molecular weight of 159.2 and an empirical formula of $C_9H_{17}NO_2$.

Brand Names
- Alzain; Axalid
- Gabafit; Gabamax; Gabanext; Gafasafe; Galinerve
- Lecaent
- Lyrica
- Maxgalin
- Neugabid; Nova; Nuramed
- Peganex; Pevesca; Pregab; Pregaba

Generics Available
- Yes

Licensed Indications for Epilepsy
- Adjunctive treatment of partial (focal) seizures with or without secondary generalization in adults (UK SPC; FDA PI)

Licensed Indications for Non-epilepsy Conditions
- Peripheral and central neuropathic pain in adults (UK SPC)
- Generalized anxiety disorders in adults (UK SPC)
- Management of pain associated with diabetic peripheral neuropathy (FDA PI)
- Management of postherpetic neuralgia (FDA PI)
- Management of fibromyalgia (FDA PI)

Non-licensed Use for Epilepsy
- There are none

Non-licensed Use for Non-epilepsy Conditions
- Panic disorder
- Social anxiety disorder

Ineffective (Contraindicated)
- Pregabalin may exaggerate myoclonus

P

- Treatment-emergent myoclonic jerks may be a warning sign against the use of pregabalin in generalized and other myoclonic epilepsies, where myoclonus is often prominent and can be unveiled or aggravated by pregabalin

Mechanism of Action
- Binds to the α2-δ protein subunit of voltage-gated calcium channels
- This closes N and P/Q presynaptic calcium channels, diminishing excessive neuronal activity and neurotransmitter release
- Although structurally related to GABA, it does not directly act on GABA or its receptors

Efficacy Profile
- The goals of treatment are to achieve complete seizure remission when possible, or at least improved frequency and severity of seizures, while also minimizing adverse effects and improving patient quality of life
- Efficacy should be apparent within 2 weeks of treatment initiation
- If it is not producing clinical benefits within 6–8 weeks, it may require a dosage increase or it may not work at all
- If pregabalin is ineffective or only partially effective, it can be replaced by or combined with another AED that is appropriate for the patient's seizure type or epilepsy syndrome

Pharmacokinetics
Absorption and Distribution
- Oral bioavailability: ≥90%
- Food co-ingestion: decreases the extent of absorption (25–30%) and absorption is delayed by ~2.5 hours
- Tmax: 1–2 hours
- Time to steady state: 1–2 days
- Pharmacokinetics: linear
- Protein binding: 0%
- Volume of distribution: 0.57 L/kg
- Salivary concentrations: it is not known whether pregabalin is secreted into saliva and whether such concentrations are similar to the unbound levels seen in plasma

Metabolism
- Pregabalin is not metabolized

Elimination
- Following a single dose, half-life values are 5–7 hours
- The renal clearance of pregabalin is proportional to the CrCl
- Renal excretion: ~98% of an administered dose is excreted unchanged in urine

PHARMACOKINETICS

P

Drug Interaction Profile
Pharmacokinetic Drug Interactions
- Interactions between AEDs: effects on pregabalin:
  - Gabapentin and phenytoin can *decrease* pregabalin plasma levels
- Interactions between AEDs: effects by pregabalin:
  - Pregabalin can *decrease* plasma levels of tiagabine
- Interactions between AEDs and non-AED drugs: effects on pregabalin:
  - To date, there have been no reports of other non-AED drugs affecting the clearance of pregabalin and affecting pregabalin plasma levels
- Interactions between AEDs and non-AED drugs: effects by pregabalin:
  - To date, there have been no reports of pregabalin affecting the clearance of other non-AED drugs and affecting their plasma levels

Pharmacodynamic Drug Interactions
- Pregabalin may potentiate the effects of ethanol and lorazepam
- Respiratory failure and coma have been reported in patients co-prescribed pregabalin and other CNS-depressant medications
- Pregabalin appears to be additive in the impairment of cognitive and gross motor function associated with oxycodone
- CNS adverse effects, particularly somnolence, can increase in patients co-prescribed antispasticity agents

Hormonal Contraception
- Pregabalin does not enhance the metabolism of oral contraceptives so as to decrease plasma levels of hormonal contraceptives and, therefore, does not compromise contraception control

Adverse Effects
How Drug Causes Adverse Effects
- CNS adverse effects may be due to excessive blockade of voltage-sensitive calcium channels

Common Adverse Effects
- Somnolence, dizziness
- Ataxia, fatigue, tremor, dysarthria, paresthesia, abnormal coordination
- Impaired attention, memory impairment, confusion, euphoric mood, irritability
- Vomiting, dry mouth, constipation, increased appetite, flatulence
- Blurred vision, diplopia
- Peripheral edema
- Libido decreased, erectile dysfunction

Life-threatening or Dangerous Adverse Effects
- Rare neutropenia, hypoglycemia, atrioventricular block, and congestive heart failure
- Some patients may experience hypersensitivity reactions, including facial, perioral, and upper-airway angioedema – pregabalin should be withdrawn immediately if these symptoms present
- Cases of renal failure have been reported; however, discontinuation of pregabalin reversed the adverse effect

Rare and not Life-threatening Adverse Effects
- Ageusia
- Amenorrhea, dysmenorrhea
- Ascites, dysphagia, pancreatitis
- Hyporeflexia, hyperesthesia
- Hyperacusis
- Myoclonus, dyskinesia
- Peripheral vision loss, oscillopsia, photopsia, strabismus
- Syncope, stupor

Weight Change
- Weight gain is common

What to do About Adverse Effects
- Discuss common and severe adverse effects with patients or parents before starting medication, including symptoms that should be reported to the physician
- Sedation is dose-related and can subside with time
- Take more of the dose at night to reduce daytime sedation
- Lower the dose

Dosing and Use
Usual Dosage Range
- Adults: 150–600 mg/day
- Children: 15–20 mg/kg/day

Available Formulations
- Capsules: 25 mg, 50 mg, 75 mg, 100 mg, 150 mg, 200 mg, 225 mg, 300 mg
- Oral solution: 20 mg/mL

How to Dose
- When initiating pregabalin treatment, start with a low dose and titrate slowly so as to minimize adverse effects
  - *For adults:* start treatment with 50 mg/day in two divided doses; subsequently at 7-day intervals increase in steps of 50 mg daily to 300 mg daily in two to three divided doses; maintenance dose

P

generally not greater than 600 mg/day given in two or three equally divided doses

Although dosage recommendations for children have not been provided, the following suggestions are based on general rules of dosage requirements in infants and children:

- In a *child less than 16 years:* start treatment with 1.5–2.0 mg/kg twice daily (3.5 mg/kg/day) for 1 week; increase by 3.0–3.5 mg/kg/day in divided doses as tolerated and as needed at weekly intervals; maximum dose 7.5 mg/kg twice daily (15 mg/kg/day)
- In an *infant:* start treatment with 2.5 mg/kg twice daily (5.0 mg/kg/day) for 1 week; increase by 5.0 mg/kg/day in divided doses as tolerated and as needed at weekly intervals; maximum dose 10 mg/kg twice daily (20 mg/kg/day)

Dosing Tips
- Titration of dose should be undertaken based on individual tolerability and response to the drug
- Patients should be informed that in the event of the need to withdraw pregabalin they may experience a variety of withdrawal symptoms (insomnia, headache, nausea, diarrhea, flu syndrome, nervousness, depression, pain, sweating, and dizziness)

How to Withdraw Drug
- There is no need to adjust dosage of concurrent medications as pregabalin is being discontinued, because plasma levels of other drugs do not change (see Pharmacokinetic Drug Interactions section)
- Taper: a gradual dose reduction over a minimum of a 1-week period should be undertaken
- Withdrawal may be associated with a variety of symptoms, including: insomnia, headache, nausea, diarrhea, flu syndrome, nervousness, depression, pain, sweating, and dizziness
- Rapid discontinuation may induce withdrawal seizures

Overdose
- In overdoses up to 15 g, no unexpected adverse effects were observed
- The most common adverse effects observed with pregabalin overdose include somnolence, confusional state, agitation, and restlessness
- If indicated, the stomach should be emptied by lavage or by induction of emesis
- Hemodialysis removes pregabalin from blood (50% over 4 hours) and, therefore, may be a useful procedure in cases of overdose

Tests and Therapeutic Drug Monitoring
- Before starting: kidney function tests may be useful in elderly or those with renal impairment to guide dosing of pregabalin
- During treatment: follow kidney function tests, which may be useful in elderly or those with renal impairment to guide dosing of pregabalin

PREGABALIN

P

- Therapeutic drug monitoring:
  - There are no data relating the plasma concentration of pregabalin with that of seizure suppression
  - Thus, although routine monitoring of pregabalin is not recommended, measurement of plasma pregabalin concentrations as a "benchmark," with sporadic re-measurement may be useful as a check on compliance/adherence
  - There are no data indicating the usefulness of monitoring pregabalin by use of saliva
- Before giving a drug that can cause weight gain to an overweight or obese patient, consider determining whether the patient already has pre-diabetes (fasting plasma glucose 100–125 mg/dL), diabetes (fasting plasma glucose greater than 126 mg/dL), or dyslipidemia (increased total cholesterol, LDL cholesterol, and triglycerides; decreased HDL cholesterol), and treat or refer such patients for treatment, including nutrition and weight management, physical activity counseling, smoking cessation, and medical management
- Monitor weight and BMI during treatment

Other Warnings/Precautions
- Some diabetic patients who gain weight on pregabalin treatment may need to adjust their hypoglycemic medications
- Some patients may experience dizziness and somnolence and thus caution needs to be exercised if patient intends to drive or use machinery

Do not Use
- If patient has a proven allergy to pregabalin or gabapentin or to any of the excipients – tablets contain lactose
- Because the tablets contain lactose, patients with rare hereditary problems of galactose intolerance, Lapp lactose deficiency, or glucose–galactose malabsorption should not take this formulation

Special Populations
Renal Impairment
- Pregabalin is renally excreted, so the dose needs to be adjusted according to CrCl as follows:
  - CrCl of ≥60 mL/min – starting dose: 150 mg/day taken twice or three times a day; maximum dose: 600 mg/day
  - CrCl of ≥30-<60 mL/min – starting dose: 75 mg/day taken twice or three times a day; maximum dose: 300 mg/day
  - CrCl of ≥15-<30 mL/min – starting dose: 25–50 mg/day taken once or twice a day; maximum dose: 150 mg/day
  - CrCl of <15 mL/min – starting dose: 25 mg/day taken once a day; maximum dose: 75 mg/day

- Because pregabalin can be removed by hemodialysis, patients receiving hemodialysis may require supplemental doses of pregabalin

Hepatic Impairment
- Because pregabalin is not metabolized and is excreted as unchanged drug in urine, dosage adjustment will not be necessary in patients with hepatic impairment

Children
- Pregabalin is not licensed for use in children

Elderly
- Elderly patients are more susceptible to adverse effects and therefore may not tolerate higher doses
- Because of an age-related reduction in renal function, lower initial and target pregabalin doses are appropriate and should be based on CrCl values
- Because pregabalin is associated with dizziness and somnolence, the elderly may be at increased risk of falls
- The elderly have an increased risk of confusion and mental impairment
- Elderly patients are often prescribed concurrent drug therapies for comorbidities and therefore may be at greater risk for pharmacokinetic and pharmacodynamic interactions; as the risk of pharmacokinetic interactions with pregabalin is low or non-existent, pregabalin may be advantageous for use in the elderly

Pregnancy
- Specialist advice should be given to women who are of childbearing potential; they should be informed about the teratogenicity of all AEDs and the importance of avoiding an unplanned pregnancy; the AED treatment regimen should be reviewed when a woman is planning to become pregnant
- Rapid discontinuation of AEDs should be avoided as this may lead to breakthrough seizures, which could have serious consequences for the woman and the unborn child
- Pregabalin was previously classified by the US FDA as risk category C (some animal studies show adverse effects, no controlled studies in humans); the current FDA Pregnancy and Lactation Rule has eliminated pregnancy risk category labels; recent data on the risk of major congenital malformations following first-trimester exposure to pregabalin monotherapy are conflicting, with one study indicating a signal of increased risk, while another suggested no increased risk with pregabalin exposure
- Use in women of childbearing potential requires weighing potential benefits to the mother against the risks to the fetus

- Use with other AEDs in combination may cause a higher risk for teratogenic effects than pregabalin monotherapy
- Taper drug if discontinuing
- Seizures, even mild seizures, may cause harm to the embryo/fetus
- During pregnancy, pregabalin pharmacokinetics do not change

Breast Feeding
- Breast milk: ~75% of maternal plasma levels
- Breastfed infants: it is not known what plasma pregabalin concentrations are achieved in breastfed infants compared with the levels of their mothers. However, the pregabalin dose from breast milk is estimated to be ~7% of the total daily maternal dose
- If drug is continued while breast feeding, infant should be monitored for possible adverse effects
- If adverse effects are observed, recommend bottle feeding

The Overall Place of Pregabalin in the Treatment of Epilepsy
Pregabalin is a narrow-spectrum AED with an expanding role in the management of partial (focal) seizures. Pregabalin is primarily used as adjunctive therapy in patients with refractory partial/focal seizures who have failed to respond to other AED combinations.

Primary Seizure Types
- Partial (focal) seizures with or without secondary generalization

Secondary Seizure Types
- None

Potential Advantages
- Pregabalin is generally well tolerated, with only mild adverse effects, although it can have more substantial adverse effects at higher doses
- Because it is not metabolized by the liver and excreted exclusively by renal elimination, pregabalin is not associated with any significant pharmacokinetic interactions
- Drug absorption and clinical efficacy may be more consistent for pregabalin compared with gabapentin because of its highly consistent and linear absorption due to transportation by more than one transport system in the gastrointestinal tract

Potential Disadvantages
- Exaggerates myoclonus
- Requires two to three times a day dosing
- Unknown teratogenic potential

P

PREGABALIN

Suggested Reading

Ben-Menachem E. Pregabalin pharmacology and its relevance to clinical practice. *Epilepsia* 2004; **45** (Suppl 6): 13–18.

Corrigan BW, Poole WF, Posvar EL, Strand JC, Alvey CW, Radulovic LL. Metabolic disposition of pregabalin in healthy volunteers. *Clinical Pharmacology and Therapeutics* 2001; **69**: P18.

Elger CE, Brodie MJ, Anhut H, Lee CM, Barrett JA. Pregabalin add-on treatment in patients with partial seizures: a novel evaluation of flexible-dose and fixed-dose treatment in a double-blind, placebo-controlled study. *Epilepsia* 2005; **46**: 1926–1936.

Lockwood PA, Pauer L, Scavone JM, Allard M, Mendes da Costa L, Alebic-Kolbah T, Plotka A, Alvey CW, Chew ML. The pharmacokinetics of pregabalin in breast milk, plasma, and urine of healthy postpartum women. *Journal of Human Lactation* 2016; **32**: NP1–NP6.

Patorno E, Bateman BT, Huybrechts KF, MacDonald SC, Cohen JM, Desai RJ, Panchaud A, Mogun H, Pennell PB, Hernandez-Diaz S. Pregabalin use early in pregnancy and the risk of major congenital malformations. *Neurology* 2017; **88**: 2020–2025.

Patsalos PN. *Antiepileptic drug interactions: a clinical guide*, 3rd edition. Springer, London, UK; 2016.

Patsalos PN, Zugman M, Lake C, James A, Ratnaraj N, Sander JW. Serum protein binding of 25 antiepileptic drugs in a routine clinical setting: a comparison of free non-protein-bound concentrations. *Epilepsia* 2017; **58**: 1234–1243.

Randnitis EJ, Posver EL, Alvey CW, Sedman AJ, Cook JA, Bockbrader HN. Pharmacokinetics of pregabalin in subjects with various degrees of renal function. *Journal of Clinical Pharmacology* 2003; **43**: 277–283.

Taylor CP, Angelotti T, Fauman E. Pharmacology and mechanism of action of pregabalin: the calcium channel α2-δ (alpha2 – delta) subunit as a target for antiepileptic drug discovery. *Epilepsy Research* 2007; **73**: 137–150.

Winterfeld U, Merlob P, Baud D, Rousson V, Panchaud A, Rothuizen LE, Bernard N, Vial T, Yates LM, Pistelli A, Ellfolk M, Eleftheriou G, de Vries LC, Jonville-Bera AP, Kadioglu M, Biollaz J, Buclin T. Pregnancy outcome following maternal exposure to pregabalin may call for concern. *Neurology* 2016; **86**: 2251–2257.

PRIMIDONE

P

Therapeutics
Chemical Name and Structure
Primidone, 5-ethyldihydro-5-phenyl-4,6(1-H,5H)pyrimidinedione, is a white crystalline substance, with a molecular weight of 218.25 and an empirical formula of $C_{12}H_{14}N_2O_2$.

Brand Names
- Apo-Primidone
- Cyral
- Liskantin
- Majsolin; Mizodin; Mutigan; Mylepsinum; Myidone; Mysoline
- Primidon; Prysoline
- Sertan

Generics Available
- Yes

Licensed Indications for Epilepsy
- Monotherapy or adjunctive therapy in the control of grand mal, psychomotor, and focal seizures in adults and children (FDA PI)
- For the management of grand mal and psychomotor (temporal lobe) epilepsy (UK SPC)
- For the management of focal and Jacksonian seizures, myoclonic jerks, and akinetic attacks (UK SPC)

Licensed Indications for Non-epilepsy Conditions
- Essential tremor (UK SPC)

Non-licensed Use for Epilepsy
- Juvenile myoclonic epilepsy
- Primarily generalized tonic–clonic seizures

Non-licensed Use for Non-epilepsy Conditions
- Holmes' tremor

Ineffective (Contraindicated)
- Absence seizures

THERAPEUTICS

P

PRIMIDONE

Mechanism of Action

Because primidone is rapidly converted to phenobarbital, it is considered that phenobarbital is the primary contributor to the pharmacological effects of primidone

- The mechanism of action of primidone itself has not been elucidated
- Primidone exerts well-demonstrated seizure protection that is independent from phenobarbital
- Mechanisms of action demonstrated for phenobarbital include:
  - Enhancement of GABA inhibition
  - Enhances postsynaptic $GABA_A$ receptor–mediated chloride currents by prolonging the opening of the chloride-ionophore
  - Concentration-dependent reduction of calcium-dependent action potentials

Efficacy Profile

- The goals of treatment are to achieve complete seizure remission when possible, or at least improved frequency and severity of seizures, while also minimizing adverse effects and improving patient quality of life
- The full therapeutic effect of primidone may not be achieved until steady-state levels of phenobarbital are reached
- Being converted to phenobarbital, primidone will have all of the efficacies of phenobarbital
- Once chronic therapy is initiated, it is usually continued for at least 2 years following the last seizure
- Used mainly for partial seizures and generalized convulsive seizures
- In contrast to phenobarbital, primidone is not used in neonates with seizure
- Although phenobarbital has proven efficacy for the prophylactic treatment of febrile seizures, primidone is not used for this indication
- Juvenile myoclonic epilepsy also responds to primidone, although it is no longer a drug of first choice because valproic acid and other AEDs have become available
- If primidone is ineffective or only partially effective, it can be replaced by or combined with another AED that is appropriate for the patient's seizure type or epilepsy syndrome

Pharmacokinetics

Absorption and Distribution

- Oral bioavailability: >90%
- Food co-ingestion: it is not known whether the rate of absorption or the extent of absorption is affected by food co-ingestion
- Tmax: 2–4 hours (adults); 4–6 hours (children)
- Time to steady state: 2–4 days (primidone); 15–29 days (for derived phenobarbital)
- Pharmacokinetics: linear

P

- Protein binding: 10%
- Volume of distribution: 0.5–0.8 L/kg
- Salivary concentrations: it is not known whether primidone is secreted into saliva and whether such concentrations are similar to the unbound levels seen in plasma

Metabolism
- Primidone is metabolized in the liver to two primary metabolites, namely phenobarbital and phenyl-ethyl-malonamide (PEMA)
- Phenobarbital subsequently undergoes metabolism to two metabolites, *p*-hydroxyphenobarbital and 9-D-glucopyranosylphenobarbital
- PEMA is pharmacologically active and can be measured in the plasma of patients taking primidone, but has a much lower potency than primidone and phenobarbital
- At steady state during chronic primidone therapy, plasma levels of primidone and phenobarbital are similar (phenobarbital:primidone ratio ~1.5), but during co-medication with an enzyme-inducing drug, phenobarbital plasma levels may be three to five times higher than primidone levels
- Phenobarbital undergoes autoinduction so that its clearance can increase and this may require an upward dosage adjustment of primidone when prescribed as monotherapy

Elimination
- In the absence of enzyme-inducing AEDs, half-life values for primidone in adults are 7–22 hours
- In the presence of enzyme-inducing co-medication, half-life values for primidone in adults are 3–12 hours
- Half-life values in children are 5–11 hours
- Half-life values in newborns are 8–80 hours
- Renal excretion: during monotherapy ~65% of an administered dose is excreted as unchanged primidone in urine; during polytherapy with enzyme-inducing AEDs only ~40% is excreted as unchanged primidone in urine

Drug Interaction Profile
Pharmacokinetic Drug Interactions
Because phenobarbital is invariably present during long-term primidone treatment, all of the effects of phenobarbital on other drugs described previously for phenobarbital can be expected with primidone, and all of the interactions affecting phenobarbital will also affect the phenobarbital derived from primidone.
- Interactions between AEDs: effects on primidone and phenobarbital:
  - See Phenobarbital section
  - Acetazolamide *decreases* the gastrointestinal absorption of primidone and can *decrease* primidone plasma levels

P

- Carbamazepine and phenytoin can accelerate the conversion of primidone to phenobarbital, which results in *decreased* primidone levels and *increased* phenobarbital levels
- Clobazam, ethosuximide, and stiripentol can *increase* plasma levels of primidone
- Methsuximide, sulthiame, and valproic acid can *increase* plasma levels of phenobarbital
- Interactions between AEDs: effects by primidone:
  - See Phenobarbital section
- Interactions between AEDs and non-AED drugs: effects on primidone and phenobarbital:
  - See Phenobarbital section
  - Isoniazid and nicotinamide inhibit primidone biotransformation, resulting in an *increase* in primidone plasma levels and a *decrease* in phenobarbital plasma levels
- Interactions between AEDs and non-AED drugs: effects by primidone:
  - See Phenobarbital section

Pharmacodynamic Drug Interactions
- Perampanel in combination with primidone can be associated with an increased risk of decreased appetite

Hormonal Contraception
- Primidone enhances the metabolism of oral contraceptives so as to decrease plasma levels of hormonal contraceptives and to reduce their effectiveness, leading to breakthrough bleeding and contraceptive failure; medium- or high-dose oral contraceptive preparations are indicated in patients taking primidone; in addition to recommendations for additional barrier contraceptives and folic acid 1,000 mg daily in all women of childbearing potential

Adverse Effects
How Drug Causes Adverse Effects
- Mechanism by which primidone causes adverse effects has not been established and is presumed to be the same as the mechanism invoked for its efficacy
- In most instances, it is not possible to separate the adverse effects caused by primidone from those caused by phenobarbital
- Because of the conversion to and significant accumulation of phenobarbital, primidone treatment can be associated with all the adverse effects of phenobarbital
- The acute initial toxicity clearly differentiates primidone and phenobarbital; even after a low initial dose of primidone, some patients experience transient adverse effects – usually drowsiness, dizziness, ataxia, nausea, and vomiting – that are so debilitating that they may

be reluctant to take another dose; because this acute toxic reaction occurs before phenobarbital or PEMA is detected in the blood, it is considered to be caused by primidone itself
• Tolerance rapidly develops to the initial acute toxicity of primidone

Common Adverse Effects
The adverse effects listed below are attributable to primidone, pheno-barbital, or both:
• Sedation and drowsiness
• Hyperactivity and irritability (especially in children)
• CNS-related adverse effects are usually dose-dependent and are reversible: dysarthria, ataxia, incoordination, and nystagmus
• Depression
• Cognitive impairment
• Decreased bone mineral density

Life-threatening or Dangerous Adverse Effects
• Stevens–Johnson syndrome, erythema multiforme, toxic epidermal necrolysis (very rare)
• Hypersensitivity reactions, may lead to hepatic failure

Rare and not Life-threatening Adverse Effects
• Movement disorders, such as dyskinesia, may be induced by phenobarbital
• Seizure exacerbation or de novo seizures
• Hematologic toxicity, mainly megaloblastic anemia
• Exacerbation of acute intermittent porphyria
• Vitamin K-deficient hemorrhagic disease in newborns of mothers treated with primidone/phenobarbital; can be prevented by adminis-tration of vitamin K to the mother before delivery
• Connective tissue disorders associated with long-term phenobarbital therapy (unusual in children), such as Dupuytren contractures, plantar fibromatosis, heel and knuckle pads, frozen shoulder, Peyronie disease, and diffuse joint pain
• Loss of libido and erectile dysfunction

Weight Change
• Not common

What to do About Adverse Effects
• Discuss common and severe adverse effects with patients or parents before starting medication, including symptoms that should be reported to the physician
• Primidone must be started at a low dose to avoid acute initial toxicity
• Dosage reduction in cases of presumably dose-related adverse effects
• Consider calcium and vitamin D supplements in cases of low 25-hydroxyvitamin D levels and/or decreased bone mineral density

P

ADVERSE EFFECTS

P

Dosing and Use

Usual Dosage Range
- Adults and children >8 years: 750–1500 mg/day (10–20 mg/kg/day)
- Children 2–8 years: 10–20 mg/kg
- Infants (<2 years of age): 10–25 mg/kg/day
- Newborns: 15–25 mg/kg/day

Available Formulations
- Tablets: 50 mg, 250 mg
- Suspension: 250 mg/5 mL

How to Dose
- *For adults and children over 8 years of age:* start treatment with 125 mg at night; the dose can then be increased every 3 days as tolerated, to a final daily maintenance dose of 10–20 mg/kg/day; some patients initially need as little as one-quarter tablet (62.5 mg) or a 50-mg tablet. Divide daily dose into two to three doses
- *Children and infants:* start treatment with 50 mg or less at night; the dose can then be increased every 3 days as tolerated, to a final maintenance dose of 10–25 mg/kg/day in infants, and 10–20 mg/kg/day in children. Divide daily dose into two to three doses
- *Newborns:* 15–25 mg/kg/day in divided doses two to four times/day; start with lower dosage and titrate upward; conversion of primidone to phenobarbital is slow in newborns, and phenobarbital levels are lower than primidone levels, even after 5 days of treatment

Dosing Tips
- Given the relatively short half-life of primidone, the daily dose of primidone is usually divided into two or more doses
- In neonates, infants, and children, it is preferable to divide the daily dose into three divided doses

How to Withdraw Drug
- May need to adjust dosage of concurrent medications as primidone is being discontinued, because plasma levels of other drugs may change (see Pharmacokinetic Drug Interactions section)
- After long-term administration, primidone should always be discontinued gradually over several weeks
- Barbiturates and benzodiazepines are the AEDs most commonly associated with withdrawal seizures upon rapid discontinuation
- Unless there is a specific reason to proceed faster, it is appropriate to taper the primidone dose linearly over 3–6 months, with reductions every 2–4 weeks

Overdose
- Similar to phenobarbital (see Phenobarbital section), but primidone overdose can specifically cause crystalluria, with possible renal failure,

especially at primidone plasma levels of 200 mg/L (920 µmol/L) or above

- Can be fatal, mostly secondary to cardiorespiratory failure
- Symptoms include: constricted pupils, nystagmus, ataxia, somnolence, stupor or coma, pulmonary edema, and respiratory failure
- In individuals who have not been previously exposed to phenobarbital, plasma levels at or above 80 mg/L are considered lethal
- Higher plasma levels may be tolerated by patients on chronic phenobarbital therapy
- Treatment consists mainly of cardiorespiratory support
- Alkalinization with sodium bicarbonate, iv hydration, and forced diuresis accelerate the elimination of phenobarbital through the kidneys
- The stomach should be emptied immediately by lavage or by induction of emesis
- Hemodialysis removes phenobarbital from blood and, therefore, serves as a useful procedure in cases of primidone overdose
- It is not known whether hemodialysis removes primidone from blood and, therefore, could serve as a useful procedure in cases of overdose

Tests and Therapeutic Drug Monitoring

- Monitoring of blood count and liver function tests usually not necessary
- Because primidone therapy can alter vitamin D metabolism and affect bone mineral density, 25-hydroxyvitamin D levels should be monitored in all patients, and vitamin D supplementation should be prescribed as needed; consider also DEXA bone scan in patients at risk for osteopenia
- Therapeutic drug monitoring:
  - Optimum seizure control in patients on monotherapy is most likely to occur at phenobarbital plasma concentrations of 10–40 mg/L (43–172 µmol/L)
  - Optimum seizure control in patients on monotherapy is most likely to occur at primidone plasma concentrations of 5–10 mg/L (23–46 µmol/L)
  - The phenobarbital conversion factor from mg/L to µmol/L is 4.31 (i.e., 1 mg/L = 4.31 µmol/L)
  - The primidone conversion factor from mg/L to µmol/L is 4.59 (1 mg/L = 4.59 µmol/L)
  - Monitoring primidone levels is of little help in clinical practice; if blood levels are used to adjust the primidone dose, then phenobarbital rather than primidone levels are preferred because, at the usual concentration ratios, the adverse effects from a high phenobarbital level are more likely to limit further dosage increases
  - The reference range of phenobarbital (and primidone) in plasma is considered to be the same for children and adults, although no data are available to support this clinical practice

P

DOSING AND USE

P

PRIMIDONE

- Phenobarbital can be monitored by use of saliva which is a measure of the free non-protein-bound plasma concentration and is pharmacologically relevant
- There are no data indicating the usefulness of monitoring primidone by use of saliva

Do not Use
- In patients with known history of allergic reaction to barbiturates
- In patients with known history of intermittent acute porphyria
- For the treatment of absence seizures

Special Populations
Renal Impairment
- Primidone and phenobarbital are renally secreted, therefore, the dose of primidone may need to be lowered

Hepatic Impairment
- Primidone is substantially metabolized and phenobarbital is extensively metabolized in the liver and consequently lower doses of primidone may be required

Children
- Children have an increased metabolic capacity and consequently higher doses on an mg/kg/day basis are usually required to achieve the equivalent therapeutic plasma levels seen in adults
- Pharmacokinetic interactions in children are usually of a greater magnitude than that seen in adults

Elderly
- Elderly patients are more susceptible to adverse effects of primidone and phenobarbital (especially somnolence) and, therefore may not tolerate higher doses
- Because of an age-related reduction in renal and hepatic function, lower primidone doses are appropriate
- Invariably the elderly are prescribed drug therapies for concurrent comorbidities and, therefore, the risk of pharmacokinetic interactions with primidone is substantial

Pregnancy
- Specialist advice should be given to women who are of childbearing potential; they should be informed about the teratogenicity of all AEDs and the importance of avoiding an unplanned pregnancy; the AED treatment regimen should be reviewed when a woman is planning to become pregnant

P

- Rapid discontinuation of AEDs should be avoided as this may lead to breakthrough seizures, which could have serious consequences for the woman and the unborn child
- Primidone was previously classified by the US FDA as risk category D (positive evidence of risk to human fetus; potential benefits may still justify its use during pregnancy); the current FDA Pregnancy and Lactation Rule has eliminated pregnancy risk category labels; analysis of a recent pregnancy registry revealed that phenobarbital was associated with a higher risk of congenital malformations than most other AEDs, in particular cardiac defects and oral clefts; because of the conversion of primidone to phenobarbital, this increased risk is likely to be associated with primidone therapy also
- Supplementation with folic acid may reduce the risk of congenital abnormalities
- Use in women of childbearing potential requires weighing potential benefits to the mother against the risks to the fetus
- Seizures, even mild seizures, may cause harm to the embryo/fetus
- Use with other AEDs in combination may cause a higher prevalence of teratogenic effects than primidone monotherapy
- Taper drug if discontinuing
- Vitamin K-deficient hemorrhagic disease in newborns of mothers treated with phenobarbital or primidone; can be prevented by administration of vitamin K to the mother before delivery
- During pregnancy primidone pharmacokinetics change significantly so that at late gestation primidone clearance increases by ~20%, whereas plasma concentrations of derived phenobarbital decrease by 50–70%, the latter due to increased clearance and reduction in albumin concentrations; an increase in primidone dose may be required in some patients

Breast Feeding
- Breast milk: 40–96% (mean, 75%) of maternal plasma levels
- Breast milk: phenobarbital: 30–50% of maternal plasma levels
- Breastfed infants: primidone can accumulate to levels that are similar to maternal plasma levels
- Breastfed infants: phenobarbital plasma levels may reach 50–>100% of maternal plasma levels
- If drug is continued while breast feeding, infant should be monitored for possible adverse effects, including sedation, poor sucking and weight gain, and vomiting
- If adverse effects are observed, recommend bottle feeding

The Overall Place of Primidone in the Treatment of Epilepsy

Primidone is currently a drug of second or third choice in patients with partial (focal) onset or generalized convulsive seizures. Because of its sedative and cognitive effects, it is never a drug of first choice. Its

THE EPILEPSY PRESCRIBER'S GUIDE TO ANTIEPILEPTIC DRUGS

P

PRIMIDONE

spectrum of use is more limited than that of phenobarbital, but it may at times be effective when other drugs have failed.

Primary Seizure Types
• Partial (focal) and secondary generalized seizures

Secondary Seizure Types
• Juvenile myoclonic epilepsy
• Primarily generalized tonic–clonic seizures

Potential Advantages
• Low systemic toxicity
• Relatively inexpensive

Potential Disadvantages
• Primidone and phenobarbital produce more sedative and behavioral adverse effects than most other AEDs
• Associated with significant pharmacokinetic interactions and usually acts as an inducer of hepatic metabolism
• Potential teratogen

Suggested Reading

Hernandez-Diaz S, Smith CR, Shen A, Mittendorf R, Hauser WA, Yerby M, Holmes LB. Comparative safety of antiepileptic drugs during pregnancy. *Neurology* 2012; **78**: 1692–1699.

Kjaer D, Horvath-Puho E, Christensen J, Vestergaard M, Czeizel AE, Sorensen HT, Olsen J. Antiepileptic drug use, folic acid supplementation, and congenital abnormalities: a population-based case-control study. *British Journal of Obstetrics and Gynaecology* 2008; **115**: 98–103.

Kuhnz W, Koch S, Helge H, Nau H. Primidone and phenobarbital during lactation period in epileptic women: total and free drug serum levels in the nursed infants and their effects on neonatal behavior. *Developmental Pharmacology and Therapeutics* 1988; **11**: 147–154.

Leppik IE, Cloyd JC, Miller K. Development of tolerance to the side effects of primidone. *Therapeutic Drug Monitoring* 1984; **6**: 189–191.

Mattson RH, Cramer JA, Collins JF, Smith DB, Delgado-Escueta AV, Browne TR, Williamson PD, Treiman DM, McNamara JO, McCutchen CB. Comparison of carbamazepine, phenobarbital, phenytoin, and primidone in partial and secondarily generalized tonic-clonic seizures. *New England Journal of Medicine* 1985; **313**: 145–151.

Nau H, Rating D, Hauser I, Jäger E, Koch S, Helge H. Placental transfer and pharmacokinetics of primidone and its metabolites phenobarbital, PEMA and hydroxyphenobarbital in neonates and infants of

264

epileptic mothers. *European Journal of Clinical Pharmacology* 1980; **18**: 31–42.

Patsalos PN. *Antiepileptic drug interactions: a clinical guide*, 3rd edition. Springer, London, UK; 2016.

Sapin JI, Riviello JJ, Grover WD. Efficacy of primidone for seizure control in neonates and young infants. *Pediatric Neurology* 1988; **4**: 292–295.

Shellhaas RA, Barks AK, Joshi SM. Prevalence and risk factors for vitamin D insufficiency among children with epilepsy. *Pediatric Neurology* 2010; **42**: 422–426.

van Heijst AN, de Jong W, Seldenrijk R, van Dijk A. Coma and crystalluria: a massive primidone intoxication treated with haemoperfusion. *Journal of Toxicology and Clinical Toxicology* 1983; **20**: 307–318.

P

SUGGESTED READING

R RUFINAMIDE

Therapeutics

Chemical Name and Structure

Rufinamide, 1-[(2,6-difluorophenyl) methyl]-1-hydro-1,23-triazole-4-carboxamide, is a white powder, with a molecular weight of 238.19 and an empirical formula of $C_{10}H_8F_2N_4O$.

Brand Names
• Banzel
• Inovelon

Generics Available
• No

Licensed Indications for Epilepsy
• Adjunctive treatment of seizures in Lennox–Gastaut syndrome in patients 4 years and older (UK SPC; FDA PI)

Licensed Indications for Non-epilepsy Conditions
• There are none

Non-licensed Use for Epilepsy
• Epileptic spasms
• Myoclonic-astatic epilepsy
• Partial (focal) seizures
• Status epilepticus

Non-licensed Use for Non-epilepsy Conditions
• There are none

Ineffective (Contraindicated)
• Data on seizure contraindications are not available

Mechanism of Action
• Acts as a blocker of voltage-sensitive sodium channels

R

- Prevents sodium channels from returning to an activated state (from an inactivated state), thereby preventing the generation of sustained bursts of high-frequency action potentials

Efficacy Profile
- The goals of treatment are to achieve complete seizure remission when possible, or at least improved frequency and severity of seizures, while also minimizing adverse effects and improving patient quality of life
- Efficacy should be apparent within 4 weeks of treatment initiation
- If it is not producing clinical benefits within 6–8 weeks, it may require a dosage increase or it may not work at all
- If rufinamide is ineffective or only partially effective, it can be replaced by or combined with another AED that is appropriate for the patient's seizure type or epilepsy syndrome

Pharmacokinetics
Absorption and Distribution
- Oral bioavailability: not determined; however, it is dose-dependent in that as dose increases the bioavailability decreases
- Food co-ingestion: substantially (mean, 44%) increases the amount of rufinamide absorbed, maximum serum concentration (Cmax) values are increased by ~100%, whereas Tmax values are shortened (6 hours vs. 8 hours when fasted)
- Tmax: 4–6 hours
- Time to steady state: 1–2 days
- Pharmacokinetics: linear up to 1600 mg/day; non-linear >1600 mg/day due to reduced oral bioavailability
- Protein binding: 35%
- Volume of distribution: 0.71–1.14 L/kg
- Salivary concentrations: rufinamide is secreted into saliva and concentrations are similar to the unbound levels seen in plasma

Metabolism
- Rufinamide is metabolized in the liver, primarily by hydrolysis which is not CYP-dependent, to CGP 47292
- CGP 47292 is excreted in urine (~70%) and feces (~9%)
- Approximately 7% is excreted in urine as minor acyl-glucuronide metabolites of CGP 47292
- The metabolites of rufinamide are not pharmacologically active
- Autoinduction is not a feature of rufinamide metabolism

Elimination
- The plasma half-life in healthy volunteers and in patients with epilepsy is 6–10 hours
- Clearance values in children can be expected to be ~50% greater

R

- Clearance values in females are lower than for males
- Renal excretion: ~4% of an administered dose is excreted unchanged in urine

Drug Interaction Profile
Pharmacokinetic Drug Interactions
- Interactions between AEDs: effects on rufinamide:
  - Carbamazepine, methsuximide, oxcarbazepine, phenobarbital, phenytoin, primidone, and vigabatrin can *increase* the clearance of rufinamide and *decrease* rufinamide plasma levels
  - Valproic acid can *decrease* the clearance of rufinamide and *increase* rufinamide plasma levels
- Interactions between AEDs: effects by rufinamide:
  - Rufinamide can *decrease* plasma levels of carbamazepine and lamotrigine
  - Rufinamide can *increase* plasma levels of phenobarbital and phenytoin
- Interactions between AEDs and non-AED drugs: effects on rufinamide:
  - To date, there have been no reports of other non-AED drugs affecting the clearance of rufinamide and affecting rufinamide plasma levels
- Interactions between AEDs and non-AED drugs: effects by rufinamide:
  - Rufinamide can *decrease* plasma levels of triazolam

Pharmacodynamic Drug Interactions
- To date, none have been reported

Hormonal Contraception
- Rufinamide enhances the metabolism of oral contraceptives so as to decrease plasma levels of hormonal contraceptives and to reduce their effectiveness, leading to breakthrough bleeding and contraceptive failure; medium- or high-dose oral contraceptive preparations are indicated in patients taking rufinamide; in addition to recommendations for additional barrier contraceptives and folic acid 1 mg daily in all women of childbearing potential

Adverse Effects
How Drug Causes Adverse Effects
- Not known

Common Adverse Effects
- Dizziness, diplopia, somnolence
- Nausea, vomiting, fatigue

RUFINAMIDE

268

Life-threatening or Dangerous Adverse Effects
- Hypersensitivity syndrome (fever, rash, lymphadenopathy, liver function test abnormalities, and hematuria)
- Decreases QTc interval, therefore, patients with congenital short QT syndrome or a family history of the syndrome may be at risk
- Increased frequency of status epilepticus

Rare and not Life-threatening Adverse Effects
- To date, there are none

Weight Change
- Weight loss may occur

What to do About Adverse Effects
- Discuss common and severe adverse effects with patients or parents before starting medication, including symptoms that should be reported to the physician
- CNS-related adverse effects are usually dose-dependent, are reversible, and are prevented by slow and upward titration following initiation of treatment
- Risk of serious adverse effects is greatest in the first few months of treatment
- Common adverse effects such as sedation often abate after a few months

Dosing and Use
Usual Dosage Range
- Weight range <30 kg: up to a maximum dose of 1000 mg/day
- Weight range 30–50 kg: up to a maximum dose of 1800 mg/day
- Weight range 50.1–70 kg: up to a maximum dose of 2400 mg/day
- Weight range >70 kg: up to a maximum dose of 3200 mg/day

Available Formulations
- Tablets: 100 mg, 200 mg, 400 mg

How to Dose
- When initiating rufinamide treatment start with a low dose and titrate slowly so as to minimize adverse effects.
  - *For children 4 years of age or older and less than 30 kg and not receiving valproic acid:* start treatment with 100 mg twice daily; every 2 days increase by 200 mg/day in divided doses; maintenance dose generally 1000 mg/day
  - *For children 4 years of age or older and less than 30 kg and receiving valproic acid:* start treatment with 100 mg twice daily; every 2 days increase by 200 mg/day in divided doses; maintenance dose generally 400–600 mg/day

R

DOSING AND USE

269

R

RUFINAMIDE

- *For adults and children 4 years or older of 30 kg or over:* start treatment with 200 mg twice daily; every 2 days increase by 400 mg/day in divided doses; maintenance dose generally 1800 mg/day (30–50 kg), 2400 mg/day (50.1–70 kg), and 3200 mg/day (>70 kg)

Dosing Tips
- Should be ingested twice daily with water in the morning and in the evening, in two equally divided doses.
- As food enhances the absorption of rufinamide, it is preferable to ingest rufinamide with food
- If patient has difficulty swallowing, tablets can be crushed and administered in half a glass of water

How to Withdraw Drug
- May need to adjust dosage of concurrent medications as rufinamide is being discontinued, because plasma levels of other drugs may change (see Pharmacokinetic Drug Interactions section)
- Taper: reduce dose by ~25% every 2 days
- Rapid discontinuation may increase the risk of seizures

Overdose
- To date, no cases have been reported
- If indicated the stomach should be emptied by lavage or by induction of emesis
- Hemodialysis removes 30% of rufinamide from blood and, therefore, may be a useful procedure in cases of overdose

Tests and Therapeutic Drug Monitoring
- Before starting: liver and kidney function tests
- Consider ECG to rule out short QT syndrome
- During treatment: liver and kidney function tests every 12 months
- Therapeutic drug monitoring:
  - Optimum seizure control in patients on monotherapy is most likely to occur at rufinamide plasma concentrations of 10–40 mg/L (42–168 µmol/L)
  - The conversion factor from mg/L to µmol/L is 4.20 (i.e., 1 mg/L = 4.20 µmol/L)
  - The reference range of rufinamide in plasma is considered to be the same for children and adults, although no data are available to support this clinical practice
  - Preliminary data suggest that rufinamide can be monitored by use of saliva, which is a measure of the free non-protein-bound plasma concentration that is pharmacologically relevant
  - There are no data indicating the usefulness of monitoring rufinamide by use of saliva

Other Warnings/Precautions
- To date, there are none

Do not Use
- If patient has congenital short QT syndrome or a family history of the syndrome
- If patient has a proven allergy to rufinamide or to any of the excipients, which include lactose
- Because formulation contains lactose, patients with rare hereditary problems of galactose intolerance, Lapp lactose deficiency, or glucose–galactose malabsorption should not take this medicine

Special Populations

Renal Impairment
- Rufinamide is renally secreted and thus the dose may need to be lowered in renally impaired patients
- Because rufinamide can be removed by hemodialysis, patients receiving hemodialysis may require supplemental doses of rufinamide

Hepatic Impairment
- Rufinamide is extensively metabolized in the liver and consequently lower doses may be required

Children
- Children have an increased metabolic capacity and consequently higher doses on a mg/kg basis are usually required to achieve the equivalent therapeutic plasma levels seen in adults
- Pharmacokinetic interactions in children are usually of a greater magnitude than that seen in adults

Elderly
- Elderly patients are more susceptible to adverse effects and, therefore, may not tolerate higher doses
- Because of an age-related reduction in hepatic function, lower rufinamide doses are appropriate
- Elderly patients frequently receive concurrent drug therapies for comorbidities, and therefore may be at greater risk for pharmacokinetic and pharmacodynamic interactions; the risk of pharmacokinetic interactions with rufinamide is moderate

Pregnancy
- Specialist advice should be given to women who are of childbearing potential; they should be informed about the teratogenicity of all AEDs and the importance of avoiding an unplanned pregnancy; the AED treatment regimen should be reviewed when a woman is planning to become pregnant
- Rapid discontinuation of AEDs should be avoided as this may lead to breakthrough seizures, which could have serious consequences for the woman and the unborn child

- Rufinamide was previously classified by the US FDA as risk category C (some animal studies show adverse effects, no controlled studies in humans); the current FDA Pregnancy and Lactation Rule has eliminated pregnancy risk category labels
- Use in women of childbearing potential requires weighing potential benefits to the mother against the risks to the fetus
- Use with other AEDs in combination may cause a higher prevalence of teratogenic effects than rufinamide monotherapy
- Taper drug if discontinuing
- Seizures, even mild seizures, may cause harm to the embryo/fetus
- Data on the pharmacokinetic changes of rufinamide during pregnancy are not available

Breast Feeding
- Breast milk: it is not known whether rufinamide is excreted in breast milk
- Breastfed infants: it is not known what plasma rufinamide concentrations are achieved in breastfed infants compared with the levels of their mothers
- If drug is continued while breast feeding, infant should be monitored for possible adverse effects (e.g., sedation)
- If adverse effects are observed, recommend bottle feeding

The Overall Place of Rufinamide in the Treatment of Epilepsy
Rufinamide is licensed by the European Medicines Agency as an orphan drug for use specifically as adjunctive treatment of seizures associated with Lennox–Gastaut syndrome in patients aged 4 years and older. Consequently it is too early to ascertain the place of rufinamide in the treatment of patients with epilepsy.

Primary Seizure Types
- Seizures associated with Lennox–Gastaut syndrome (absences, myoclonic, tonic, and atonic (drop attacks))

Secondary Seizure Types
- Partial (focal) seizures
- Epileptic spasms
- Myoclonic-astatic epilepsy

Potential Advantages
- Rufinamide is effective in Lennox–Gastaut syndrome, a difficult-to-treat syndromic epilepsy

Potential Disadvantages
- Non-linear bioavailability
- Need to co-ingest food so as to optimize bioavailability

- Associated with pharmacokinetic interactions
- Potential teratogen, but not more than most other AEDs

R

Suggested Reading
Arroyo S. Rufinamide. *Neurotherapeutics* 2007; **4**: 155–162.
Cardot JM, Lecaillon JB, Czendlik C, Godbillon J. The influence of food on the disposition of the antiepileptic rufinamide in healthy volunteers. *Biopharmacy and Drug Disposition* 1998; **19**: 259–262.
Coppola G, Besag F, Cusmai R, Dulac O, Kluger G, Moavero R, Nabbout R, Nikanorova M, Pisani F, Verrotti A, von Stulpnagel C, Curatolo P. Current role of rufinamide in the treatment of childhood epilepsy: literature review and treatment guidelines. *European Journal of Paediatric Neurology* 2014; **18**: 685–690.
Coppola G, Zamponi N, Kluger G, Mueller A, Anna Rita M, Parisi P, Isone C, Santoro E, Curatolo P, Verrotti A. Rufinamide for refractory focal seizures: an open-label, multicenter European study. *Seizure* 2013; **22**: 33–36.
Glauser T, Kluger G, Sachdeo R, Krauss G, Perdomo C, Arroyo S. Rufinamide for generalized seizures associated with Lennox–Gastaut syndrome. *Neurology* 2008; **70**: 1950–1958.
Mazzucchelli I, Rapetti M, Fattore C, Franco V, Gatti G, Perucca E. Development and validation of an HPLC-UV detection assay for the determination of rufinamide in human plasma and saliva. *Analytical and Bioanalytical Chemistry* 2011; **401**: 1013–1021.
Mourand I, Crespel A, Gelisse P. Dramatic weight loss with rufinamide. *Epilepsia* 2013; **54**: e5–e8.
Olson HE, Loddenkemper T, Vendrame M, Poduri A, Takeoka M, Bergin AM, Libenson MH, Duffy FH, Rotenberg A, Coulter D, Bourgeois BF, Kothare SV. Rufinamide for the treatment of epileptic spasms. *Epilepsy and Behavior* 2011; **20**: 344–348.
Perucca E, Cloyd J, Critchley D, Fuseau E. Rufinamide: clinical pharmacokinetics and concentration–response relationships in patients with epilepsy. *Epilepsia* 2008; **49**: 1123–1141.
Stülpnagel C von, Coppola G, Striano P, Müller A, Staudt M, Kluger G. First long-term experience with the orphan drug rufinamide in children with myoclonic-astatic epilepsy (Doose syndrome). *European Journal of Paediatric Neurology* 2012; **16**: 459–463.
Vendrame M, Loddenkemper T, Gooty VD, Takeoka M, Rotenberg A, Bergin AM, Eksioglu YZ, Poduri A, Duffy FH, Libenson M, Bourgeois BF, Kothare SV. Experience with rufinamide in a pediatric population: a single center's experience. *Pediatric Neurology* 2010; **43**: 155–158.

SUGGESTED READING

STIRIPENTOL

S (margin)

Therapeutics

Chemical Name and Structure

Stiripentol, 4,4-dimethyl-1[3,4(methylenedioxy)-phenyl]-1-pentan-3-ol, is a pale pink crystalline powder, with a molecular weight of 234 and an empirical formula of $C_{14}H_{18}O_3$.

Brand Names
• Diacomit

Generics Available
• No

Licensed Indications for Epilepsy
• Adjunctive treatment of seizures in children with severe myoclonic epilepsy in infancy (Dravet syndrome)
• Has been authorized under a "conditional approval" scheme by the European Medicines Agency (i.e., further evidence on stiripentol is awaited, in particular about its efficacy in combination with the maximum safe dose of the add-on therapy)

Licensed Indications for Non-epilepsy Conditions
• There are none

Non-licensed Use for Epilepsy
• Adjunctive treatment with carbamazepine in children with refractory partial (focal) seizures

Non-licensed Use for Non-epilepsy Conditions
• There are none

Ineffective (Contraindicated)
• Carbamazepine, phenytoin, and phenobarbital should not be used in conjunction with stiripentol in the management of Dravet syndrome

Mechanism of Action
• Increases brain GABA levels by inhibition of synaptic uptake of GABA and/or inhibition of GABA transaminase

S

- Enhances $GABA_A$ receptor-mediated transmission and increases the mean duration (but not the frequency) of $GABA_A$ receptor chloride channels by a barbiturate-like mechanism
- Most of the actions of stiripentol during adjunctive treatment are probably indirect and mediated by inhibition of CYP enzymes and increasing concurrent AED blood levels

Efficacy Profile
- The goals of treatment are to achieve complete seizure remission when possible, or at least improved frequency and severity of seizures, while also minimizing adverse effects and improving patient quality of life
- Efficacy should be apparent within 2–4 weeks of treatment initiation
- If it is not producing clinical benefits within 6–8 weeks, it may require a dosage increase or it may not work at all
- If stiripentol is ineffective or only partially effective, it can be replaced by or combined with another AED that is appropriate for the patient's seizure type or epilepsy syndrome

Pharmacokinetics
Absorption and Distribution
- Oral bioavailability: not determined
- Food co-ingestion: food co-ingestion is essential because stiripentol degrades rapidly in the acidic environment of an empty stomach
- Tmax: 1.5 hours
- Time to steady state: <7 days
- Pharmacokinetics: non-linear (due to saturable metabolism) so that clearance decreases with increasing dose
- Protein binding: 99%
- Volume of distribution: not known
- Salivary concentrations: it is not known whether stiripentol is secreted into saliva and whether such concentrations are similar to the unbound levels seen in plasma

Metabolism
- Stiripentol is metabolized in the liver, primarily by desmethylation and glucuronidation, to 13 different metabolites
- Precise identification of enzymes involved in metabolism not known but the principal enzymes are considered to be CYP1A2, CYP2C19, and CYP3A4
- The metabolites of stiripentol are not considered to be pharmacologically active
- Autoinduction is not a feature of stiripentol metabolism

S

STIRIPENTOL

Elimination
- Plasma half-life and clearance are dose-dependent, with clearance values decreasing with increasing dose
- Renal excretion: ~73% of an administered dose is excreted in urine as metabolites

Drug Interaction Profile
Pharmacokinetic Drug Interactions
- Interactions between AEDs: effects on stiripentol:
  - Carbamazepine, phenobarbital, phenytoin, and primidone can *increase* the clearance of stiripentol and *decrease* stiripentol plasma levels
  - Clobazam can *decrease* the clearance of stiripentol and *increase* stiripentol plasma levels
- Interactions between AEDs: effects by stiripentol:
  - Stiripentol can *increase* plasma levels of carbamazepine, ethosuximide, phenobarbital, phenytoin, primidone, valproic acid, and clobazam and its pharmacologically active metabolite N-desmethylclobazam
- Interactions between AEDs and non-AED drugs: effects on stiripentol:
  - To date, there have been no reports of other non-AED drugs affecting the clearance of stiripentol and affecting stiripentol plasma levels
- Interactions between AEDs and non-AED drugs: effects by stiripentol:
  - To date, there have been no reports of stiripentol affecting the clearance of other non-AED drugs and affecting their plasma levels
  - However, because stiripentol is a potent inhibitor of CYP2C19, CYP3A4, and CYP2D6, caution needs to be exercised if clinical circumstances require combining stiripentol with drugs that are metabolized by these isoenzymes (e.g., citalopram, omeprazole (CYP2C19); astemizole, chlorpheniramine, calcium channel blockers, statins, codeine (CYP3A4); propranolol, fluoxetine, sertraline, haloperidol, tramadol (CYP2D6))

Pharmacodynamic Drug Interactions
- Enhances anorexia and loss of appetite associated with valproic acid
- Chlorpromazine enhances its central depressant effects

Hormonal Contraception
- It is not known whether stiripentol affects hormonal contraception but theoretically it can increase plasma levels of hormonal contraceptives and thus necessitate lower doses to be prescribed

S

Adverse Effects
How Drug Causes Adverse Effects
• Not known

Common Adverse Effects
• Anorexia, loss of appetite, nausea, vomiting
• Drowsiness, ataxia, hypotonia and dystonia, hyperkinesias
• Insomnia, aggressiveness, irritability, behavior disorders, hyperexcitability

Life-threatening or Dangerous Adverse Effects
• Cutaneous photosensitivity, rash, and urticaria

Rare and not Life-threatening Adverse Effects
• To date there are none

Weight Change
• Weight gain is common (especially when co-administered with valproic acid)

What to do About Adverse Effects
• Discuss common and severe adverse effects with patients or parents before starting medication, including symptoms that should be reported to the physician
• Risk of serious adverse effects is greatest in the first few months of treatment
• Many of the adverse effects associated with stiripentol are often due to an increase in plasma levels of concomitant AEDs and usually regress when the dose of these AEDs is reduced

Dosing and Use
Usual Dosage Range
• Initially 50 mg/kg/day (in combination with clobazam and valproic acid) but up to a maximum of 4 g

Available Formulations
• Capsules: 250 mg, 500 mg
• Sachets: 250 mg, 500 mg

How to Dose
When initiating stiripentol treatment start with a low dose and titrate slowly so as to minimize adverse effects.

• The initial dose should be 50 mg/kg/day administered either twice daily or thrice daily; every 3 days increase by 100 mg/kg/day in divided doses to a maximum dose of 4 g
• It should be noted that the pivotal clinical evaluation of stiripentol was in children of 3 years of age and over with Dravet syndrome. The

DOSING AND USE

clinical decision for use of stiripentol in children <3 years of age needs to be made on an individual patient basis taking into consideration the potential clinical benefit and risks

Dosing Tips
• Bioequivalence between the capsule and oral suspension (sachet) formulations has not been determined and, therefore, clinical supervision is recommended if changing stiripentol formulation
• Should be ingested twice or thrice daily with water
• Because of the inhibitory interactions with clobazam and valproic acid, daily dosage of these AEDs may need to be reduced by 25–30%
• Because acid exposure, as occurs with gastric acid on an empty stomach, rapidly degrades stiripentol, it must always be ingested with food
• If patient has difficulty swallowing, the sachet powder formulation can be mixed in a glass of water and ingested immediately after mixing
• Stiripentol should not be ingested with milk, dairy products (yogurt, soft cream cheeses, etc.), or carbonated drinks

How to Withdraw Drug
• May need to adjust dosage of concurrent medications as stiripentol is being discontinued, because plasma levels of other drugs may change (see Pharmacokinetic Drug Interactions section)
• Taper: reduce dose by 50 mg/kg/day every 3 days
• Rapid discontinuation may increase the risk of seizures

Overdose
• To date, no cases have been reported
• If indicated the stomach should be emptied by lavage or by induction of emesis
• It is not known whether hemodialysis removes stiripentol from blood and, therefore, serves as a useful procedure in cases of overdose

Tests and Therapeutic Drug Monitoring
• Before starting: blood count and liver and renal function tests
• During treatment: blood count and liver and renal function tests every 12 months
• Therapeutic drug monitoring:
  – Stiripentol plasma concentrations associated with optimum seizure control in patients prescribed stiripentol have not been identified
  – Monitoring of concomitant AEDs is essential because stiripentol inhibits the metabolism of many AEDs
  – There are no data indicating the usefulness of monitoring stiripentol by use of saliva
• Before giving a drug that can cause weight gain to an overweight or obese patient, consider determining whether the patient already has pre-diabetes (fasting plasma glucose 100–125 mg/dL), diabetes (fasting plasma glucose greater than 126 mg/dL), or dyslipidemia (increased total cholesterol, LDL cholesterol, and triglycerides; decreased HDL

cholesterol), and treat or refer such patients for treatment, including nutrition and weight management, physical activity counseling, smoking cessation, and medical management
• Monitor weight and BMI during treatment

Other Warnings / Precautions
• Given the frequency of gastrointestinal adverse reactions to treatment with stiripentol and valproic acid (anorexia, loss of appetite, nausea, vomiting), children co-administered these AEDs should have their growth rate carefully monitored
• Because stiripentol is a potent inhibitor of hepatic enzymes, the following drug combinations require particular caution:
  – Rye ergot alkaloids (ergotamine, dihydroergotamine): ergotism with possibility of necrosis of the extremities
  – Immunosuppressants (tacrolimus, cyclosporine, sirolimus): nephrotoxicity
  – Statins (atorvastatin, simvastatin, etc.): rhabdomyolysis
  – Theophylline, caffeine: toxicity

Do not Use
• If patient is hypersensitive to the stiripentol or its excipients
• If patient has a history of psychoses in the form of episodes of delirium

Special Populations
Renal Impairment
• In the absence of specific clinical data in patients with impaired renal function, stiripentol should not be prescribed to such patients

Hepatic Impairment
• In the absence of specific clinical data in patients with impaired hepatic function, stiripentol should not be prescribed to such patients
• However, because stiripentol is extensively metabolized in the liver, lower doses would be required

Children
• Stiripentol is licensed for exclusive use in children
• Pharmacokinetic interactions in children are usually of a greater magnitude than that seen in adults

Elderly
• Stiripentol should not be prescribed to elderly patients

Pregnancy
• In view of the indication for stiripentol, its administration during pregnancy and in women of childbearing potential would not be expected; however, if it occurs specialist advice should be given to women who are of childbearing potential; they should be informed

S

about the teratogenicity of all AEDs and the importance of avoiding an unplanned pregnancy; the AED treatment regimen should be reviewed when a woman is planning to become pregnant

- Rapid discontinuation of AEDs should be avoided as this may lead to breakthrough seizures, which could have serious consequences for the woman and the unborn child
- Stiripentol was not previously classified by the US FDA for pregnancy risk category, but likely would have been rated as risk category C (some animal studies show adverse effects, no controlled studies in humans); the current FDA Pregnancy and Lactation Rule has eliminated pregnancy risk category labels
- Use in women of childbearing potential requires weighing potential benefits to the mother against the risks to the fetus
- Use with other AEDs in combination may cause a higher prevalence of teratogenic effects than stiripentol monotherapy
- Taper drug if discontinuing
- Seizures, even mild seizures, may cause harm to the embryo/fetus
- Data on the pharmacokinetic changes of stiripentol during pregnancy are not available

Breast Feeding
- Breast milk: it is not known whether stiripentol is excreted in breast milk
- Breastfed infants: it is not known what plasma stiripentol concentrations are achieved in breastfed infants compared with the levels of their mothers
- If drug is continued while breast feeding, infant should be monitored for possible adverse effects (e.g., sedation)
- If adverse effects are observed, recommend bottle feeding

The Overall Place of Stiripentol in the Treatment of Epilepsy
Stiripentol is licensed for use as adjunctive treatment of seizures associated with Dravet syndrome in patients aged 3 years and older. It is unlikely that stiripentol will be licensed for adult patients with other types of epilepsy and, therefore, stiripentol is not expected to have a significant role in epilepsy management.

Primary Seizure Types
- Seizures associated with Dravet syndrome (clonic and tonic–clonic attacks)

Secondary Seizure Types
- None

Potential Advantages
- Effective in Dravet syndrome, a difficult-to-treat syndromic epilepsy

Potential Disadvantages
- Associated with non-linear pharmacokinetics so that plasma levels increase disproportionately to dose
- Need to co-ingest food so as to optimize bioavailability
- Associated with pharmacokinetic interactions and usually acts as an inhibitor of hepatic metabolism
- Potential teratogen

S

SUGGESTED READING

Suggested Reading

Balestrini S, Sisodiya SM. Audit of use of stiripentol in adults with Dravet syndrome. *Acta Neurological Scandinavica* 2016; **135**: 73–79.

Cazali N, Tran A, Treluyer JM, Rey E, d'Athis P, Vincent J, Pons G. Inhibitory effect of stiripentol on carbamazepine and saquinavir metabolism in human. *British Journal of Clinical Pharmacology* 2003; **56**: 526–536.

Chiron C. Stiripentol. *Neurotherapeutics* 2007; **4**: 123–125.

Chiron C, Marchand MC, Tran A, d'Athis P, Vincent J, Dulac O, Pons G. Stiripentol in severe myoclonic epilepsy in infancy: a randomised placebo-controlled syndrome-dedicated trial. STICLO study group. *Lancet* 2000; **356**: 1638–1642.

Chiron C, Tonnelier S, Rey E, Brunet ML, Tran A, d'Athis P, Vincent J, Dulac O, Pons G. Stiripentol in childhood partial epilepsy: randomized placebo-controlled trial with enrichment and withdrawal design. *Journal of Child Neurology* 2006; **21**: 496–502.

Giraud C, Treluyer JM, Rey E, Chiron C, Vincent J, Pons G, Tran A. In vitro and in vivo inhibitory effect of stiripentol on clobazam metabolism. *Drug Metabolism and Disposition* 2006; **34**: 608–611.

Kassai B, Chiron C, Augier S, Cucherat M, Rey E, Gueyffier F, Guerrini R, Vincent J, Dulac O, Pons G. Severe myoclonic epilepsy in infancy: a systematic review and meta-analysis of individual patient data. *Epilepsia* 2008; **49**: 343–348.

May TW, Boor R, Mayer T, Jurgens U, Rambeck B, Holert N, Korn-Merker E, Brandt C. Concentrations of stiripentol in children and adults with epilepsy: the influence of dose, age, and comedication. *Therapeutic Drug Monitoring* 2012; **34**: 390–397.

Patsalos PN, Zugman M, Lake C, James A, Ratnaraj N, Sander JW. Serum protein binding of 25 antiepileptic drugs in a routine clinical setting: a comparison of free non-protein-bound concentrations. *Epilepsia* 2017; **58**: 1234–1243.

Wilmshurst JM, Gaillard WD, Vinayan KP, Tsuchida TN, Plouin P, Van Bpgaert P, Carrizosa J, Elia M, Craiy D, Jovic MJ, Nordli D, Hirtz D, Wong V, Glauser T, Mizrahi EM, Cross JH. Summary of recommendations for the management of infantile seizures: task force reports for the ILAE Commission on Pediatrics. *Epilepsia* 2015; **56**: 1185–1197.

SULTHIAME

Therapeutics

Chemical Name and Structure

Sulthiame, 4(1,1-diozothiazinan-2-yl)benzenesulfonamide, is a white powder, with a molecular weight of 290.04 and an empirical formula of $C_{10}H_{14}N_2O_4S_2$.

Brand Names
• Ospolot

Generics Available
• None

Licensed Indications for Epilepsy
• Treatment of rolandic epilepsy when treatment with other AEDs has failed (licensed in Argentina, Australia, Austria, Czech Republic, Denmark, Finland, Germany, Hungary, Israel, Japan, Norway, Slovakia, Sweden, and Switzerland)

Licensed Indications for Non-epilepsy Conditions
• Behavioral disorders associated with epilepsy, hyperkinetic behavior, temporal lobe epilepsy, myoclonic seizures, generalized tonic–clonic seizures, Jacksonian seizures (licensed in Australia)

Non-licensed Use for Epilepsy
• Partial seizures with or without secondary generalization
• Benign childhood epilepsies and epileptic encephalopathies, particularly those with EEG continuous spike wave during sleep (e.g., pseudo-Lennox syndrome, bioelectric status epilepticus in non-rapid eye movement (REM) sleep, Landau–Kleffner syndrome)
• Infantile spasms (West syndrome)

Non-licensed Use for Non-epilepsy Conditions
• There are none

Ineffective (Contraindicated)
- Data on seizure contraindications are not available

Mechanism of Action
- Inhibits voltage-gated sodium channels
- Inhibits release of glutamate
- Inhibits the enzyme carbonic anhydrase in glial cells which increases CO_2 concentrations leading to acidification of the extracellular space; this results in a reduction in inward currents associated with NMDA calcium receptors and causes depression of intrinsic neuronal excitability

Efficacy Profile
- The goals of treatment are to achieve complete seizure remission when possible, or at least improved frequency and severity of seizures, while also minimizing adverse effects and improving patient quality of life
- Efficacy should be apparent within 2 weeks of treatment initiation
- If it is not producing clinical benefits within 6–8 weeks, it may require a dosage increase or it may not work at all
- If sulthiame is ineffective or only partially effective, it can be replaced by or combined with another AED that is appropriate for the patient's seizure type or epilepsy syndrome

Pharmacokinetics
Absorption and Distribution
- Oral bioavailability: 100%
- Food co-ingestion: it is not known whether food co-ingestion affects absorption
- Tmax: 1–5 hours
- Time to steady state: ~3 days (adults); ~2 days (children)
- Pharmacokinetics: linear
- Protein binding: 29%
- Volume of distribution: not determined
- Salivary concentrations: it is not known whether sulthiame is secreted into saliva and whether such concentrations are similar to the unbound levels seen in plasma

Metabolism
- Sulthiame undergoes moderate metabolism in the liver by means of unknown isoenzymes to unknown metabolites
- The metabolites of sulthiame are not considered to be pharmacologically active
- Autoinduction is not a feature of sulthiame metabolism

S

SULTHIAME

Elimination
- Half-life values in adults are 8–15 hours
- Half-life values in children are 5–7 hours
- Renal excretion: 80–90% of an administered dose is excreted in urine, of which 32% is as unchanged sulthiame

Drug Interaction Profile
Pharmacokinetic Drug Interactions
- Interactions between AEDs: effects on sulthiame:
  - Carbamazepine and primidone can *increase* the clearance of sulthiame and *decrease* sulthiame plasma levels
- Interactions between AEDs: effects by sulthiame:
  - Sulthiame can *increase* plasma levels of lamotrigine, phenobarbital, and phenytoin
- Interactions between AEDs and non-AED drugs: effects on sulthiame:
  - Antacids containing magnesium trisilicate, bismuth oxycarbonate, and magnesium oxide may reduce sulthiame gastrointestinal absorption and *decrease* plasma sulthiame levels
- Interactions between AEDs and non-AED drugs: effects by sulthiame:
  - To date, there have been no reports of sulthiame affecting the clearance of other non-AED drugs and affecting their plasma levels

Pharmacodynamic Drug Interactions
- Concomitant administration with primidone, particularly in children, is associated with a profound pharmacodynamic interaction whereby the intensity of undesirable adverse effects such as dizziness, uncertain gait, and drowsiness may be exacerbated
- Because sulthiame is a sulfonamide derivative, concomitant administration with alcohol will result in similar adverse pharmacodynamic interactions to that observed with disulfiram and secondary to vasodilatation, namely: pulsating headache, nausea, vomiting, respiratory depression, tachycardia, hypotension, amblyopia, arrhythmias, excitation, impairment of consciousness
- Concomitant administration with other AEDs (e.g., acetazolamide, topiramate, zonisamide) that inhibit carbonic anhydrase could potentially increase kidney stone formation, metabolic acidosis, hemodilution, and blood electrolyte changes

Hormonal Contraception
- It is not known whether sulthiame affects the metabolism of oral contraceptives but theoretically it can increase plasma levels of hormonal contraceptives and thus necessitate lower doses to be prescribed

Adverse Effects

How Drug Causes Adverse Effects
• CNS adverse effects theoretically due to actions secondary to inhibition of carbonic anhydrase activity

Common Adverse Effects
• Paresthesias of the extremities and face
• Tachypnea, hyperpnea, dyspnea
• Dizziness, headache, diplopia
• Stenocardia, tachycardia
• Loss of appetite

Life-threatening or Dangerous Adverse Effects
• Rare induction of renal failure
• Rare serious rash, including Stevens–Johnson syndrome and toxic epidermal necrolysis (Lyell syndrome) or polyneuritis
• As a carbonic anhydrase inhibitor, sulthiame is associated with adverse effects associated with such inhibition and include nephrolithiasis, metabolic acidosis, and hemodilution with changed electrolytes
• In a single case sulthiame administration was associated with progressive weakness of the limbs, hypersalivation, slurred speech, and increasing drowsiness ending up in a coma
• Increased seizure activity

Rare and not Life-threatening Adverse Effects
• Anxiety
• Hallucinations
• Joint pain
• Myesthetic phenomena

Weight Change
• Weight loss can occur

What to do About Adverse Effects
• Discuss common and severe adverse effects with patients or parents before starting medication, including symptoms that should be reported to the physician
• Many of the adverse effects are dose-dependent and will subside and disappear with dose reduction
• Patients and their carers must be informed that if fever, sore throat, allergic skin reactions with swelling of lymph nodes, or flu-like symptoms occur, they should contact their physician immediately
• It is advisable to perform regular checks of blood count and renal function so that if the above clinical symptoms are accompanied by thrombocytopenia or leukopenia, sulthiame should be discontinued
• Sulthiame should be discontinued immediately if a severe allergic reaction occurs or if creatinine levels show a constant increase

S

ADVERSE EFFECTS

285

- Sulthiame should generally not be administered to patients who are already receiving acetazolamide, topiramate, zonisamide, or the ketogenic diet, because these treatments also predispose to metabolic acidosis and to kidney stones
- Consider calcium and vitamin D supplements in case of low 25-hydroxyvitamin D levels and/or decreased bone mineral density

Dosing and Use

Usual Dosage Range
- Adults: 200–600 mg/day
- Children (2–12 years of age): 5–10 mg/kg/day

Available Formulations
- Tablets: 50 mg, 200 mg

How to Dose
- When initiating sulthiame treatment start with a low dose and titrate slowly so as to minimize adverse effects
  - *For adults:* start treatment with 50 mg twice daily; each week increase by 100 mg/day in divided doses until an optimum response is achieved; maintenance dose generally 200–600 mg/day given in two equally divided doses
  - *Children:* start treatment with 5 mg/kg/day; after 1 week increase to 10 mg/kg/day; maintenance dose generally 5–10 mg/kg/day given in two equally divided doses

Dosing Tips
- Slow dose titration may reduce the incidence of adverse effects
- Tablets should only be administered as whole tablets with plenty of water; dose should be rounded down to the nearest whole tablet
- If therapy is not successful within 1–2 months, sulthiame should be discontinued

How to Withdraw Drug
- May need to adjust dosage of concurrent medications as sulthiame is being discontinued, because plasma levels of other drugs may change (see Pharmacokinetic Drug Interactions section)
- Taper: a gradual dose reduction over a period of 2 weeks should be undertaken
- Rapid discontinuation may induce withdrawal seizures and should only be undertaken if there are safety concerns (e.g., a rash)

Overdose
- Doses of 4–5 g have been associated with headache, dizziness, ataxia, impairment of consciousness, metabolic acidosis, and crystals in urine

- A dose of 20 g resulted in a fatality in one case and in another case the patient survived with full recovery
- Sodium bicarbonate may be administered as an infusion to treat the acidosis
- If indicated the stomach should be emptied by lavage or by induction of emesis
- It is not known whether hemodialysis removes sulthiame from blood and, therefore, serves as a useful procedure in cases of overdose

Tests and Therapeutic Drug Monitoring
- Before starting: blood count and kidney function test and serum electrolytes
- During treatment: serum electrolytes at weekly intervals for the first month of treatment and thereafter at monthly intervals; after 6 months of treatment these checks should be undertaken at 3–6-month intervals
- Because sulthiame can alter vitamin D metabolism and affect bone mineral density, 25-hydroxyvitamin D levels should be monitored in all patients, and vitamin D supplementation should be prescribed as needed; consider also DEXA bone scan in patients at risk for osteopenia
- Therapeutic drug monitoring:
  - Optimum seizure control in adult patients on polytherapy is most likely to occur at plasma sulthiame concentrations of 2–10 mg/L (7–34 µmol/L)
  - Optimum seizure control in children on polytherapy is most likely to occur at sulthiame plasma concentrations of 1–3 mg/L (3–10 µmol/L)
  - The conversion factor from mg/L to µmol/L is 3.45 (i.e., 1 mg/L = 3.45 µmol/L)
  - There are no data indicating the usefulness of monitoring sulthiame by use of saliva

Other Warnings/Precautions
- In some children seizure suppression and reduction in spike frequency by sulthiame may be associated with concurrent deterioration in cognitive function (e.g., memory decline, reduction in attention skill and mathematics ability)

Do not Use
- If patient has a proven allergy to sulthiame or other sulfonamides or to any of the excipients, which include lactose monohydrate
- Because formulation contains lactose, patients with rare hereditary problems of galactose intolerance, Lapp lactose deficiency, or glucose–galactose malabsorption should not take this medicine
- In patients with acute porphyria, hyperthyroidism, arterial hypertension, or a history of psychiatric disease

S

DOSING AND USE

S

SULTHIAME

Special Populations
Renal Impairment
- Sulthiame is renally excreted and the dose may need to be lowered in renally impaired patients
- Because it is not known whether sulthiame can be removed by hemodialysis, it is not known whether patients receiving hemodialysis require supplemental doses of sulthiame

Hepatic Impairment
- Sulthiame undergoes moderate metabolism in the liver and consequently lower doses will be required in patients with hepatic impairment

Children
- Children have an increased metabolic capacity and consequently higher doses on a mg/kg basis are usually required to achieve the equivalent therapeutic plasma levels seen in adults
- Pharmacokinetic interactions in children are usually of a greater magnitude than that seen in adults

Elderly
- Elderly patients are more susceptible to adverse effects and, therefore may not tolerate higher doses
- Because of an age-related reduction in hepatic function, lower sulthiame doses are appropriate
- Because sulthiame is associated with impaired alertness and reaction capacity, the elderly may have reduced ability to drive a car, operate machinery, or perform other activities requiring increased alertness
- Elderly patients frequently receive concurrent drug therapies for comorbidities, and therefore may be at greater risk for pharmacokinetic and pharmacodynamic interactions; the risk of pharmacokinetic interactions with sulthiame is substantial

Pregnancy
- Specialist advice should be given to women who are of childbearing potential; they should be informed about the teratogenicity of all AEDs and the importance of avoiding an unplanned pregnancy; the AED treatment regimen should be reviewed when a woman is planning to become pregnant
- Rapid discontinuation of AEDs should be avoided as this may lead to breakthrough seizures, which could have serious consequences for the woman and the unborn child
- Sulthiame has not been formally classified by the US FDA for pregnancy risk category, but would likely have been rated category C (some animal studies show adverse effects, no controlled studies in humans); the current FDA Pregnancy and Lactation Rule has eliminated pregnancy risk category labels

S

- Use in women of childbearing potential requires weighing potential benefits to the mother against the risks to the fetus
- Use with other AEDs in combination may cause a higher prevalence of teratogenic effects than sulthiame monotherapy
- Taper drug if discontinuing
- Seizures, even mild seizures, may cause harm to the embryo/fetus
- It is unknown whether the pharmacokinetics of sulthiame change during pregnancy

Breast Feeding
- Breast milk: it is not known whether sulthiame is excreted in breast milk
- Breastfed infants: it is not known what plasma sulthiame concentrations are achieved in breastfed infants compared with the levels of their mothers
- If drug is continued while breast feeding, infant should be monitored for possible adverse effects
- If adverse effects are observed, recommend bottle feeding

The Overall Place of Sulthiame in the Treatment of Epilepsy
The good tolerability, significant efficacy, and convenience of use suggest that sulthiame could become a first-line drug in the treatment of benign partial epilepsies of childhood and juvenile myoclonic epilepsy. There appears to be no significant difference between carbamazepine and sulthiame in the treatment of benign childhood epilepsy with centrotemporal spikes. It also has a role as add-on treatment in other partial and myoclonic epilepsies. With regard to seizures secondary to Rett syndrome, sulthiame may be a good alternative to carbamazepine, particularly in those patients where carbamazepine is not effective or not well tolerated. Sulthiame has comparable efficacy to vigabatrin in the management of West syndrome.

Primary Seizure Types
- Benign childhood epilepsies: rolandic epilepsy, pseudo-Lennox syndrome, Landau–Kleffner syndrome
- Epileptic encephalopathies, particularly those with EEG continuous spike wave during sleep

Secondary Seizure Types
- None

Potential Advantages
- Particularly useful in various childhood epilepsies
- Not associated with significant adverse effects

S

SULTHIAME

Potential Disadvantages
- Associated with significant pharmacokinetic interactions, particularly with phenytoin, and usually acts as an inhibitor of hepatic metabolism
- Has limited licensed indications in only a few countries worldwide
- Potential teratogen

Suggested Reading

Ben-Zeev B, Watemberg N, Lerman P, Barash I, Brand N, Lerman-Sagie T. Sulthiame in childhood epilepsy. *Pediatric International* 2004; **46**: 521–524.

Borusiak P, Langer T, Heruth M, Karenfort M, Bettendorf U, Jenke AC. Antiepileptic drugs and bone metabolism in children: data from 128 patients. *Journal of Child Neurology* 2013; **28**: 176–183.

Debus OM, Kurlemann G; Study group. Sulthiame in the primary therapy of West syndrome: a randomized double-blind placebo-controlled add-on trial on baseline pyridoxine medication. *Epilepsia* 2004; **45**: 103–108.

Doose H, Baier WK, Ernst JP, Tuxhorn I, Volzke E. Benign partial epilepsy: treatment with sulthiame. *Developmental Medicine and Child Neurology* 1988; **30**: 683–684.

Fejerman N, Caraballo R, Cersósimo R, Ferraro SM, Galicchio S, Amartino H. Sulthiame add-on therapy in children with focal epilepsies associated with encephalopathy related to electrical status epilepticus during slow sleep (ESES). *Epilepsia* 2012; **53**: 1156–1161.

Freilinger M, Seidl R, Hauser E. Carbamazepine, oxcarbazepine and sulthiame in newly diagnosed benign epilepsy of childhood with rolandic spikes. *Epilepsia* 1997; **38**(Suppl 3): 97–98.

Houghton GW, Richens A. Inhibition of phenytoin metabolism by sulthiame. *British Journal of Pharmacology* 1973; **49**: 157–158.

Huppke P, Kohler K, Brockmann K, Stettner GM, Gartner J. Treatment of epilepsy in Rett syndrome. *European Journal of Paediatric Neurology* 2007; **11**: 10–16.

Koepp MJ, Patsalos PN, Sander JWAS. Sulthiame in adults with refractory epilepsy and learning disability: an open trial. *Epilepsy Research* 2002; **50**: 277–282.

Kramer U, Shahar E, Zelnik N, Lerman-Sagie T, Watemberg N, Nevo Y, Ben-Zeev B. Carbamazepine versus sulthiame in treating benign childhood epilepsy with centrotemporal spikes. *Journal of Child Neurology* 2002; **17**: 914–916.

Lerman P, Nussbaum E. The use of sulthiame in myoclonic epilepsy of childhood and adolescence. *Acta Neurologica Scandinavica* 1975: **60** (Suppl): 7–12.

May TW, Korn-Merker E, Rambeck B, Boenigk HE. Pharmacokinetics of sulthiame in epileptic patients. *Therapeutic Drug Monitoring* 1994; **16**: 251–257.

Rating D, Wolf C, Bast T. Sulthiame as monotherapy in children with benign childhood epilepsy with centrotemporal spikes: a 6-month randomized, double-blind, placebo-controlled study. Sulthiame Study Group. *Epilepsia* 2000; **41**: 1284–1288.

Shamdeen MG, Jost W, Frohnhöfer M, Gortner L, Meyer S. Effect of sulthiame on EEG pathology, behavior and school performance in children with Rolandic epileptiform discharges. *Pediatric International* 2012; **54**: 798–800.

Tan HJ, Singh J, Gupta R, de Gpede C. Comparison of antiepileptic drugs, no treatment, or placebo for children with benign epilepsy with centro temporal spikes. *Cochrane Database Systematic Reviews* 2014; (9): CS06779

Wirrell E, Sherman EM, Vanmastigt R, Hamiwka L. Deterioration in cognitive function in children with benign epilepsy of childhood with centro temporal spikes treated with sulthiame. *Journal of Child Neurology* 2008; **23**: 14–21.

S

T

TIAGABINE

Therapeutics

Chemical Name and Structure

Tiagabine HCl, R-n-(4,4-di(3-methyl-thien-2-yl)-but-3-enyl)-nipecotic acid hydrochloride, is a white odorless crystalline powder, with a molecular weight of 375.5 and an empirical formula of $C_{20}H_{25}NO_2S_2$.

Brand Names

- Gabitril
- Tigatel

Generics Available

- Yes

Licensed Indications for Epilepsy

- Adjunctive treatment of partial (focal) seizures with or without secondary generalization where seizure control is not achieved by optimum doses of at least one other AED (UK SPC; FDA PI)

Licensed Indications for Non-epilepsy Conditions

- There are none

Non-licensed Use for Epilepsy

- There are none

Non-licensed Use for Non-epilepsy Conditions

- Anxiety disorders
- Bipolar disorder
- Insomnia
- Neuropathic pain/chronic pain

Ineffective (Contraindicated)

- Induces absence seizures
- Provokes absence status epilepticus, often ending in generalized tonic–clonic seizures

T

Mechanism of Action
• Selectively blocks reuptake of GABA by presynaptic and glial GABA transporter-1 (GAT-1)

Efficacy Profile
• The goals of treatment are to achieve complete seizure remission when possible, or at least improved frequency and severity of seizures, while also minimizing adverse effects and improving patient quality of life
• Continue treatment until all symptoms are gone or until improvement is stable and then continue treating indefinitely as long as improvement persists
• Efficacy should be apparent within 2 weeks of treatment initiation
• If it is not producing clinical benefits within 6–8 weeks, it may require a dosage increase or it may not work at all
• If tiagabine is ineffective or only partially effective, it can be replaced by or combined with another AED that is appropriate for the patient's seizure type or epilepsy syndrome

Pharmacokinetics
Absorption and Distribution
• Oral bioavailability: ≥90%
• Food co-ingestion: delays the rate but does not decrease the extent of absorption
• Tmax: 0.5–2 hours
• Time to steady state: 1–2 days
• Pharmacokinetics: linear
• Protein binding: 96%
• Volume of distribution: 1.0 L/kg
• Salivary concentrations: it is not known whether tiagabine is secreted into saliva and whether such concentrations are similar to the unbound levels seen in plasma

Metabolism
• Metabolized in the liver, primarily by CYP3A4, to two 5-oxo-tiagabine isomers (E5 and Z-5) which represent ~60% of metabolism
• The remaining 40% of metabolites have yet to be identified
• The metabolites of tiagabine are not pharmacologically active
• Autoinduction is not a feature of tiagabine metabolism

Elimination
• During tiagabine monotherapy half-life values in adults are 7–9 hours
• During tiagabine polytherapy with enzyme-inducing AEDs half-life values in adults are 2–3 hours
• Renal excretion: 25% of tiagabine is eliminated in urine and <2% of an administered dose is excreted unchanged; 63% of an administered dose is excreted in feces as metabolites

PHARMACOKINETICS

T

TIAGABINE

Drug Interaction Profile
Pharmacokinetic Drug Interactions
- Interactions between AEDs: effects on tiagabine:
  - Carbamazepine, phenobarbital, phenytoin, pregabalin, and primidone can *increase* the clearance of tiagabine and *decrease* tiagabine plasma levels
  - Valproic acid can displace tiagabine from its albumin protein-binding sites in blood and *increases* free pharmacologically active tiagabine levels
- Interactions between AEDs: effects by tiagabine:
  - Tiagabine can *decrease* valproic acid plasma levels
- Interactions between AEDs and non–AED drugs: effects on tiagabine:
  - Cimetidine and gemfibrozil can *increase* tiagabine plasma levels
  - Naproxen and salicylic acid can displace tiagabine from its albumin protein-binding sites in blood and *increases* free pharmacologically active tiagabine levels
- Interactions between AEDs and non–AED drugs: effects by tiagabine:
  - To date, there have been no reports of tiagabine affecting the clearance of other non–AED drugs and affecting their plasma levels

Pharmacodynamic Drug Interactions
- Co-medication with vigabatrin: enhanced seizure control may occur
- Co-medication with triazolam: may slightly prolong the CNS-depressant effect of triazolam

Hormonal Contraception
- Tiagabine does not enhance the metabolism of oral contraceptives so as to decrease plasma levels of hormonal contraceptives and, therefore, does not compromise contraception control

Adverse Effects
How Drug Causes Adverse Effects
- CNS adverse effects may be due to excessive actions of GABA

Common Adverse Effects
- Sedation, dizziness, asthenia, nervousness
- Depression, difficulty concentrating, speech/language problems, confusion, tremor
- Nausea, vomiting, diarrhea
- Ecchymosis (bruising)

Life-threatening or Dangerous Adverse Effects
- Concerns that tiagabine, like the GABAergic-acting vigabatrin, may cause visual field defects have not been substantiated
- Suicidal ideation and behavior may occur

T

Rare and not Life-threatening Adverse Effects
• Delusion
• Hallucinations

Weight Change
• Not common; weight gain reported but not expected

What to do About Adverse Effects
• Discuss common and severe adverse effects with patients or parents before starting medication, including symptoms that should be reported to the physician
• Take more of the dose at night or all of the dose at night to reduce daytime sedation
• Lower the dose

Dosing and Use

Usual Dosage Range
• Adults: 30–45 mg/day (with enzyme-inducing AEDs)
• Adults: 15–30 mg/day (without enzyme-inducing AEDs)
• Children: 0.5–2 mg/kg/day

Available Formulations
• Tablets: 5 mg, 10 mg, 15 mg (UK)
• Tablets: 2 mg, 4 mg, 12 mg, 16 mg (USA)

How to Dose
• When initiating tiagabine treatment start with a low dose and titrate slowly so as to minimize adverse effects
   – *For adults co-prescribed enzyme-inducing AEDs:* start treatment with 5–10 mg twice daily for 1 week; each week increase by 5–10 mg/day; maintenance dose generally 30–45 mg/day and at doses greater than 30 mg administration should be thrice daily
   – *For adults co-prescribed non-enzyme-inducing AEDs:* start treatment with 5–10 mg twice daily for 1 week; each week increase by 5–10 mg/day; maintenance dose generally 15–30 mg/day
   – *Children over 12 years old:* start treatment with 0.1 mg/kg/day and titrate in increments of 0.1 mg/kg/day every 1 or 2 weeks; maintenance dose generally 0.5–2 mg/kg/day

Dosing Tips
• Because for a given dose patients on non-enzyme-inducing AEDs achieve tiagabine blood levels that are double that of patients receiving enzyme-inducing AEDs, these patients often require lower and less frequent doses of tiagabine; these patients may also require a slower titration schedule compared with that of induced patients

DOSING AND USE

T

- Gastrointestinal absorption is markedly slowed by the concomitant intake of food, which also lessens peak plasma levels; thus, for improved tolerability and consistent therapeutic response, patients should be instructed to always take tiagabine with food
- The manner of dose administration (high dosage, fast titration rate) may increase tiagabine-associated status epilepticus and new-onset seizures

How to Withdraw Drug
- There is no need to adjust dosage of concurrent medications as tiagabine is being discontinued, because plasma levels of other drugs do not change (see Pharmacokinetic Drug Interactions section)
- Taper: over a period of 2–3 weeks
- Rapid discontinuation may increase the risk of withdrawal seizures

Overdose
- No fatalities have been reported (doses up to 720 mg); symptoms include: coma, sedation, agitation, confusion, speech difficulty, hostility, depression, weakness, myoclonus, spike and wave stupor, tremors, vomiting
- If indicated the stomach should be emptied by lavage or by induction of emesis
- It is not known whether hemodialysis removes tiagabine from blood and, therefore, serves as a useful procedure in cases of overdose

Tests and Therapeutic Drug Monitoring
- Before starting: blood count, including platelet count, and liver and kidney function tests
- During treatment: blood count, including platelet count (particularly if bruising is observed), liver and kidney function tests every 6–12 months
- Rare cases of visual field defects have been reported with tiagabine; if visual field symptoms develop the patient should be referred to an ophthalmologist for further evaluation, including perimetry
- Therapeutic drug monitoring:
  - Overall, in patients treated with therapeutic doses of tiagabine, plasma tiagabine concentrations are in the order of 20–200 ng/mL (53–532 nmol/L)
  - The conversion factor from ng/mL to nmol/L is 2.66 (i.e., 1 ng/L = 2.66 nmol/L)
  - The reference range of tiagabine in plasma is considered to be the same for children and adults, although no data are available to support this clinical practice
  - There are no data indicating the usefulness of monitoring tiagabine by use of saliva

TIAGABINE

T

Other Warnings/Precautions
- Some patients may experience dizziness and somnolence and thus caution needs to be exercised if patient intends to drive or use machinery
- Accidental injury was an adverse effect reported by 2.8% of patients administered tiagabine during its clinical evaluation
- Low white blood cell count ($<2.5 \times 10^9$ per liter) was more frequent with tiagabine (4.1%) compared with placebo (1.5%)
- Patients with a history of serious behavioral problems have an increased risk of recurrence of these symptoms

Do not Use
- If patient has a proven allergy to gabapentin or pregabalin or to any of the excipients: tablets contain lactose
- Because formulation contains lactose, patients with rare hereditary problems of galactose intolerance, Lapp lactose deficiency, or glucose–galactose malabsorption should not take this medicine

Special Populations
Renal Impairment
- Although tiagabine undergoes moderate renal excretion, its pharmacokinetics are unaffected in patients with renal impairment, so the dose need not be changed

Hepatic Impairment
- Tiagabine is extensively metabolized and consequently lower doses and/or reduced dose intervals should be used and patients should be monitored closely for adverse effects such as dizziness and tiredness
- In patients with mild to moderate hepatic impairment (Child–Pugh score 5–9), Cmax and AUC values are 50% and 70% higher respectively; consequently the initial daily maintenance dose should be 5–10 mg, administered twice daily
- The fraction of unbound tiagabine is up to twofold greater in patients with moderate hepatic impairment compared to patients with normal hepatic function
- Tiagabine should not be used in patients with severe hepatic impairment

Children
- Children have an increased metabolic capacity and consequently higher doses on a mg/kg basis are usually required to achieve the equivalent therapeutic plasma levels seen in adults
- Pharmacokinetic interactions in children are usually of a greater magnitude than that seen in adults
- There is no experience with tiagabine in children under the age of 12 years and, therefore, tiagabine should not be used in this age group

SPECIAL POPULATIONS

T

TIAGABINE

Elderly
- Elderly patients are more susceptible to adverse effects and, therefore, may not tolerate higher doses
- Because of an age-related reduction in renal and hepatic function, lower tiagabine doses are appropriate
- Elderly patients frequently receive concurrent drug therapies for comorbidities, and therefore may be at greater risk for pharmacokinetic and pharmacodynamic interactions; the risk of pharmacokinetic interactions with tiagabine is moderate

Pregnancy
- Specialist advice should be given to women who are of childbearing potential; they should be informed about the teratogenicity of all AEDs and the importance of avoiding an unplanned pregnancy; the AED treatment regimen should be reviewed when a woman is planning to become pregnant
- Rapid discontinuation of AEDs should be avoided as this may lead to breakthrough seizures, which could have serious consequences for the woman and the unborn child
- Tiagabine was previously classified by the US FDA as risk category C (some animal studies show adverse effects, no controlled studies in humans); the current FDA Pregnancy and Lactation Rule has eliminated pregnancy risk category labels
- Use in women of childbearing potential requires weighing potential benefits to the mother against the risks to the fetus
- Use with other AEDs in combination may cause a higher prevalence of teratogenic effects than tiagabine monotherapy
- Taper drug if discontinuing
- Seizures, even mild seizures, may cause harm to the embryo/fetus
- Data on the pharmacokinetic changes of tiagabine during pregnancy are not available. However, because tiagabine is highly protein-bound (96%) and its elimination is the consequence of extensive metabolism, significant changes in the pharmacokinetics of tiagabine can be expected during pregnancy

Breast Feeding
- Breast milk: it is not known whether tiagabine is excreted into breast milk
- Breastfed infants: it is not known what plasma tiagabine concentrations are achieved in breastfed infants compared with the levels of their mothers
- If drug is continued while breast feeding, infant should be monitored for possible adverse effects
- If adverse effects are observed, recommend bottle feeding

THE EPILEPSY PRESCRIBER'S GUIDE TO ANTIEPILEPTIC DRUGS

T

The Overall Place of Tiagabine in the Treatment of Epilepsy
The efficacy of tiagabine is limited to partial (focal) seizures and its role is limited to adjunctive medication in severe forms of partial (focal) seizures that failed to respond to other AED combinations. It may also be effective in epileptic spasms of epileptic encephalopathies.

Primary Seizure Types
• Severe partial (focal) epilepsies with or without secondary generalized tonic–clonic seizures

Secondary Seizure Types
• None

Potential Advantages
• Does not affect the pharmacokinetics of other drugs

Potential Disadvantages
• Narrow spectrum of efficacy against focal seizures only
• It is a pro-absence drug; its use is prohibited in idiopathic generalized epilepsy with absences
• May require two to four times a day dosing
• Needs to be taken with food
• Associated with significant pharmacokinetic interactions in that its metabolism is readily induced
• Potential teratogen

SUGGESTED READING

Suggested Reading

Ben-Menachem E. International experience with tiagabine add-on therapy. *Epilepsia* 1995; **36** (Suppl 6): S14–S21.

Brodie MJ. Tiagabine pharmacology in profile. *Epilepsia* 1995; **36** (Suppl 6): S7–S9.

Brodie MJ. Tiagabine in the management of epilepsy. *Epilepsia* 1997; **38** (Suppl 2): S23–S27.

Leppik IE. Tiagabine: the safety landscape. *Epilepsia* 1995; **36** (Suppl 6): S10–S13.

Patsalos PN. *Antiepileptic drug interactions: a clinical guide*, 3rd edition. Springer, London, UK; 2016.

Patsalos PN, Zugman M, Lake C, James A, Ratnaraj N, Sander JW. Serum protein binding of 25 antiepileptic drugs in a routine clinical setting: a comparison of free non-protein-bound concentrations. *Epilepsia* 2017; **58**: 1234–1243.

Pulman J, Marson AG, Hutton JL. Tiagabine add-on for drug-resistant partial epilepsy. *Cochrane Database Systematic Review* 2012; **5**: CD001908.

So EJ, Wolff D, Graves NM, Leppik IE, Cascino GD, Pixton GC, Gustavson LE. Pharmacokinetics of tiagabine as add-on therapy

T

in patients taking enzyme-inducing antiepilepsy drugs. *Epilepsy Research* 1995; **22**: 221–226.

Uthman BM, Rowan J, Ahmann PA, Leppik IE, Schachter SC, Sommerville KW, Shu V. Tiagabine for complex partial seizures. A randomized, add-on, dose-response trial. *Archives of Neurology* 1998; **55**: 56–62.

Walker MC. The mechanism of action of tiagabine. *Reviews in Contemporary Pharmacotherapy* 2002; **12**: 213–224.

Wang X, Patsalos PN. The pharmacokinetic profile of tiagabine. *Reviews in Contemporary Pharmacotherapy* 2002; **12**: 225–234.

TIAGABINE

TOPIRAMATE

Therapeutics

Chemical Name and Structure

Topiramate, 2,3:4,5-bis-O-(1-methylethylidene)-β-D-fructopyranose sulfamate, is a sulfamate-substituted monosaccharide derived from the D-enantiomer of fructose. Its molecular weight is 339.37, and its empirical formula is $C_{12}H_{21}NO_8S$.

Brand Names
- Epilramate; Epitomax; Epitop
- Gabatopa
- Nuromate
- Qsymia; Quedexy XR
- Topamac; Topamax; Topamax Sprinkle; Topamed; Topilex; Topimax; Topinmate; Topiragen; Topirid; Topitrim; Topival; Topper; Trokendi XR

Generics Available
- Yes

Licensed Indications for Epilepsy
- Monotherapy (in patients 10 years or older) or adjunctive therapy (in patients 2 years or older) of partial/focal and secondary generalized seizures (FDA PI)
- Monotherapy (in patients 10 years or older) or adjunctive therapy (in patients 2 years or older) of primary generalized tonic–clonic seizures in patients 10 years or older (FDA PI)
- Adjunctive treatment of seizures associated with Lennox–Gastaut syndrome in patients 2 years or older (FDA PI)
- Monotherapy in adults, adolescents, and children over 6 years of age who have generalized tonic–clonic seizures or partial/focal seizures with or without secondary generalized seizures (UK SPC)
- Adjunctive therapy for adults, adolescents, and children over 2 years of age for partial/focal seizures with or without secondary generalized seizures and for primary generalized tonic–clonic seizures and for the treatment of seizures associated with Lennox–Gastaut syndrome (UK SPC)

Licensed Indications for Non-epilepsy Conditions
• Migraine prophylaxis in adults (UK SPC) and in patients 12 years of age and older (FDA PI)

Non-licensed Use for Epilepsy
• Infantile spasms (West syndrome)
• Juvenile myoclonic epilepsy
• Myoclonic astatic epilepsy (Doose syndrome)
• Myoclonic seizures
• Progressive myoclonic epilepsy
• Severe myoclonic epilepsy of infancy (Dravet syndrome)

Non-licensed Use for Non-epilepsy Conditions
• Binge-eating disorder
• Bipolar disorder
• Chronic daily headache
• Cluster headaches
• Essential tremor
• Idiopathic intracranial hypertension (pseudotumor cerebri)
• Neuropathic pain
• Posttraumatic stress disorder
• Psychotropic drug-induced weight gain
• Sleep-related eating disorder

Ineffective (Contraindicated)
• Topiramate is potentially effective against all seizure types and is not contraindicated for any seizure type or epilepsy; however, topiramate efficacy for absence seizures is weak, and possibly ineffective

Mechanism of Action
• Enhances GABA-mediated inhibition
• Inhibits voltage-dependent sodium channels
• Enhances potassium channel conduction
• Inhibition of L-type high voltage-activated calcium channels
• Decreases glutamate-mediated excitatory neurotransmission
• Carbonic anhydrase inhibition, but the potency of topiramate is much lower than that of acetazolamide; topiramate probably does not exert its anticonvulsant effect through inhibition of carbonic anhydrase, but this mechanism may cause some of the clinical adverse effects

Efficacy Profile
• The goals of treatment are to achieve complete seizure remission when possible, or at least improved frequency and severity of seizures, while also minimizing adverse effects and improving patient quality of life
• Therapeutic effect usually evident within 2–4 weeks
• If topiramate is ineffective or only partially effective, it can be replaced by or combined with another AED that is appropriate for the patient's seizure type or epilepsy syndrome

TOPIRAMATE

Pharmacokinetics
Absorption and Distribution
- Oral bioavailability: >80%
- Food co-ingestion: neither delays the rate of absorption nor decreases the extent of absorption
- Tmax: 2–4 hours
- Time to steady state: 4–5 days
- Pharmacokinetics: linear
- Protein binding: 15%
- Volume of distribution: 0.6–0.8 L/kg
- Salivary concentrations: topiramate is secreted into saliva and concentrations are similar to the unbound levels seen in plasma

Metabolism
- Topiramate is not extensively metabolized in patients who are not receiving concurrent enzyme-inducing AED co-medications, and typically 40–50% of a topiramate dose is excreted unchanged by means of the kidneys
- Metabolites thus far identified include two hydroxy and two diol metabolites, as well as several glucuronide conjugates, none of which constitutes more than 5% of an administered dose
- Although the specific CYP isoenzymes for the metabolism of topiramate have not been identified, it is evident that isoenzymes induced by carbamazepine and phenytoin play a major role
- Metabolites are not pharmacologically active
- Topiramate may undergo tubular reabsorption
- Autoinduction is not a feature of topiramate metabolism

Elimination
- During maintenance topiramate monotherapy, half-life values in adults are 20–30 hours
- Compared with adults, topiramate clearance is approximately 50% higher in older children, and twice the adult value in infants
- During maintenance topiramate polytherapy with enzyme-inducing AEDs, half-life values in adults are 10–15 hours
- Renal excretion: ~20–60% of an administered topiramate dose is eliminated unchanged in urine

Drug Interaction Profile
Pharmacokinetic Drug Interactions
- Interactions between AEDs: effects on topiramate:
  – Carbamazepine, eslicarbazepine acetate, oxcarbazepine, phenobarbital, phenytoin, primidone, and valproic acid can *increase* the clearance of topiramate and *decrease* topiramate plasma levels

T

- Interactions between AEDs: effects by topiramate:
  - Topiramate can *decrease* the clearance of phenytoin and *increase* phenytoin plasma levels
  - Topiramate can *increase* the clearance of eslicarbazepine acetate, perampanel, and valproic acid and *decrease* their plasma levels
- Interactions between AEDs and non-AED drugs: effects on topiramate:
  - Amitriptyline, Atkins diet (modified), diltiazem, hydrochlorothiazide, lithium, metformin, posaconazole, propranolol, and sumatriptan can *decrease* the clearance of topiramate and *increase* topiramate plasma levels
- Interactions between AEDs and non-AED drugs: effects by topiramate:
  - Topiramate can *increase* the clearance and *decrease* the plasma levels of amitriptyline, digoxin, glibenclamide, imatinib, lithium, pioglitazone, risperidone, and sumatriptan
  - Topiramate can *decrease* the clearance and *increase* the plasma levels of diltiazem, flunarizine, gamma-hydroxybutyrate, haloperidol, lithium, and metformin

Pharmacodynamic Drug Interactions
- Topiramate and lamotrigine can have a synergistic anticonvulsant effect consequent to a pharmacodynamic interaction
- Topiramate may enhance the risk of valproate-associated adverse effects, including elevated ammonium, hyperammonemic encephalopathy, elevated transaminases, apathy, and hypothermia
- It has been proposed that the hyperammonemic encephalopathy may be due to an increase in the presence of topiramate of a potentially toxic metabolite of valproate, 4-ene-valproate
- Symptoms of decreased appetite, weight loss, and nervousness by topiramate can be exacerbated by levetiracetam, particularly in children
- Topiramate may interact with other carbonic anhydrase inhibitors (e.g., acetazolamide, sulthiame, zonisamide) to increase the risk of kidney stones

Hormonal Contraception
- Crucially, at doses higher than 200 mg, topiramate enhances the metabolism of oral contraceptives so as to decrease plasma levels of hormonal contraceptives, potentially leading to breakthrough bleeding and contraceptive failure; medium- or high-dose oral contraceptive preparations are indicated in women of childbearing potential; in addition to recommendations for additional barrier contraceptives and folic acid 1000 mg daily in all women of child-bearing potential

TOPIRAMATE

Adverse Effects

How Drug Causes Adverse Effects
- Mechanism by which topiramate causes adverse effects has not been established
- Carbonic anhydrase inhibition by topiramate, although not or only minimally involved in its antiepileptic activity, may be the mechanism responsible for some of the clinical adverse effects, such as metabolic acidosis, paresthesias, kidney stones, and hypohydrosis

Common Adverse Effects
- Psychomotor slowing
- Fatigue
- Change in cognition
- Impairment of language and verbal memory, slurred speech
- Decreased attention, change in behavior and mood
- CNS-related adverse effects are often not dose-dependent but they are reversible
- Anorexia, nausea, taste perversion, and weight loss
- Metabolic acidosis (lowered serum bicarbonate or CO_2, especially in children)
- Hypohydrosis (decreased sweating, especially in children, may lead to hyperthermia)
- Sedation, asthenia, dizziness, ataxia, nervousness, nystagmus, tremor
- Blurred or double vision

Life-threatening or Dangerous Adverse Effects
- Metabolic acidosis
- Oligohydrosis and hyperthermia (more common in children)

Rare and not Life-threatening Adverse Effects
- Nephrolithiasis (1–2%)
- Paresthesias, mostly tingling in the fingers and toes
- Acute bilateral secondary narrow angle-closure glaucoma
- Enhancement of the risk of valproate-associated hyperammonemic encephalopathy
- Dysguesia

Weight Change
- Weight loss is common; usually seen within 3 months and with a peak effect within 12–18 months, is dose-related with more weight loss at high doses (mean, 6.5 kg or 7.3% decline) and less weight loss at lower doses (mean, 1.6 kg or 2.5% decline)

What to do About Adverse Effects
- Discuss common and severe adverse effects with patients or parents before starting medication, including symptoms that should be reported to the physician

T

- Discuss symptoms associated with kidney stones, glaucoma, and hypohydrosis
- Some CNS-related adverse effects may be lessened by slow titration, but sometimes persist even at low doses
- Cognitive adverse effects may be pronounced in some patients even at low doses, but totally absent even at relatively high doses in others
- Metabolic acidosis is usually compensated, but patients may be treated with oral bicarbonate for CO_2 values of 15–18 mEq/L or less
- Topiramate should generally not be administered to patients who are already receiving acetazolamide, sulthiame, zonisamide, or the ketogenic diet, because these treatments also predispose to metabolic acidosis and to kidney stones
- Patients should be encouraged to drink fluids (especially water) liberally (encouraging 8–10 10-oz. (2400–3000-mL) glasses/bottles daily) while on topiramate to reduce the risk of kidney stones
- Anorexia and weight loss may improve with dosage reduction
- Children who benefit from topiramate treatment but experience hypohydrosis should avoid hot ambient temperatures, be promptly removed from hot environments when exhibiting symptoms or signs of heat stroke, and if symptomatic may experience improvement with cool wet sponge baths or being wrapped in a cool wet towel

TOPIRAMATE

Dosing and Use

Usual Dosage Range
- Adults: 100–400 mg/day (without enzyme-inducing AEDs)
- Adults: 200–600 mg/day (with enzyme-inducing AEDs)
- Children (2–16 years): 3 mg/kg/day (monotherapy)
- Children (2–16 years): 6–9 mg/kg/day (with enzyme-inducing AEDs)

Available Formulations
- Capsules: 15 mg, 25 mg, 50 mg
- Tablets: 25 mg, 50 mg, 100 mg, 200 mg
- Sprinkle capsules: 15 mg, 25 mg, 50 mg

How to Dose
- *For adults and children over 12 years of age:* start treatment with 25–50 mg/day, twice daily; at intervals of 1–2 weeks increase as needed and as tolerated by 25–50 mg/day; maintenance dose generally 100–600 mg/day
- *Children less than 12 years and infants:* start treatment with approximately 0.5–1.0 mg/kg/day, two or three times daily; at intervals of 1–2 weeks increase as needed and as tolerated by approximately 0.5–1.0 mg/kg/day; maintenance dose generally 3–9 mg/kg/day; doses of >20 mg/kg/day may be necessary and well tolerated, especially in infants; dosage requirements increase twofold in children co-prescribed enzyme-inducing AEDs

T

Dosing Tips
- Slow dose titration may delay onset of therapeutic action but enhance tolerability to sedating and cognitive adverse effects
- Some patients may do very well at relatively low doses of topiramate, such as 50–100 mg/day in adults or 2–3 mg/kg/day in children; the response to treatment should be assessed at these doses before increasing the dose further
- If there has been no evidence of seizure reduction at doses of 10–15 mg/kg/day in children, increasing the dose further is unlikely to be beneficial, but if there has been a gradual reduction in the seizure frequency, further dosage increases may be beneficial and well tolerated
- Topiramate is available in a sprinkle capsule formulation, which can be swallowed whole or sprinkled over approximately a teaspoon of soft food (e.g., apple sauce); the mixture should be consumed immediately

How to Withdraw Drug
- May need to adjust dosage of concurrent medications as topiramate is being discontinued, because plasma levels of other drugs may change (see Pharmacokinetic Drug Interactions section)
- No data are available on potential for withdrawal seizures or symptoms upon rapid discontinuation
- Rapid discontinuation may increase the risk of seizures
- If possible, taper dose over a period of several weeks
- Women of childbearing potential who are taking a medium- or high-dose oral contraceptive preparation while on topiramate can be switched to a regular contraceptive if they are not taking another enzyme-inducing AED, and should be counseled to use barrier contraceptives and receive folic acid 1000 mg daily

Overdose
- A patient who ingested 96–110 g of topiramate was admitted to hospital with coma lasting 20–24 hours followed by full recovery after 3–4 days; another patient who ingested 8 g of topiramate was admitted to hospital with non-convulsive status epilepticus, but fully recovered after being administered 4 mg of lorazepam iv
- Signs and symptoms of topiramate overdoses include: severe metabolic acidosis, convulsions, drowsiness, speech disturbance, blurred vision, diplopia, impaired mentation, lethargy, abnormal coordination, stupor, hypotension, abdominal pain, agitation, dizziness, and depression
- Deaths have been reported after polydrug overdoses involving topiramate
- The stomach should be emptied immediately by lavage or by induction of emesis
- Hemodialysis removes topiramate from blood and therefore serves as a useful procedure in cases of overdose

DOSING AND USE

Tests and Therapeutic Drug Monitoring
- Routine laboratory testing is not necessary
- Periodic serum bicarbonate levels can be considered to monitor for topiramate-related hyperchloremic non-anion gap metabolic acidosis (i.e., decreased serum bicarbonate in the absence of chronic respiratory alkalosis) in children or non-verbal patients who may not be able to describe symptoms well or readily demonstrate clinical signs of metabolic acidosis (i.e., hyperventilation, fatigue, anorexia, cardiac arrhythmias, stupor)
- Therapeutic drug monitoring:
  - Optimum seizure control in adult patients on monotherapy is most likely to occur at topiramate plasma concentrations of 5–20 mg/L (15–59 μmol/L)
  - Optimum seizure control in children aged 6–12 years on topiramate monotherapy is most likely to occur at topiramate plasma concentrations of 2–21 mg/L (6–59 μmol/L)
  - Optimum seizure control in children 5 years and younger on topiramate monotherapy is most likely to occur at topiramate plasma concentrations of 3–29 mg/L (9–86 μmol/L)
  - The conversion factor from mg/L to μmol/L is 2.95 (i.e., 1 mg/L = 2.95 μmol/L)
  - Topiramate can be monitored by use of saliva, which is a measure of the free non-protein-bound plasma concentration that is pharmacologically relevant

Other Warnings/Precautions
- Patients should be monitored carefully for evidence of cognitive adverse effects
- Patients should be monitored carefully for evidence of kidney stones; in those with symptoms of kidney stones (i.e., flank or pelvic pain, hematuria), urinary straining for diagnostic stone capture and renal ultrasound should be considered
- If symptoms of metabolic acidosis develop (hyperventilation, fatigue, anorexia, cardiac arrhythmias, stupor), then dose may need to be reduced or treatment may need to be discontinued
- Depressive effects may be increased by other CNS depressants (alcohol, MAOIs, other AEDs, etc.)
- Use with caution when combining with other drugs that predispose patients to heat-related disorders, including carbonic anhydrase inhibitors and anticholinergics

Do not Use
- Avoid use or use only with great caution in patients undergoing treatments that are associated with an increase in risk of kidney stones, such as acetazolamide, sulthiame, zonisamide, and the ketogenic diet
- Use with caution in patients taking valproic acid

T

- If there is a proven allergy to topiramate or to any of the excipients: tablets contain lactose
- Because formulations contain lactose, patients with rare hereditary problems of galactose intolerance, Lapp lactose deficiency, or glucose–galactose malabsorption should not take this medicine

Special Populations

Renal Impairment
- Topiramate is renally excreted and consequently lower doses may be required
- In renal failure (CrCl <30 mL/min/1.73 m^2) approximately 50% of the usual dose is recommended
- After hemodialysis, an additional dose (approximately half of the daily dose, in addition to the full daily dose) of topiramate may be necessary, because topiramate is cleared from plasma during dialysis at a rate which is approximately nine times higher than in patients with normal renal function

Hepatic Impairment
- Topiramate is extensively metabolized in the liver (particularly when co-prescribed with enzyme-inducing AEDs), and consequently lower doses may be necessary to avoid adverse effects

Children
- Children have an increased metabolic capacity and consequently higher mg/kg/day doses are usually required to achieve the equivalent therapeutic plasma levels
- Pharmacokinetic interactions in children are usually of a greater magnitude than that seen in adults
- Children receiving topiramate are at higher risk of developing metabolic acidosis and symptoms related to hypohydrosis

Elderly
- Elderly patients are more susceptible to adverse effects (especially somnolence), and therefore often are unable to tolerate higher doses
- Because of an age-related reduction in renal and hepatic function, lower initial and target topiramate doses with slower titration may be appropriate
- Elderly patients are often prescribed concurrent drug therapies for comorbidities and therefore may be at greater risk for pharmacokinetic and pharmacodynamic interactions; the risk of pharmacokinetic interactions with topiramate is substantial

Pregnancy
- Specialist advice should be given to women who are of childbearing potential; they should be informed about the teratogenicity of all

SPECIAL POPULATIONS

309

T

TOPIRAMATE

AEDs and the importance of avoiding an unplanned pregnancy; the AED treatment regimen should be reviewed when a woman is planning to become pregnant
• Rapid discontinuation of AEDs should be avoided as this may lead to breakthrough seizures, which could have serious consequences for the woman and the unborn child
• Topiramate is classified by the US FDA as risk category C (some animal studies show adverse effects); the current FDA Pregnancy and Lactation Rule has eliminated pregnancy risk category labels; analysis of pregnancy registry data has revealed that topiramate may be associated with a higher risk of congenital malformations than several other AEDs, in particular cleft lip; hypospadias has also been associated with topiramate
• Use in women of childbearing potential requires weighing potential benefits to the mother against the risks to the fetus
• Use with other AEDs in combination may cause a higher risk for teratogenic effects than topiramate monotherapy
• Taper drug over several weeks if discontinuing
• Seizures, even mild seizures, may cause harm to the embryo/fetus
• During pregnancy, topiramate pharmacokinetics change significantly, so that topiramate plasma concentrations decrease by ~40% due to increased clearance; an increase in topiramate dose is usually required as pregnancy progresses, so monitoring of serum topiramate levels at least once per trimester, with dosage adjustment as appropriate to ensure similar concentrations to historical benchmark levels, should be considered

Breast Feeding
• Breast milk: 70–110% of maternal plasma levels
• Breastfed infants: topiramate plasma levels are 9–17% of maternal plasma levels
• If drug is continued while breast feeding, the infant should be monitored for possible adverse effects (irritability or sedation)
• If adverse effects are observed, recommend bottle feeding

The Overall Place of Topiramate in the Treatment of Epilepsy
Topiramate is a broad-spectrum AED, and is a first- or second-line therapy in partial (focal) epilepsies and idiopathic generalized epilepsies with generalized tonic–clonic seizures, as well as juvenile myoclonic epilepsy. It has a particular place in the treatment of refractory partial (focal) and symptomatic generalized epilepsies such as Lennox–Gastaut syndrome.

Primary Seizure Types
• Partial/focal seizures with or without secondary generalization

- Idiopathic generalized seizures (with generalized tonic–clonic seizures, as well as juvenile myoclonic epilepsy)
- Lennox–Gastaut syndrome

Secondary Seizure Types
- Juvenile myoclonic epilepsy
- Infantile spasms (West syndrome)
- Severe myoclonic epilepsy of infancy (Dravet syndrome)
- Myoclonic astatic epilepsy (Doose syndrome)
- Myoclonic seizures
- Progressive myoclonic epilepsy

Potential Advantages
- Topiramate has a broad spectrum of seizure protection and is not associated with seizure aggravation
- Demonstrates a favorable pharmacokinetic profile with linear pharmacokinetics
- Topiramate has a well-defined adverse event profile with limited potential for serious or irreversible adverse effects

Potential Disadvantages
- The main limitations for the use of topiramate have been its negative effect on cognitive functions, and several other potential adverse effects
- Problematic for patients at risk for kidney stones, metabolic acidosis, or hypohidrosis
- Children may suffer from predictable detrimental reductions in growth rate and bone-related sequelae in long-term use
- Associated with significant pharmacokinetic interactions
- Potential teratogen

Suggested Reading

Ben-Menachem E, Axelsen M, Johanson EH, Stagge A, Smith U. Predictors of weight loss in adults with topiramate-treated epilepsy. *Obesity Research* 2003; **11**: 556–562.

Biton V, Bourgeois BF. Topiramate in patients with juvenile myoclonic epilepsy. *Archives of Neurology* 2005; **62**: 1705–1708.

Biton V, Montouris GD, Ritter F, Riviello JJ, Reife R, Lim P, Pledger G. A randomized, placebo-controlled study of topiramate in primary generalized tonic-clonic seizures. Topiramate YTC Study Group. *Neurology* 1999; **52**: 1330–1337.

Faught E, Wilder BJ, Ramsay RE, Reife RA, Kramer LD, Pledger GW, Karim RM. Topiramate placebo-controlled dose-ranging trial in refractory partial epilepsy using 200-, 400-, and 600-mg daily dosages. Topiramate YD Study Group. *Neurology* 1996; **46**: 1684–1690.

T

Glauser TA, Clark PO, Strawsburg R. A pilot study of topiramate in the treatment of infantile spasms. *Epilepsia* 1998; **39**: 1324–1328.

Groeper K, McCann ME. Topiramate and metabolic acidosis: a case series and review of the literature. *Paediatric Anaesthesia* 2005; **15**: 167–170.

Hamer HM, Knake S, Schomburg U, Rosenow F. Valproate-induced hyperammonemic encephalopathy in the presence of topiramate. *Neurology* 2000; **54**: 230–232.

Hernandez-Diaz S, Smith CR, Shen A, Mittendorf R, Hauser WA, Yerby M, Holmes LB. Comparative safety of antiepileptic drugs during pregnancy. *Neurology* 2012; **78**: 1692–1699.

Johannessen Landmark C, Patsalos PN. Drug interactions involving the new second- and third-generation antiepileptic drugs. *Expert Reviews in Neurotherapeutics* 2010; **10**: 119–140.

Marson AG, Al-Kharusi AM, Alwaidh M, et al.; SANAD Study group. The SANAD study of effectiveness of carbamazepine, gabapentin, lamotrigine, oxcarbazepine, or topiramate for treatment of partial epilepsy: an unblinded randomised controlled trial. *Lancet* 2007; **369**: 1000–1015.

Marson AG, Al-Kharusi AM, Alwaidh M, et al.; SANAD Study group. The SANAD study of effectiveness of valproate, lamotrigine, or topiramate for generalised and unclassifiable epilepsy: an unblinded randomised controlled trial. *Lancet* 2007; **369**: 1016–1026.

Meador KJ, Loring DW, Hulihan JF, Kamin M, Karim R. Differential cognitive and behavioral effects of topiramate and valproate. *Neurology* 2003; **60**: 1483–1488.

Meador KJ, Loring DW, Vahle VJ, Ray PG, Werz MA, Fessler AJ, Ogrocki P, Schoenberg MR, Miller JM, Kustra RP. Cognitive and behavioral effects of lamotrigine and topiramate in healthy volunteers. *Neurology* 2005; **64**: 2108–2114.

Mirza N, Marson AG, Pirmohamed M. Effect of topiramate on acid–base balance: extent, mechanism and effects. *British Journal of Clinical Pharmacology* 2009; **68**: 655–661.

Mula M, Trimble MR, Thompson P, Sander JW. Topiramate and word-finding difficulties in patients with epilepsy. *Neurology* 2003; **60**: 1104–1107.

Nallani SC, Glauser TA, Hariparsad N, Setchell K, Buckley DJ, Buckley AR, Desai PB. Dose-dependent induction of cytochrome P450 (CYP) 3A4 and activation of pregnane X receptor by topiramate. *Epilepsia* 2003; **44**: 1521–1528.

Ohman I, Sabers A, de Flon P, Luef G, Tomson T. Pharmacokinetics of topiramate during pregnancy. *Epilepsy Research* 2009; **87**: 124–129.

Patsalos PN. *Antiepileptic drug interactions: a clinical guide*, 3rd edition. Springer, London, UK; 2016.

Patsalos PN, Berry DJ. Therapeutic drug monitoring of antiepileptic drugs by use of saliva. *Therapeutic Drug Monitoring* 2013; **35**: 4–29.

Privitera M, Fincham R, Penry J, Reife R, Kramer L, Pledger G, Karim R. Topiramate placebo-controlled dose-ranging trial in refractory

TOPIRAMATE

partial epilepsy using 600-, 800-, and 1,000-mg daily dosages. Topiramate YE Study Group. *Neurology* 1996; **46**: 1678–1683.

Pulman J, Jette N, Dykeman J, Hemming K, Hutton JL, Marson AG. Topiramate add-on for drug-resistant partial epilepsy. *Cochrane Database Systematic Review* 2014; **2**: CD001417.

Sachdeo R C, Glauser TA, Ritter F, Reife R, Lim P, Pledger G. A double-blind, randomized trial of topiramate in Lennox–Gastaut syndrome. *Neurology* 1999; **52**: 1882–1887.

St. Louis EK, Gidal BE, Henry TR, Kaydanova Y, Krumholz A, McCabe PH, Montouris GD, Rosenfeld WE, Smith BJ, Stern JM, Waterhouse EJ, Schulz RM, Garnett WR, Bramley T. Conversions between monotherapies in epilepsy: expert consensus. *Epilepsy and Behavior* 2007; **11**: 222–234.

T

VALPROATE

Therapeutics

Chemical Name and Structure

Valproic acid, *N*-dipropylacetic acid, is a short-chain branched fatty acid that occurs as a colorless liquid, with a molecular weight of 144.21 and an empirical formula of $C_8H_{16}O_2$. Because most formulations are salts (e.g., sodium valproate, magnesium valproate, and sodium divalproate), valproic acid is often called valproate.

COOH

Brand Names
- Absenor; Apilepsin; Atemperator
- Convulex
- Depacon; Dapakan; Depakene; Depakene-R; Depakin; Depakine; Depakine Chrono; Depakote; Depakote ER; Depakote Sprinkles; Depalept; Depalept Chrono; Depamag; Deprakine; Deproic; Desorate; Diproex ER; Dipromal; Divalproex
- Epilex; Epilim; Epilim Chrono; Epilim Chronosphere; Episenta; Epival; Ergenyl; Everiden
- Leptilan; Logical; Logical Jarabe
- Orfiril; Orfiril Retard
- Petilin; Pragmaten
- Valcote; Valnex; Valpakine; Valparin; Valporal; Valprax; Valpro; Vematina; Vupral

Generics Available
- Yes

Licensed Indications for Epilepsy
- Complex partial (focal dyscognitive) seizures that occur either in isolation or in association with other types of seizures (monotherapy and adjunctive) (FDA PI)
- Simple and complex absence seizures (monotherapy and adjunctive) (FDA PI)
- Multiple seizure types which include absence seizures (adjunctive) (FDA PI)
- Monotherapy or adjunctive therapy for any form of epilepsy in patients of any age (UK SPC)

Licensed Indications for Non-epilepsy Conditions
- Mania (Divalproex only) (FDA PI)
- Mania in bipolar disorder (all formulations) (UK SPC)
- Migraine prophylaxis (Divalproex, Divalproex ER) (FDA PI)
- Migraine prophylaxis (all formulations) (UK SPC)

V

Non-licensed Use for Epilepsy
- Febrile seizures
- Infantile spasms (West syndrome)
- Juvenile myoclonic epilepsy
- Lennox–Gastaut syndrome
- Neonatal seizures
- Refractory status epilepticus

Non-licensed Use for Non-epilepsy Conditions
- Psychosis, schizophrenia (adjunctive)

Ineffective (Contraindicated)
- Valproic acid is potentially effective against all seizure types and is not contraindicated for any seizure type or epilepsy
- Adverse effect profile may not justify use for prophylaxis of febrile seizures

Mechanism of Action
- Raises brain levels of GABA, possibly through inhibition of GABA transaminase, or through inhibition of succinic semialdehyde dehydrogenase, or through an increase in glutamic acid decarboxylase activity; these changes occur at higher than usual therapeutic doses and their time course lags behind the anticonvulsant effect
- Can reduce sustained repetitive high-frequency firing by blocking voltage-sensitive sodium channels or by activating calcium-dependent potassium conductance
- Decreases brain levels of the excitatory amino acid aspartate
- Decreases the expression of hippocampal glutamate transporter-1
- None of the identified actions are widely accepted as the predominant relevant mechanism

Efficacy Profile
- The goals of treatment are to achieve complete seizure remission when possible, or at least improved frequency and severity of seizures, while also minimizing adverse effects and improving patient quality of life
- Onset of action may occur within a few days, but maximal efficacy may not be seen until several weeks after initiation of therapy
- Goal of therapy in idiopathic generalized epilepsies is not only full seizure control, but also normalization of EEG
- No unusual incidence of loss of efficacy
- If ineffective or only partially effective, consider replacing by or co-prescribing with lamotrigine, ethosuximide, levetiracetam, topiramate, or zonisamide for generalized epilepsies, or another appropriate drug in patients with focal-onset seizures

THERAPEUTICS

Pharmacokinetics

Absorption and Distribution

- Oral bioavailability: >90% (8–20% lower for extended-release formulations)
- Food co-ingestion: delays the rate of absorption but has no effect on the extent of absorption
- Tmax: 1–2 hours (syrup and uncoated immediate-release tablets); 3–7 hours (enteric-coated tablets and sprinkles); extended-release formulations have prolonged Tmax values
- Time to steady state: 2–4 days
- Pharmacokinetics: non-linear due to saturable protein binding
- Protein binding: 90%; saturable at therapeutic concentrations: free (unbound) fraction 7% at 50 mg/L, 9% at 75 mg/L, 15% at 100 mg/L, 22% at 125 mg/L, and 30% at 150 mg/L
- The free fraction of valproic acid is also higher in newborns, as well as in the elderly
- Volume of distribution: 0.13–0.19 L/kg (adults); 0.20–0.30 L/kg (children)
- Salivary concentrations: valproic acid is secreted into saliva but concentrations do not reflect the unbound levels seen in plasma

Metabolism

- The metabolism of valproic acid in the liver is extensive and complex in that it involves multiple metabolic pathways, including O-glucuronidation, β-oxidation, Ω-oxidation, hydroxylation, ketone formation, and desaturation
- To date in excess of 25 metabolites have been identified
- Valproic acid glucuronide and 3-oxo-valproic acid are by far the most abundant metabolites (~40% and 33% of an administered dose respectively)
- Hydroxylation to form 4-ene-valproic acid and other metabolites is by means of the action of CYP2A6, CYP2C9, CYP2C19, and CYP2B6 isoenzymes, whereas O-glucuronidation is mediated by UGT1A3 and UGT2B7 isoforms
- Some metabolites are pharmacologically active; 2-ene-valproic acid and 4-ene-valproic acid have anticonvulsant activity that is similar in potency to that of valproic acid itself
- Autoinduction is not a feature of valproic acid metabolism

Elimination

- In the absence of enzyme-inducing AEDs, half-life values for valproic acid in adults are 12–16 hours
- In the presence of enzyme-inducing AEDs, half-life values for valproic acid in adults are 5–9 hours
- In the absence of enzyme-inducing AEDs in children, half-life values are 8.4–12.5 hours in infants, and 8.6–12.3 hours in older children
- In the presence of enzyme-inducing AEDs in children, half-life values are 4–8 hours in infants, and 7–9.4 hours in older children

- Newborns eliminate valproic acid slowly, with half-life values of 20–40 hours
- Renal excretion: ~97% of an administered dose is excreted as metabolites in urine; 40% as valproic acid glucuronide and 33% as 3-oxo-valproic acid; 20% comprise ~22 other minor metabolites
- Renal excretion: 1–3% of an administered dose is excreted as unchanged valproic acid in urine

Drug Interaction Profile
Pharmacokinetic Drug Interactions

- Interactions between AEDs: effects on valproic acid:
  - Carbamazepine, ethosuximide, eslicarbazepine acetate, lamotrigine, perampanel, phenobarbital, phenytoin, primidone, tiagabine, and topiramate can *increase* the clearance of valproic acid and *decrease* valproic acid plasma levels
  - Clobazam, felbamate, and stiripentol can *decrease* the clearance of valproic acid and *increase* valproic acid plasma levels
- Interactions between AEDs: effects by valproic acid:
  - Valproic acid can *decrease* the clearance and *increase* plasma levels of carbamazepine-10,11-epoxide (pharmacologically active metabolite of carbamazepine), ethosuximide, felbamate, lamotrigine, lorazepam, midazolam, phenobarbital, and rufinamide
  - Valproic acid can *increase* the clearance and *decrease* plasma levels of topiramate
  - Valproic acid can *increase* the free fraction of phenytoin by displacing phenytoin from its plasma protein (albumin) binding site and by a concurrent inhibition of phenytoin clearance
  - Valproic acid can *increase* the free fraction of 10-hydroxycarbazepine (pharmacologically active metabolite of oxcarbazepine) and diazepam by displacing them from their plasma protein (albumin) binding sites
- Interactions between AEDs and non-AED drugs: effects on valproic acid:
  - Amikacin, cimetidine, diflunisal, doripenem, ertapenem, imipenem, meropenem, naproxen, panipenem, rifampicin, ritonavir, and tebipenem can *increase* the clearance of valproic acid and *decrease* valproic acid plasma levels
  - Oral contraceptives can *increase* the clearance of valproic acid and *decrease* valproic acid plasma levels
  - Acyclovir, Atkins diet (modified), cholestyramine, cisplatin, efavirenz, and methotrexate can *decrease* valproic acid plasma levels by means of an unknown mechanism
  - Bupropion, chlorpromazine, erythromycin, guanfacine, isoniazid, lithium, sertraline, and verapamil can *decrease* the clearance and *increase* valproic acid plasma levels

– Acetylsalicylic acid can *increase* the free fraction of valproic acid by displacing valproic acid from its plasma protein (albumin) binding site and by a concurrent inhibition of valproic acid clearance
• Interactions between AEDs and non-AED drugs: effects by valproic acid:
  – Valproic acid can *decrease* the clearance and *increase* the plasma levels of amitriptyline, clomipramine, clozapine, doxepin, lersivirine, lopinavir, lorazepam, naproxen, nimodipine, nortriptyline, paclitaxel, quetiapine, and zidovudine
  – Valproic acid can *increase* the free fraction of warfarin by displacing warfarin from its plasma protein (albumin) binding site and leads to an increase in international normalized ratio
  – Valproic acid can *increase* the clearance and *decrease* the plasma levels of aripiprazole, clozapine, moclobemide, olanzapine, oxiracetam, propofol, and rocuronium

Pharmacodynamic Drug Interactions
• Patients who fail to respond to maximally tolerated doses of either valproic acid or lamotrigine alone can achieve better seizure control when the two agents are combined. This pharmacodynamic interaction also entails a risk of reciprocal potentiation of adverse effects, particularly tremor, and a reduction in the dosage of both drugs is usually required
• The combination of ethosuximide with valproic acid can also lead to a favorable pharmacodynamic interaction which may allow the control of absence seizures in patients not responsive to monotherapy with either drug
• Use of valproate with clonazepam may cause absence status
• Topiramate may enhance the risk of valproate-associated adverse effects, including elevated ammonium, hyperammonemic encephalopathy, elevated transaminases, apathy, and hypothermia
• It has been proposed that the hyperammonemic encephalopathy may be due to an increase in the presence of topiramate of a potentially toxic metabolite of valproate, 4-ene-valproate
• Valproic acid in combination with lithium is associated with a pharmacodynamic interaction, leading to lithium neurotoxicity
• Valproic acid in combination with cisplatin is associated with three-fold higher incidence of thrombopenia, neutropenia, or both; this is considered to be a consequence of a pharmacodynamic interaction
• Delirium can occur when quetiapine is added to valproic acid consequent to a pharmacodynamic interaction
• Delirium can occur when zotepine is added to valproic acid consequent to a pharmacodynamic interaction
• Adverse effects comprising dyskinesia and bruxism can occur during methylphenidate and valproic acid combination therapy consequent to a pharmacodynamic interaction
• A pharmacodynamic interaction has been suggested between zolpidem and valproic acid whereby somnambulism occurs

VALPROATE

V

Hormonal Contraception
- Valproic acid does not enhance the metabolism of oral contraceptives so as to decrease plasma levels of hormonal contraceptives and, therefore, does not compromise contraception control; however, given the significant risk of teratogenesis with valproic acid, physicians should consider providing additional recommendations for use of barrier methods and supplemental folic acid 1000 mg in all women of childbearing potential who are using valproic acid (despite the possibility that valproic acid mediates teratogenesis via folate-independent mechanisms)

Adverse Effects
How Drug Causes Adverse Effects
- Mechanism by which valproic acid causes adverse effects has not been established, but CNS adverse effects are likely due to same mechanism as seizure protection
- Metabolite 4-ene-valproic acid has pronounced embryotoxicity and hepatotoxicity

Common Adverse Effects
- Tremor, drowsiness, lethargy, dizziness, ataxia, asthenia, headache
- Nausea, vomiting, anorexia, constipation, dyspepsia, diarrhea, gastro-intestinal distress
- Alopecia
- Hyperammonemia
- Hypocarnitinemia
- Decreased bone mineral density

Life-threatening or Dangerous Adverse Effects
- Rare hepatotoxicity with liver failure, sometimes severe and fatal, particularly in children under 2 years of age
- Rare pancreatitis, sometimes fatal
- Reversible dementia, brain atrophy, encephalopathy, extrapyramidal symptoms
- Neutropenia, bone marrow suppression

Rare and not Life-threatening Adverse Effects
- Facial and limb edema
- Nocturnal enuresis
- Hyperinsulinism (debated)
- Menstrual irregularities (debated)
- Polycystic ovaries (controversial)

Weight Change
- Weight gain is common; can be a health problem in some patients, with weight gains up to 50 kg reported

ADVERSE EFFECTS

V

What to do About Adverse Effects
- Discuss common and severe adverse effects with patients or parents before starting medication, including symptoms that should be reported to the physician
- CNS-related adverse effects are usually dose-dependent and are reversible
- Risk of serious adverse effects is greatest in the first few months of treatment
- Thrombocytopenia is usually dose-related and platelet counts between 100,000 and 200,000 are common and can be monitored without intervention
- Tremor may improve with dosage reduction and with propranolol treatment
- Mild to moderate hyperammonemia is usually asymptomatic and does require intervention
- L-carnitine supplementation is strongly suggested in the following groups of patients: those with certain secondary carnitine deficiency syndromes, symptomatic valproic acid-associated hyperammonemia, multiple risk factors for valproic acid hepatotoxicity or renal-associated syndromes, infants and young children taking valproic acid, patients with epilepsy using the ketogenic diet who have hypocarnitinemia, patients receiving dialysis, and premature infants who are receiving total parenteral nutrition
- Consider calcium (600–1000 mg/day) and vitamin D supplements (2000 IU/day) in cases of decreased bone mineral density
- Obtain liver function tests in cases of symptoms suggestive of valproic acid hepatotoxicity, which include nausea, vomiting, anorexia, lethargy, jaundice, edema, and at times loss of seizure control
- Obtain serum amylase and lipase in cases of symptoms suggestive of pancreatitis, which include mostly vomiting and abdominal pain
- Multivitamins fortified with zinc and selenium may help reduce alopecia
- Sedation can be problematic and not tolerated by some patients; can wear off over time but can re-emerge as dose increases and then wear off again over time
- Consider calcium and vitamin D supplements in case of low 25-hydroxyvitamin D levels and/or decreased bone mineral density

Dosing and Use
Usual Dosage Range
- Adults: 500–2500 mg/day
- Children under 20 kg: 20–40 mg/kg/day
- Children over 20 kg: 20–30 mg/kg/day

Available Formulations
- Enteric-coated tablets: 200 mg, 500 mg
- Crushable tablets: 100 mg

VALPROATE

- Capsules: 150 mg, 300 mg, 500 mg
- Solution (sugar-free) or syrup: 200 mg/5 mL, 250 mg/5 mL
- Sustained-release tablets: 200 mg, 300 mg, 500 mg
- Depakote tablets: 250 mg, 500 mg
- Divalproex tablets: 125 mg, 300 mg, 500 mg (as valproic acid equivalents)
- Divalproex tablets, delayed-release: 125 mg, 250 mg, 500 mg (as valproic acid equivalents)
- Divalproex sprinkles: 125 mg (as valproic acid equivalents)
- Divalproex tablets, extended-release: 250 mg, 500 mg (as valproic acid equivalents)
- Chronospheres sachet (modified-release granules):
  - 50 mg (sodium valproate, 33.33 mg; valproic acid, 14.51 mg; overall equivalent to 50 mg sodium valproate)
  - 100 mg (sodium valproate, 66.66 mg; valproic acid, 29.03 mg; overall equivalent to 100 mg sodium valproate)
  - 250 mg (sodium valproate, 166.76 mg; valproic acid, 72.6 mg; overall equivalent to 250 mg sodium valproate)
  - 500 mg (sodium valproate, 333.30 mg; valproic acid, 145.14 mg; overall equivalent to 500 mg sodium valproate)
  - 750 mg (sodium valproate, 500.06 mg; valproic acid, 217.75 mg; overall equivalent to 750 mg sodium valproate)
  - 1000 mg (sodium valproate, 666.60 mg; valproic acid, 290.27 mg; overall equivalent to 1000 mg sodium valproate)
- Powder and solution for iv injection: 400 mg/4 mL
- Liquid for oral administration: 200 mg/5 mL

How to Dose
- *For adults and children over 12 years of age:* start treatment with 500 mg/day, twice daily; at intervals of 5–7 days increase as needed and as tolerated by 500 mg/day; maintenance dose generally 1000–2500 mg/day
- *Children:* start treatment with approximately 15 mg/kg/day, twice daily or three times daily; at intervals of 5–7 days increase as needed and as tolerated by up to 15 mg/kg/day; maintenance dose generally 20–30 mg/kg/day; doses of up to 100 mg/kg/day may be necessary, especially in younger children; dosage requirements increase twofold in children co-prescribed enzyme-inducing AEDs

Dosing Tips
- Higher peak valproic acid levels occur with the regular enteric-coated and suspension formulation than with the same dose of the extended-release formulation
- Regular enteric-coated formulations are not extended-release but merely delayed-release formulations; absorption of valproic acid is delayed but rapid
- Use enteric-coated formulation to avoid gastrointestinal effects

DOSING AND USE

V

- Do not break or chew enteric-coated tablets as this will defeat the purpose of the enteric coating
- Modified-release granules should be sprinkled on a small amount of soft food or in drinks, which should be cold or at room temperature
- A mixture of modified-release granules with soft food or drinks should not be stored for future use
- Slow dose titration may delay onset of therapeutic action but enhance tolerability to sedating effects
- Daily doses of the extended-release formulations should be 8–20% higher than for the other formulations to achieve the same plasma levels of valproic acid because of the slightly reduced bioavailability of the extended-release formulations
- Given the half-life of immediate-release valproate (e.g., Depakene, Depakote), twice-daily dosing is probably ideal
- Extended-release valproate (e.g., Depakote ER) can be given once daily
- However, extended-release valproate is only 80% as bioavailable as immediate-release valproate, producing plasma drug levels 10–20% lower than with immediate-release valproate
- Thus, the dose of extended-release valproate may need to be higher (by approximately one-third) when converting patients to ER formulation
- Divalproex ER improves gastrointestinal adverse effects and alopecia compared with immediate-release Divalproex or generic valproate
- The amide of valproic acid is available in Europe (valpromide (Depamide)) and has a more profound interaction with carbamazepine epoxide compared with other formulations

How to Withdraw Drug
- May need to adjust dosage of concurrent medications as valproic acid is being discontinued, because plasma levels of other drugs may change (see Pharmacokinetic Drug Interactions section)
- Rapid discontinuation may increase the risk of seizures
- If possible, taper dose over a period of 1–3 months

Overdose
- Can be fatal, but patients have survived valproic acid levels as high as 2120 mg/L
- Symptoms include: somnolence, heart block, coma
- If indicated the stomach should be emptied by lavage or by induction of emesis
- Hemodialysis removes valproic acid from blood and, therefore, serves as a useful procedure in cases of overdose

Tests and Therapeutic Drug Monitoring
- Before starting: obtain CBC and transaminases
- Inform all female patients of childbearing age about the teratogenicity (spina bifida) and the importance of avoiding an unplanned pregnancy

V

- During treatment: blood count and liver function tests at the latest after 2 months, then at least every 6 months throughout treatment
- Because valproic acid can alter vitamin D metabolism and affect bone mineral density, 25-hydroxyvitamin D levels should be monitored in all patients, and vitamin D supplementation should be prescribed as needed; consider also DEXA bone scan in patients at risk for osteopenia
- Monitor weight and BMI during treatment
- Therapeutic drug monitoring:
  - Optimum seizure control in patients on monotherapy is most likely to occur at valproic acid plasma concentrations of 50–100 mg/L (350–700 μmol/L)
  - The conversion factor from mg/L to μmol/L is 6.93 (i.e., 1 mg/L = 6.93 μmol/L)
  - Because enteric-coated valproic acid is a delayed-release formulation, the lowest plasma level of a 24-hour period may not be before the morning dose, but rather in the late morning or early afternoon
  - The reference range of valproic acid in plasma is considered to be the same for children and adults, although no data are available to support this clinical practice
  - Valproic acid can be monitored by use of saliva; however, concentrations are not a good reflection of the free non-protein-bound plasma concentration that is pharmacologically relevant
- Before giving a drug that can cause weight gain to an overweight or obese patient, consider determining whether the patient already has pre-diabetes (fasting plasma glucose 100–125 mg/dL), diabetes (fasting plasma glucose greater than 126 mg/dL), or dyslipidemia (increased total cholesterol, LDL cholesterol, and triglycerides; decreased HDL cholesterol), and treat or refer such patients for treatment, including nutrition and weight management, physical activity counseling, smoking cessation, and medical management

Other Warnings/Precautions
- Patients should be monitored carefully for signs of unusual bleeding or bruising
- Obtain liver function tests in cases of symptoms suggestive of valproic acid hepatotoxicity, which include nausea, vomiting, anorexia, lethargy, jaundice, edema (predominantly facial), and at times loss of seizure control
- Obtain serum amylase and lipase in cases of symptoms suggestive of pancreatitis, which include vomiting, abdominal pain, nausea, and anorexia
- Somnolence may be more common in the elderly and may be associated with dehydration, reduced nutritional intake, and weight loss, requiring slower dosage increases, lower doses, and monitoring of fluid and nutritional intake
- Evaluate for urea cycle disorders, as hyperammonemic encephalopathy, sometimes fatal, has been associated with valproate administration

DOSING AND USE

in these uncommon disorders; urea cycle disorders such as ornithine transcarbamylase deficiency are associated with unexplained encephalopathy, mental retardation, elevated plasma ammonia, cyclical vomiting, and lethargy

Do not Use
* In patients with known urea cycle disorder (severe hyperammonemia)
* In patients with hepatic disease or significant hepatic dysfunction
* In patients with a history of pancreatitis
* In patients with pre-existing thrombocytopenia
* In patients with suspected mitochondrial disorder
* Use with great caution in infants 2 years old or younger, especially in combination with other AEDs
* If there is a proven allergy to valproic acid, sodium valproate, or any excipients

Special Populations
Renal Impairment
* Renal disease has little or no impact on valproic acid pharmacokinetics, although protein binding may be reduced
* Because valproic acid can be removed by hemodialysis, patients receiving hemodialysis may require supplemental doses of valproic acid

Hepatic Impairment
* Valproic acid is extensively metabolized and consequently lower doses will be required in patients with hepatic impairment
* Liver cirrhosis may lead to decreased protein binding and decreased clearance of valproic acid

Children
* Children have an increased metabolic capacity and consequently higher doses on a mg/kg/day basis are usually required to achieve the equivalent therapeutic plasma levels
* Pharmacokinetic interactions in children are usually of a greater magnitude than that seen in adults
* Risk of fatal hepatotoxicity is highest in infants 2 years of age and younger, especially in AED polytherapy
* Use in children requires close medical supervision

Elderly
* Elderly patients are more susceptible to adverse effects (especially somnolence) and, therefore, often do better at lower doses
* Because of an age-related reduction in renal and hepatic function, lower valproate doses are appropriate
* Elderly patients are often prescribed concurrent drug therapies for comorbidities and therefore may be at greater risk for pharmacokinetic

V

and pharmacodynamic interactions; the risk of pharmacokinetic interactions with valproic acid is substantial
- Because of a tendency for lower serum albumin values, elderly patients may have a higher free (unbound) fraction of valproic acid
- Sedation in the elderly may be more common and associated with dehydration, reduced nutritional intake, and weight loss
- Monitor fluid and nutritional intake

Pregnancy
- Specialist advice should be given to women who are of childbearing potential; they should be informed about the teratogenicity of all AEDs and the importance of avoiding an unplanned pregnancy; the AED treatment regimen should be reviewed when a woman is planning to become pregnant
- Rapid discontinuation of AEDs should be avoided as this may lead to breakthrough seizures, which could have serious consequences for the woman and the unborn child
- Valproate was previously classified by the US FDA as risk category D (positive evidence of risk to human fetus); potential benefits may still justify its use during pregnancy; the current FDA Pregnancy and Lactation Rule has eliminated pregnancy risk category labels
- When taken during pregnancy, valproic acid can cause major malformations, including neural tube defects, and cognitive delay in offspring; this may be dose-related; analysis of a recent pregnancy registry revealed that valproic acid was associated with the highest risk of congenital malformations compared to several other AEDs, in particular neural tube defects, hypospadias, cardiac defects, and oral clefts
- Use in women of childbearing potential requires weighing potential benefits to the mother against the risks to the fetus; if a pregnancy is planned, valproic acid should be preferably discontinued beforehand, whenever possible; in general, a woman should not become pregnant while taking valproic acid and, if she does, an attempt should be made to replace and discontinue the medication as soon as possible
- If a patient becomes pregnant while taking valproic acid, careful and early monitoring with fetal ultrasound should be undertaken
- If possible, start on folate 1 mg/day before pregnancy to reduce risk of neural tube defects
- If drug is continued, consider vitamin K during the last 6 weeks of pregnancy to reduce risks of bleeding
- Seizures, even mild seizures, may cause harm to the embryo/fetus
- Use with other AEDs in combination may cause a higher prevalence of teratogenic effects than valproic acid monotherapy
- Taper drug if discontinuing
- During pregnancy valproic acid pharmacokinetics change significantly so that valproic acid plasma concentrations can decrease by up to 40% and free valproic acid plasma concentrations decrease by 29% due to increased clearance; binding is significantly decreased during pregnancy, resulting in an increased free fraction of the drug,

SPECIAL POPULATIONS

V

particularly at higher plasma concentrations; an increase in valproate dose may be required in some patients

Breast Feeding
- Breast milk: 4–20% of maternal plasma levels
- Breastfed infants: valproic acid plasma levels are 4–12% of maternal plasma levels
- The potential benefit to the mother should be weighed against the potential risk to the infant when considering recommendations regarding nursing
- If drug is continued while breast feeding, infant should be monitored for possible adverse effects, including hematological effects
- If adverse effects are observed, recommend bottle feeding

The Overall Place of Valproate in the Treatment of Epilepsy
Valproate is considered to be a broad-spectrum AED, effective against all types of seizures and epilepsies. It is generally considered the first-line therapy for all types of generalized seizures (idiopathic and symptomatic, e.g., childhood and juvenile absence epilepsy, juvenile myoclonic epilepsy, benign myoclonic epilepsy in infants, myoclonic astatic epilepsy, epilepsy with myoclonic absences, eyelid myoclonus with absences), progressive myoclonic epilepsy, and photosensitive epilepsy. However, valproate is possibly slightly less effective than carbamazepine against partial seizures and is more efficacious than lamotrigine and better tolerated than topiramate in patients with generalized and unclassified epilepsies. Seizure aggravation is not a feature of valproate but when it occurs it is usually in a specific clinical context such as overdose, encephalopathy, or hepatic or metabolic disorders. The serious adverse effects, particularly in women of childbearing potential and in patients in early childhood, should always be considered.

Primary Seizure Types
- Juvenile myoclonic epilepsy (myoclonic, absence, and generalized tonic–clonic seizures)
- Absence seizures
- Myoclonic seizures
- Cryptogenic or symptomatic generalized epilepsies
- Lennox–Gastaut syndrome

Secondary Seizure Types
- Partial (focal) seizures
- Infantile spasms (West syndrome)

V

Potential Advantages
- Valproate has a broad spectrum of seizure protection
- It is among the best or is the best AED for the treatment of idiopathic generalized epilepsies
- No other AED has better efficacy than valproate in primarily generalized seizures, although some of the new AEDs (such as levetiracetam or lamotrigine) are better tolerated
- Also potentially effective in the more therapy-resistant cryptogenic or symptomatic generalized epilepsies
- Available in oral formulations of various strengths and as a parenteral formulation

Potential Disadvantages
- Idiosyncratic and other adverse effects, some potentially severe
- Requires frequent blood testing and close monitoring
- Pharmacokinetics are not linear due to saturable protein binding
- Associated with significant pharmacokinetic interactions and usually acts as an inhibitor of hepatic metabolism
- Potential teratogen, perhaps more substantive than any other AED

Suggested Reading

Asconapé JJ, Penry JK, Dreifuss FE, Riela A, Mirza W. Valproate-associated pancreatitis. *Epilepsia* 1993; **34**: 177–183.

Biton V, Mirza W, Montouris G, Vuong A, Hammer AE, Barrett PS. Weight change associated with valproate and lamotrigine monotherapy in patients with epilepsy. *Neurology* 2001; **56**: 172–177.

Bryant AE, Dreifuss FE. Valproic acid hepatic fatalities. III. U.S. experience since 1986. *Neurology* 1996; **46**: 465–469.

Glaucer TA, Cnaan A, Shinnar S, Hirtz DG, Dlugos D, Masur D, Clark PO, Capparelli EV, Adamson PC. for the Childhood Absence Epilepsy Study Group. Ethosuximide, valproic acid, and lamotrigine in childhood absence epilepsy. *New England Journal of Medicine* 2010; **362**: 790–799.

Hernandez-Diaz S, Smith CR, Shen A, Mittendorf R, Hauser WA, Yerby M, Holmes LB. Comparative safety of antiepileptic drugs during pregnancy. *Neurology* 2012; **78**: 1692–1699.

Limdi NA, Shimpi AV, Faught E, Gomez CR, Burneo JG. Efficacy of rapid IV administration of valproic acid for status epilepticus. *Neurology* 2005; **64**: 353–355.

Marson AG, Al-Kharusi AM, Alwaidh M, et al. The SANAD study of effectiveness of valproate, lamotrigine, or topiramate for generalised and unclassifiable epilepsy: an unblinded randomised controlled trial. *Lancet* 2007; **369**: 1016–1026.

Marson AG, Williamson PR, Clough H, Hutton JL, Chadwick DW; Epilepsy Monotherapy Trial Group. Carbamazepine versus

SUGGESTED READING

valproate monotherapy for epilepsy: a meta-analysis. *Epilepsia* 2002; **43**: 505–513.

Mattson RH, Cramer JA, Collins JF; Dept. of VA Epilepsy Cooperative Study No. 264 Group. A comparison of valproate with carbamazepine for the treatment of complex partial seizures and secondarily generalized tonic-clonic seizures in adults. *New England Journal of Medicine* 1992; **327**: 765–771.

Meador KJ, Baker GA, Browning N, Clayton-Smith J, Combs-Cantrell DT, Cohen M, Kalayjian LA, Kanner A, Liporace JD, Pennell PB, Privitera M, Loring DW. Cognitive function at 3 years of age after fetal exposure to antiepileptic drugs. *New England Journal of Medicine* 2009; **360**: 1597–1605.

Patsalos PN. *Antiepileptic drug interactions: a clinical guide*, 3rd edition. Springer, London, UK; 2016.

Patsalos PN, Berry DJ, Bourgeois BF, Cloyd JC, Glauser TA, Johannessen SI, Leppik IE, Tomson T, Perucca E. Antiepileptic drugs – best practice guidelines for therapeutic drug monitoring: a position paper by the Subcommission on Therapeutic Drug Monitoring, ILAE Commission on Therapeutic Strategies. *Epilepsia* 2008; **49**: 1239–1276.

Patsalos PN, Zugman M, Lake C, James A, Ratnaraj N, Sander JW. Serum protein binding of 25 antiepileptic drugs in a routine clinical setting: a comparison of free non-protein-bound concentrations. *Epilepsia* 2017; **58**: 1234–1243.

Ramsey RE, Wilder BJ, Murphy JV, Holmes GL, Uthman B. Efficacy and safety of valproic acid versus phenytoin as sole therapy for newly diagnosed primary generalized tonic-clonic seizures. *Journal of Epilepsy* 1992; **5**: 55–60.

Shallcross R, Bromley RL, Irwin B, Bonnett LJ, Morrow J, Baker GA. Child development following in utero exposure. Levetiracetam vs sodium valproate. *Neurology* 2011; **76**: 383–389.

Sommerville KS, Dutta S, Biton V, Zhang Y, Cloyd JC, Uthman B. Bioavailability of a Divalproex extended-release formulation versus the conventional Divalproex formulation in adult patients receiving enzyme-inducing antiepileptic drugs. *Clinical Drug-Investigation* 2003; **23**: 661–670.

Vestergaard P, Rejnmark L, Mosekilde L. Fracture risk associated with use of antiepileptic drugs. *Epilepsia* 2004; **45**: 1330–1337.

Villareal HJ, Wilder BJ, Willmore LJ, Bauman AW, Hammond EJ, Bruni J. Effect of valproic acid on spike and wave discharges in patients with absence seizures. *Neurology* 1978; **28**: 886–891.

Wyszynski DF, Nambisan M, Surve T, Alsdorf RM, Smith CR, Holmes LB. Antiepileptic drug pregnancy registry. Increased rate of major malformations in offspring exposed to valproate during pregnancy. *Neurology* 2005; **64**: 961–965.

VIGABATRIN

Therapeutics

Chemical Name and Structure

Vigabatrin, (±)-amino-hex-5-enoic acid, is supplied as a racemic mixture of two enantiomers in equal proportions: the (S+)-enantiomer and the R(–)-enantiomer, with only the (S+)-enantiomer being pharmacologically active. It is a white to off-white crystalline solid, with a molecular weight of 129.2 and an empirical formula of $C_6H_{11}NO_2$.

Brand Names
- Sabril; Sabrilan; Sabrilex

Generics Available
- No

Licensed Indications for Epilepsy
- Adjunctive treatment of partial (focal) seizures with and without secondary generalization not satisfactorily controlled with other AEDs (UK SPC)
- Monotherapy in the treatment of infantile spasms (West syndrome) (UK SPC)
- Adjunctive therapy for adult patients with refractory complex partial (focal dyscognitive) seizures who have inadequately responded to several alternative treatments (FDA PI)
- Monotherapy for pediatric patients 1 month to 2 years of age with infantile spasms (FDA PI)

Licensed Indications for Non-epilepsy Conditions
- There are none

Non-licensed Use for Epilepsy
- There are none

Non-licensed Use for Non-epilepsy Conditions
- There are none

Ineffective (Contraindicated)
- Aggravates typical absence seizures and provokes absence status epilepticus
- Idiopathic generalized epilepsies with absences

V

VIGABATRIN

- May exaggerate atypical absences such as those occurring in Lennox–Gastaut syndrome
- May exaggerate myoclonic seizures such as those occurring in progressive and non-progressive myoclonic epilepsies
- In the USA, vigabatrin can be obtained only through the manufacturer and only with proper documentation that the patient fulfills the licensed indication criteria; accordingly, children older than 2 years will not receive vigabatrin

Mechanism of Action
- As an analog of GABA, it was specifically developed to increase brain GABA
- Binds irreversibly and covalently to GABA transaminase, causing permanent inactivation
- Inactivation of GABA transaminase, which is responsible for the breakdown of GABA in neurons and glia, results in an increase in brain (synaptic) GABA

Efficacy Profile
- The goals of treatment are to achieve complete seizure remission when possible, or at least improved frequency and severity of seizures, while also minimizing adverse effects and improving patient quality of life
- Efficacy should be apparent within 3 months of treatment initiation
- Discontinuation should occur in the absence of definitive, meaningful seizure reduction during this period to eliminate the potential for developing peripheral visual field defects

Pharmacokinetics
Absorption and Distribution
- Oral bioavailability: 60–80%
- Food co-ingestion: neither delays the rate of absorption nor decreases the extent of absorption
- Tmax: 1–2 hours
- Time to steady state: 1–2 days
- Pharmacokinetics: linear
- Protein binding: 0%
- Volume of distribution: 0.8 L/kg
- Salivary concentrations: vigabatrin is secreted into saliva but it is not known whether such concentrations are similar to the unbound levels seen in plasma

Metabolism
- Vigabatrin is not metabolized

V

Elimination
- Following a single dose, half-life values in adults are 5–8 hours
- The renal clearance of vigabatrin is proportional to the CrCl
- Renal excretion: ~100% of an administered dose is excreted unchanged in urine

Drug Interaction Profile
Pharmacokinetic Drug Interactions
- Interactions between AEDs: effects on vigabatrin:
  - Felbamate *increases* the excretion of vigabatrin and *decreases* vigabatrin plasma levels
- Interactions between AEDs: effects by vigabatrin:
  - Vigabatrin can *decrease* plasma levels of carbamazepine, phenytoin, and rufinamide
  - Vigabatrin can *increase* plasma levels of carbamazepine
- Interactions between AEDs and non-AED drugs: effects on vigabatrin:
  - To date, there have been no reports of other non-AED drugs affecting the clearance of vigabatrin and affecting vigabatrin plasma levels
- Interactions between AEDs and non-AED drugs: effects by vigabatrin:
  - To date, there have been no reports of vigabatrin affecting the clearance of other non-AED drugs and affecting their plasma levels

Pharmacodynamic Drug Interactions
- Co-medication with carbamazepine: enhanced seizure control (partial seizures) may occur
- Co-medication with lamotrigine: enhanced seizure control (partial and secondary generalized tonic–clonic seizures) may occur
- Co-medication with phenobarbital, particularly in patients with tuberous sclerosis: phenobarbital appears to delay or prevent the onset of seizure control by vigabatrin
- Co-medication with tiagabine: enhanced seizure control may occur

Hormonal Contraception
- Vigabatrin does not enhance the metabolism of oral contraceptives so as to decrease plasma levels of hormonal contraceptives and, therefore, does not compromise contraception control

Adverse Effects
How Drug Causes Adverse Effects
- It is possible that the peripheral visual field defects associated with vigabatrin are the consequence of specific accumulation of vigabatrin in the retina

ADVERSE EFFECTS

V

- The visual field defects may be the consequence of an idiosyncratic adverse drug reaction, although dose- and duration-dependent toxicity have also been documented

Common Adverse Effects
- Visual field defects (males have a twofold greater risk than females), diplopia, nystagmus
- Sedation, dizziness, headache, ataxia
- Memory, cognitive, mental (thought disturbances), and behavioral disturbances (e.g., excitation and agitation, especially in children)
- Psychosis, mania, depression
- Paresthesia
- Nausea, abdominal pain
- Fatigue
- Vigabatrin commonly causes conspicuous magnetic resonance imaging abnormalities seen most prominently in the basal ganglia and the upper brainstem; these abnormalities tend to be reversible, even without discontinuation of the drug

Life-threatening or Dangerous Adverse Effects
- May cause an increase in seizure frequency, including status epilepticus – patients with myoclonic or absence seizures may be particularly at risk of status epilepticus
- Rare encephalopathic symptoms such as marked sedation, stupor, and confusion

Rare and not Life-threatening Adverse Effects
- Angioedema
- Urticaria
- Hallucinations
- Rash
- Retinal atrophy, optic neuritis

Weight Change
- Weight gain is common

What to do About Adverse Effects
- Discuss common and severe adverse effects with patients or parents before starting medication, including symptoms that should be reported to the physician
- Visual field defects, which usually present at 6 months to 2 years, are not usually reversible; therefore, if the patient is not responding to treatment (within 3 months), vigabatrin should be withdrawn

VIGABATRIN

Dosing and Use

Usual Dosage Range
- Adults: 1000–3000 mg/day
- Children: 1000–3000 mg/day
- Infants (monotherapy for infantile spasms): 150–200 mg/kg/day

Available Formulations
- Tablets: 500 mg
- Sachet: 500 mg (sugar-free powder)

How to Dose
- When initiating vigabatrin treatment start with a low dose and titrate slowly so as to minimize adverse effects
  - *For adults:* start treatment with 500 mg/day; each week increase by 500 mg/day; maintenance dose generally 1000–3000 mg/day given either as a single dose or in two equally divided doses
  - *Children:* start treatment with 40 mg/kg/day in one or two divided doses and increase at weekly intervals depending on body weight; maintenance dose of 500–1000 mg/day, 1000–1500 mg/day, 1500–3000 mg/day, and 2000–3000 mg/day for infants weighing 10–15 kg, 15–30 kg, 30–50 kg, and >50 kg, respectively, is often required
  - *Infants (monotherapy for infantile spasms):* start treatment with 50 mg/kg/day and titrate according to response over 7 days to a maximum of 150–200 mg/kg/day given as a single dose or in divided doses; maintenance dose generally 150–200 mg/kg/day

Dosing Tips
- The powder (sachet) formulation can be added to water, fruit juice, or milk and ingested immediately as a solution
- If the patient does not respond within 3 months of initiation of treatment, vigabatrin should be withdrawn so as to avoid induction of visual field defects, which occurs in 30% of patients
- Adverse effects in adults, such as sedation, drowsiness, fatigue, and impaired concentration, and in children, such as excitation and agitation, generally present at the beginning of treatment and decrease with time

How to Withdraw Drug
- May need to adjust dosage of concurrent medication as vigabatrin is being discontinued, because plasma levels of other drugs may change (see Pharmacokinetic Drug Interactions section)
- Taper: a gradual dose reduction over a 2–4-week period should be undertaken
- Rapid discontinuation may increase the risk of rebound seizures

Overdose
- To date, no fatalities have been reported
- Most common overdoses range from 7.5 to 30 g; however, ingestions up to 90 g have been reported

DOSING AND USE

- Most common symptoms include drowsiness and coma
- Other less frequently reported symptoms include: vertigo, headache, psychosis, respiratory depression or apnea, bradycardia, hypotension, agitation, irritability, confusion, abnormal behavior, and speech disorder
- If indicated the stomach should be emptied by lavage or by induction of emesis
- Hemodialysis removes 40–60% of vigabatrin from blood and, therefore, serves as a useful procedure in cases of overdose

Tests and Therapeutic Drug Monitoring
- Before starting: blood count, liver, and kidney function tests
- Before starting: all patients should have ophthalmological consultation with visual field examination using static perimetry, or electroretinography in those who cannot cooperate
- During treatment: blood count, liver and kidney function tests every 6–12 months
- During treatment: systematic perimetry (for adults) or visual evoked potentials (for children aged <9 years) every 6 months; electroretinography should be used in adults who are unable to cooperate with perimetry, and in the very young; however, it should be kept in mind that electroretinography has been shown not to be fully reliable
- In the USA, vigabatrin can be obtained only through the manufacturer and only with proper documentation of mandatory ophthalmological monitoring
- Therapeutic drug monitoring:
  - At doses between 1000 and 3000 mg/day, the expected trough vigabatrin plasma concentrations are in the range of 0.8–36 mg/L (6–279 μmol/L)
  - The conversion factor from mg/L to μmol/L is 7.74 (i.e., 1 mg/L = 7.74 μmol/L)
  - Overall, the rationale for monitoring does not apply to vigabatrin because there is no correlation between plasma concentrations and clinical efficacy, and the duration of vigabatrin's action long outlasts its plasma half-life. This is attributable to the mechanism of action of vigabatrin whereby the inactivation of the enzyme GABA transaminase is irreversible and the duration of the effect of the drug is dependent on the rate of GABA transaminase resynthesis, which requires many days
  - Measurement of plasma vigabatrin concentrations may be useful as a check on recent compliance
  - The reference range of vigabatrin in plasma is considered to be the same for children and adults, although no data are available to support this clinical practice
  - There are no data indicating the usefulness of monitoring vigabatrin by use of saliva

V

- Before giving a drug that can cause weight gain to an overweight or obese patient, consider determining whether the patient already has pre-diabetes (fasting plasma glucose 100–125 mg/dL), diabetes (fasting plasma glucose greater than 126 mg/dL), or dyslipidemia (increased total cholesterol, LDL cholesterol, and triglycerides; decreased HDL cholesterol), and treat or refer such patients for treatment, including nutrition and weight management, physical activity counseling, smoking cessation, and medical management
- Monitor weight and BMI during treatment

Other Warnings/Precautions
- Because visual field defects are irreversible even after discontinuation of vigabatrin, vigabatrin should only be prescribed after a careful assessment of the balance of benefits and risks compared with alternative treatments
- The usual pattern of visual field defects entails a concentric constriction of the visual field of both eyes, which is generally more marked nasally than temporally; in the central visual field (within 30 degrees of eccentricity) an annular nasal defect is frequently seen but central visual acuity is not impaired – however, the visual field defects reported in patients receiving vigabatrin have ranged from mild to severe, with the latter potentially disabling
- Should not be used concomitantly with other retinotoxic drugs
- Use with caution in patients with a history of psychosis, depression, or behavioral problems
- Many patients may experience reductions in their alanine transferase and aspartate transferase activities, which is considered to be the result of vigabatrin, and is usually asymptomatic; reductions in hemoglobin concentrations can also occur and may on occasion attain clinical significance

Do not Use
- If patient has any pre-existing clinically significant visual field defect
- If patient has a proven allergy to vigabatrin or to any excipient

Special Populations
Renal Impairment
- Vigabatrin is renally excreted, so the dose may need to be lowered – particularly in patients with a CrCl of <60 mL/min
- Because vigabatrin can be removed by hemodialysis, patients receiving hemodialysis may require supplemental doses of vigabatrin

Hepatic Impairment
- Vigabatrin is not metabolized in the liver and consequently dose adjustment will not be necessary

SPECIAL POPULATIONS

V

Children
- Children have an increased metabolic capacity and consequently higher doses on a mg/kg basis are usually required to achieve the equivalent therapeutic plasma levels seen in adults – specific dosing recommendations are in place for children

Elderly
- Elderly patients are more susceptible to adverse effects and, therefore, may not tolerate higher doses
- Because of an age-related reduction in renal function, lower vigabatrin doses are appropriate and patients should be monitored for undesirable effects such as sedation and confusion
- Elderly patients frequently receive concurrent drug therapies for comorbidities, and therefore may be at greater risk for pharmacokinetic and pharmacodynamic interactions; as the risk of pharmacokinetic interactions with vigabatrin is low or non-existent, vigabatrin may be advantageous for use in the elderly

Pregnancy
- Specialist advice should be given to women who are of childbearing potential; they should be informed about the teratogenicity of all AEDs and the importance of avoiding an unplanned pregnancy; the AED treatment regimen should be reviewed when a woman is planning to become pregnant
- Rapid discontinuation of AEDs should be avoided as this may lead to breakthrough seizures, which could have serious consequences for the woman and the unborn child
- Vigabatrin was previously classified by the US FDA as risk category C (some animal studies show adverse effects, no controlled studies in humans); the current FDA Pregnancy and Lactation Rule has eliminated pregnancy risk category labels, but evidence available so far does not suggest that it is more teratogenic than most other AEDs
- Use in women of childbearing potential requires weighing potential benefits to the mother against the risks to the fetus
- Use with other AEDs in combination may cause a higher prevalence of teratogenic effects than vigabatrin monotherapy
- Taper drug if discontinuing
- Seizures, even mild seizures, may cause harm to the embryo/fetus
- There are no available data on the pharmacokinetic changes of vigabatrin during pregnancy

Breast Feeding
- Breast milk: 4–20% of maternal plasma levels
- Breastfed infants: it is not known what plasma vigabatrin concentrations are achieved in breastfed infants compared with the levels of their mothers
- If drug is continued while breast feeding, infant should be monitored for possible adverse effects
- If adverse effects are observed, recommend bottle feeding

The Overall Place of Vigabatrin in the Treatment of Epilepsy

Vigabatrin is effective for the treatment of infantile spasms (West syndrome), particularly in patients with cryptogenic etiology, tuberous sclerosis, or localized cortical dysplasia, although, in the short term, it appears to be somewhat less effective than ACTH. It is also effective in simple partial and complex partial (focal) seizures with or without secondary generalization, including those caused by tuberous sclerosis. Because spasm cessation can occur within 2 weeks following initiation of vigabatrin treatment and because of the desirability of rapid seizure control to reduce secondary psychomotor regression or transition to other catastrophic seizure types (e.g., Lennox–Gastaut syndrome), vigabatrin is becoming a drug of choice for the management of infantile spasms. Furthermore, given the catastrophic nature of infantile spasms, the risk of peripheral visual field defects may be acceptable if appropriate seizure control can be achieved, thus providing an improved opportunity for normal development. Since response to treatment can usually be established within a short time, vigabatrin can be discontinued early in those patients who do not respond, thus eliminating the risk of retinal damage

Primary Seizure Types
- Simple partial or complex partial (focal) epilepsy with or without secondary generalization
- Infantile spasms (West syndrome)

Secondary Seizure Types
- None

Potential Advantages
- Vigabatrin is an effective AED for the treatment of focal epilepsies of any type (idiopathic or symptomatic) with or without secondary generalized tonic–clonic seizures
- Although corticotropin/corticosteroids are efficacious in 50–75% of patients with infantile spasms, relapse rates are high and adverse effects are substantial
- Because it is excreted exclusively by renal elimination, vigabatrin is not associated with any significant pharmacokinetic interactions

Potential Disadvantages
- Visual field defects which require frequent monitoring
- Potential teratogen

Suggested Reading
Conway M, Cubbidge R.P, Hoskings SL. Visual field severity indices demonstrate dose-dependent visual loss from vigabatrin therapy. *Epilepsia* 2008; **49**: 108–116.

V

Friedman D, Bogner M, Parker-Menzer K, Devinsky O. Vigabatrin for partial-onset seizure treatment in patients with tuberous sclerosis complex. *Epilepsy and Behavior* 2013; **27**: 118–120.

Go CY, Mackay MT, Weiss SK, Stephens D, Adams-Webber T, Ashwal S, Snead OC 3rd; Child Neurology Society; American Academy of Neurology. Evidence-based guideline update: medical treatment of infantile spasms. Report of the Guideline Development Subcommittee of the American Academy of Neurology and the Practice Committee of the Child Neurology Society. *Neurology* 2012; **78**: 1974–1980.

Johannessen Landmark C, Patsalos PN. Drug interactions involving the new second- and third-generation antiepileptic drugs. *Expert Reviews in Neurotherapeutics* 2010; **10**: 119–140.

Moskowitz A, Hansen RM, Eklund SE, Fulton AB. Electroretinographic (ERG) responses in pediatric patients using vigabatrin. *Doc Ophthalmology* 2012; **124**: 197–209.

Patsalos PN. *Antiepileptic drug interactions: a clinical guide*, 3rd edition. Springer, London, UK; 2016.

Patsalos PN, Duncan J S. The pharmacology and pharmacokinetics of vigabatrin. *Reviews in Contemporary Pharmacotherapy* 1995; **6**: 447–456.

Ryan MF, Samy A, Young J. Vigabatrin causes profound reduction in serum alanine transferase activity. *Annals of Clinical Biochemistry* 1996; **33**: 257–258.

Shields WD. Infantile spasms: little seizures, big consequences. *Epilepsy Currents* 2006; **6**:63–69.

Sills GJ, Patsalos PN, Butler E, Forrest G, Ratnaraj N, Brodie MJ. Visual field constrictions. Accumulation of vigabatrin but not tiagabine in the retina. *Neurology* 2001; **57**: 196–200.

Wheless JW, Carmant L, Bebin M, Conry JA, Chiron C, Elterman RD, Frost M, Paolicchi JM, Donald Shields W, Thiele EA, Zupanc ML, Collins SD. Magnetic resonance imaging abnormalities associated with vigabatrin in patients with epilepsy. *Epilepsia* 2009; **50**: 195–205.

Wheless JW, Clarke DF, Arzimanoglou A, Carpenter D. Treatment of pediatric epilepsy: European expert opinion, 2007. *Epileptic Disorders* 2007; **9**: 353–412.

Wheless JW, Ramsey RE, Collins SD. Vigabatrin. *Neurotherapeutics* 2007; **4**: 163–172.

Willmore LJ, Abelson MB, Ben-Menachem E, Pellock JM, Shields WD. Vigabatrin: 2008 update. *Epilepsia* 2009; **50**: 163–173.

VIGABATRIN

ZONISAMIDE

Therapeutics

Chemical Name and Structure

Zonisamide, 1,2-benzisoxazole-3-methanesulfonamide, is a white to pale yellow crystalline powder, with a molecular weight of 212.23 and an empirical formula of $C_8H_8N_2O_3S$.

Brand Names
- Excegran
- Zonegran; Zonicare; Zonimid; Zonisep; Zonit

Generics Available
- Yes

Licensed Indications for Epilepsy
- Monotherapy for partial (focal) and secondary generalized seizures in adults with newly diagnosed epilepsy (UK SPC)
- Adjunctive therapy for partial (focal) and secondary generalized seizures in adolescents, and children aged 6 years and above (UK SPC)
- Adjunctive therapy for partial (focal) and secondary generalized seizures in adults (FDA PI)

Licensed Indications for Non-epilepsy Conditions
- Parkinson disease (licensed in Japan)

Non-licensed Use for Epilepsy
- Absence seizures
- Infantile spasms (West syndrome)
- Juvenile myoclonic epilepsy
- Lennox–Gastaut syndrome
- Myoclonic astatic epilepsy (Doose syndrome)
- Myoclonic seizures
- Progressive myoclonus epilepsy (Unverricht–Lundborg and Lafora disease)

Non-licensed Use for Non-epilepsy Conditions
- Binge-eating disorder
- Bipolar disorder
- Migraine
- Neuropathic pain
- Psychotropic drug-induced weight gain

Z

Ineffective (Contraindicated)
- Zonisamide is potentially effective against all seizure types and is not contraindicated for any seizure type or epilepsy
- There is no evidence to support its use for the prophylaxis of febrile seizures
- Zonisamide does not commonly exacerbate seizures

Mechanism of Action
- Partial blockade of activity-dependent sodium channels
- Blockade of T-type calcium channels
- Inhibition of potassium-mediated glutamate release
- Increase in extracellular levels of dopamine and serotonin
- Up-regulation of excitatory amino-acid carrier-1 (EAAC-1)
- Down-regulation of the expression of GAT-1
- Carbonic anhydrase inhibition, but potency is much lower than that of acetazolamide

Efficacy Profile
- The goals of treatment are to achieve complete seizure remission when possible, or at least improved frequency and severity of seizures, while also minimizing adverse effects and improving patient quality of life
- Therapeutic effect usually evident within 2–4 weeks
- If zonisamide is ineffective or only partially effective, it can be replaced by or combined with another AED that is appropriate for the patient's seizure type or epilepsy syndrome

Pharmacokinetics
Absorption and Distribution
- Oral bioavailability: >90%
- Food co-ingestion: delays the rate of absorption (Tmax, 4–6 hours) but does not decrease the extent of absorption
- Tmax: 2–5 hours
- Time to steady state: 10–15 days
- Pharmacokinetics: linear
- Protein binding: ~40%
- Volume of distribution: 1.0–1.9 L/kg
- Salivary concentrations: zonisamide is secreted into saliva, and concentrations are similar to the unbound levels seen in plasma

Metabolism
- Zonisamide undergoes acetylation to form *N*-acetyl zonisamide and reduction to form 2-sulfamoylacetylphenol – the latter being subsequently glucuronidated
- The reduction of zonisamide to 2-sulfamoylacetylphenol is mediated by the CYP3A4 isoenzyme

- Metabolites are not pharmacologically active
- Autoinduction is not a feature of zonisamide metabolism

Elimination
- In the absence of enzyme-inducing AEDs, half-life values for zonisamide are 50–70 hours
- In the presence of enzyme-inducing AEDs, half-life values for zonisamide are 25–35 hours
- No data are available regarding the elimination half-life of zonisamide in children; however, young children (≤4 years) have a significantly increased zonisamide clearance compared with older children (5–17 years)
- Renal excretion: ~65% of an administered dose is excreted as metabolites in urine; 50% as the 2-sulfamoylacetylphenol glucuronide, and 15% as *N*-acetyl zonisamide
- Renal excretion: ~35% of an administered dose is excreted as unchanged zonisamide in urine

Drug Interaction Profile
Pharmacokinetic Drug Interactions
- Interactions between AEDs: effects on zonisamide:
  - Carbamazepine, phenobarbital, phenytoin, and primidone can *increase* the clearance of zonisamide and *decrease* zonisamide plasma levels
- Interactions between AEDs: effects by zonisamide:
  - Zonisamide can *decrease* the clearance of carbamazepine-epoxide (pharmacologically active metabolite of carbamazepine) and *increase* carbamazepine-epoxide plasma levels
- Interactions between AEDs and non-AED drugs: effects on zonisamide:
  - Atkins diet (modified) and risperidone can *decrease* zonisamide plasma levels
- Interactions between AEDs and non-AED drugs: effects by zonisamide:
- To date, there have been no reports of zonisamide affecting the clearance of other non-AED drugs and affecting their plasma levels

Pharmacodynamic Drug Interactions
- To date, none have been reported

Hormonal Contraception
- Zonisamide does not enhance the metabolism of oral contraceptives and therefore does not compromise contraception control

Adverse Effects

How Drug Causes Adverse Effects
- Mechanism by which zonisamide causes adverse effects has not been established
- Carbonic anhydrase inhibition by zonisamide, although not or only minimally involved in its antiepileptic activity, may be the mechanism responsible for some of the clinical adverse effects, such as metabolic acidosis, paresthesias, kidney stones, and hypohydrosis

Common Adverse Effects
Unlike sulfonamide antibiotic compounds, zonisamide does not contain an arylamine group at the N4-position, which contributes to allergic reactions to sulfonamide antibiotics
- Drowsiness, fatigue
- Ataxia
- Psychomotor slowing
- Impairments in verbal learning (may be transient)
- Behavioral adverse effects (e.g., aggression, agitation, irritability, poor attention, hyperactivity, dysphoria)
- Psychiatric adverse effects (i.e., hallucinations, paranoia, and psychosis)
- Anorexia, nausea, abdominal pain, vomiting, and weight loss
- Metabolic acidosis (lowered serum bicarbonate or CO_2, especially in children)
- Hypohydrosis (decreased sweating, especially in children, may lead to hyperthermia)
- Allergic rash (risk lower than for antibiotic sulfonamides)

Life-threatening or Dangerous Adverse Effects
- Very rarely, Stevens–Johnson syndrome, toxic epidermic necrolysis, hepatic necrosis
- Rare blood dyscrasias (aplastic anemia, agranulocytosis)
- Rare oligohydrosis and hyperthermia (pediatric patients)

Rare and not Life-threatening Adverse Effects
- Nephrolithiasis (1–2%)
- Paresthesias, mostly tingling in the fingers and toes
- Mild elevation of serum creatinine and BUN values

Weight Change
- Weight loss is common

What to do About Adverse Effects
- Discuss common and severe adverse effects with patients or parents before starting medication, including symptoms that should be reported to the physician
- Discuss symptoms associated with kidney stones, glaucoma, and hypohydrosis

- Some CNS-related adverse effects may be avoided or reduced by slow titration, but these sometimes persist even at low doses and despite slow titration
- Metabolic acidosis is usually compensated, but patients may be treated with oral bicarbonate for values of 15–18 mEq/L or less
- If possible, zonisamide should not be administered to patients who are already receiving acetazolamide, sulthiame, topiramate, or the ketogenic diet, because these treatments also predispose to metabolic acidosis and to kidney stones
- Patients should be encouraged to drink water liberally while on zonisamide to reduce risk of kidney stones
- Anorexia and weight loss may improve with dosage reduction
- Children who benefit from zonisamide treatment but also experience hypohydrosis should avoid exposure to hot environments, be removed from hot environments if developing symptoms or signs of heat stroke, and may experience improvement following cool/tepid sponge baths or wrapping in a cool wet towel
- Cognitive and behavioral adverse effects often improve following reduction of the dose of zonisamide, and resolve following cessation of zonisamide

Dosing and Use

Usual Dosage Range
- Adults: 100–600 mg/day (lower doses may be sufficient in monotherapy, while higher doses may be necessary with enzyme-inducing AEDs)
- Children: 8 mg/kg/day (monotherapy); 12 mg/kg/day (with enzyme-inducing AEDs)

Available Formulations
- Capsules (hard): 25 mg, 50 mg, 100 mg

How to Dose
- *For adults:* start treatment with 100 mg/day, once or twice daily; at intervals of 2 weeks, increase as needed and as tolerated by 100 mg/day; maintenance dose generally 100–600 mg/day
- For *children over 6 years of age:* start treatment with 1.0–2.0 mg/kg/day, once or twice daily; at intervals of 1–2 weeks, increase as needed and as tolerated by 1.0–2.0 mg/kg/day; maintenance dose generally 8–12 mg/kg/day; doses of 20 mg/kg/day may be necessary and well tolerated, especially in infants; dosage requirements may increase two-fold in children co-prescribed enzyme-inducing AEDs

Dosing Tips
- Slow dose titration may enhance tolerability to sedating effects, and is necessary for zonisamide to reach steady state given its long half-life

Z

ZONISAMIDE

- For intolerable sedation, may give zonisamide dosage once daily exclusively at night, or divide most of the dose given at night and a smaller dose during the day
- Adverse effects may increase notably at doses greater than 300 mg/day
- Some patients may do very well at relatively low doses of zonisamide, such as 100–200 mg/day in adults or 4–6 mg/kg/day in children; the response to treatment should be assessed at these doses before increasing the dose further
- In view of the long elimination half-life, zonisamide can be administered once or twice daily

How to Withdraw Drug
- There is no need to adjust dosage of concurrent medications as zonisamide is being discontinued, because plasma levels of other drugs do not change (see Pharmacokinetic Drug Interactions section)
- There appears to be a very low potential for withdrawal seizures or symptoms upon rapid discontinuation given the long half-life of zonisamide
- Rapid discontinuation may increase the risk of seizures, however, so when possible, taper dose over a period of several weeks to months

Overdose
- No fatalities have been reported to date
- A patient who ingested an overdose of zonisamide and had a serum level of 100.1 mg/L (471.5 μmol/L) after 31 hours developed coma, bradycardia, hypotension, and respiratory depression; the outcome was good following supportive care
- Severe metabolic acidosis could develop
- The stomach should be emptied immediately by lavage or by induction of emesis
- Hemodialysis removes zonisamide from blood, and therefore serves as a useful procedure in cases of overdose

Tests and Therapeutic Drug Monitoring
- Consider measuring serum bicarbonate (CO_2) before treatment and periodically in children or those with severe cognitive impairment in whom reporting of symptoms or recognition of signs of metabolic acidosis or hypohydrosis may be difficult
- Other routine laboratory testing is not necessary
- Therapeutic drug monitoring:
  - Optimum seizure control in patients on monotherapy is most likely to occur at zonisamide plasma concentrations of 10–40 mg/L (47–188 μmol/L)
  - The conversion factor from mg/L to μmol/L is 4.71 (i.e., 1 mg/L = 4.71 μmol/L)
  - Drowsiness is more likely to occur at levels >40 mg/L (>188 μmol/L)

- Because zonisamide has a high binding affinity to the intracellular compartment of erythrocytes, this may lead to a false elevation of the plasma zonisamide level in hemolyzed blood samples
- The reference range of zonisamide in plasma is considered to be the same for children and adults, although no data are available to support this clinical practice
- Zonisamide can be monitored by use of saliva, which is a measure of the free non-protein-bound plasma concentration that is pharmacologically relevant

Other Warnings / Precautions
- Patients should be monitored carefully for evidence of cognitive or psychiatric adverse effects
- Patients should be monitored carefully for evidence of kidney stones; in those who develop symptoms or signs of kidney stones, urinary straining and renal ultrasound should be considered to document nephrocalcinosis that may prompt zonisamide discontinuation
- Depressive effects may be increased by other CNS depressants (alcohol, MAOIs, other AEDs)
- Use with caution when combining with other drugs that predispose patients to hypohydrosis and heat-related disorders, including carbonic anhydrase inhibitors and anticholinergics
- Life-threatening rashes have developed in association with zonisamide use; zonisamide should generally be discontinued at the first sign of serious rash
- Patients should be instructed to report any symptoms of hypersensitivity immediately (fever; flu-like symptoms; rash; blisters on skin or in eyes, mouth, ears, nose, or genital areas; swelling of eyelids, conjunctivitis, lymphadenopathy)
- Patients should be monitored for signs of unusual bleeding or bruising, mouth sores, infections, fever, and sore throat, as there may be an increased risk of aplastic anemia and agranulocytosis with zonisamide

Do not Use
- If patient has a proven allergy to zonisamide or to any of the excipients
- Use with caution in patients undergoing treatments that are associated with an increase in risk of kidney stones, such as acetazolamide, sulthiame, topiramate, and the ketogenic diet
- There does not appear to be specific allergic cross-reactivity between antibiotic sulfonamides and the sulfonamide contained within zonisamide, so a history of allergic reaction to an antibiotic sulfonamide is a relative, although not absolute, contraindication for the use of zonisamide

DOSING AND USE

Z

Special Populations

Renal Impairment
- Zonisamide is renally excreted (35%), therefore, the dose may need to be lowered
- At a CrCl of <20 mL/min, the clearance of zonisamide is reduced by 35%
- Because zonisamide can be removed by hemodialysis, patients receiving hemodialysis may require supplemental doses of zonisamide

Hepatic Impairment
- Zonisamide is substantially metabolized (65%), and consequently lower doses may be required
- No studies on the effect of hepatic failure on the pharmacokinetics of zonisamide have been reported

Children
- Children have an increased metabolic capacity and consequently higher mg/kg/day doses are usually required to achieve the equivalent therapeutic plasma levels seen in adults
- Pharmacokinetic interactions in children are usually of a greater magnitude than that seen in adults
- Children are at higher risk of developing metabolic acidosis and hypohydrosis

Elderly
- The pharmacokinetics of zonisamide in elderly patients do not differ from those in adults
- Elderly patients are more susceptible to adverse effects and may therefore be intolerant of higher doses
- Because of an age-related reduction in renal and hepatic function, lower initial and target zonisamide doses with slower titration may be appropriate
- Elderly patients are often prescribed concurrent drug therapies for comorbidities and therefore may be at greater risk for pharmacokinetic and pharmacodynamic interactions; the risk of pharmacokinetic interactions with zonisamide is minimal

Pregnancy
- Specialist advice should be given to women who are of childbearing potential; they should be informed about the teratogenicity of all AEDs and the importance of avoiding an unplanned pregnancy; the AED treatment regimen should be reviewed when a woman is planning to become pregnant
- Rapid discontinuation of AEDs should be avoided as this may lead to breakthrough seizures, which could have serious consequences for the woman and the unborn child
- Zonisamide was previously classified by the US FDA as risk category C (some animal studies show adverse effects, no controlled studies

in humans), the current FDA Pregnancy and Lactation Rule has eliminated pregnancy risk category labels; evidence does not suggest that zonisamide has significant teratogenic potential
- Use in women of childbearing potential requires weighing potential benefits to the mother against the risks to the fetus
- Seizures may cause harm to the embryo/fetus
- Use with other AEDs in combination may raise the risk for teratogenic effects compared with zonisamide monotherapy
- Taper drug if discontinuing
- During pregnancy, zonisamide pharmacokinetics change significantly; zonisamide plasma concentrations decrease by 40–50% due to increased clearance consequent to enhanced metabolism; an increase in zonisamide dose may be required; monitoring plasma concentrations with comparison to historical benchmark plasma concentrations to guide further zonisamide dose adjustments at least once per trimester is reasonable; during the postpartum period, zonisamide metabolism may revert to normal, so zonisamide concentrations may subsequently increase, requiring dosage decrease to avoid adverse effects

Breast Feeding
- Breast milk: 90% of maternal plasma levels
- Breastfed infants: zonisamide plasma levels are ~100% of maternal plasma levels
- The potential benefit to the mother should be weighed against the potential risk to the infant when considering recommendations regarding nursing
- If drug is continued while breast feeding, the infant should be monitored for possible adverse effects, including sedation and irritation
- If adverse effects are observed, recommend bottle feeding

The Overall Place of Zonisamide in the Treatment of Epilepsy
Zonisamide appears to be an effective broad-spectrum AED in partial (focal) seizures with or without generalized tonic–clonic seizures, primary and secondary generalized seizures including epileptic spasms of West syndrome, other epileptic encephalopathies such as Ohtahara syndrome, and progressive and probably other myoclonic epilepsies such as Unverricht syndrome. Zonisamide is second-line therapy for partial (focal) seizures, is the drug of choice in progressive myoclonic epilepsy, and is a drug of second choice for idiopathic generalized epilepsies with generalized tonic–clonic seizures, juvenile myoclonic epilepsy, or Lennox–Gastaut syndrome.

Primary Seizure Types
- Partial (focal) epilepsies
- Progressive myoclonic epilepsy

Z

ZONISAMIDE

Secondary Seizure Types
- Myoclonic seizures
- Idiopathic generalized epilepsies with generalized tonic–clonic seizures
- Juvenile myoclonic epilepsy
- Lennox–Gastaut syndrome
- Myoclonic astatic epilepsy (Doose syndrome)
- Infantile spasms (West syndrome)

Potential Advantages
- Broad spectrum of seizure protection
- Zonisamide causes only one pharmacokinetic interaction
- Does not exacerbate seizures

Potential Disadvantages
- In contrast to topiramate, zonisamide can cause an allergic rash
- Hypohydrosis can cause hyperthermia in children
- Cognitive and psychotic episodes may be problematic
- Nephrolithiasis is a concern
- Potential teratogen

Suggested Reading

Ando H, Matsubara S, Oi A, Usai R, Suzuki M, Fujimuru A. Two nursing mothers treated with zonisamide: should breast feeding be avoided? *Journal of Obstetrics and Gynaecological Research* 2014; **40**: 275–278.

Brackett CC, Singh H, Block JH. Likelihood and mechanisms of cross-allergenicity between sulfonamide antibiotics and other drugs containing a sulfonamide functional group. *Pharmacotherapy* 2004; **24**: 856–870.

Brodie MJ, Duncan R, Vespignani H, Solyom A, Bitenskyy V, Lucas C. Dose-dependent safety and efficacy of zonisamide: a randomized, double-blind, placebo-controlled study in patients with refractory partial seizures. *Epilepsia* 2005; **46**: 31–41.

Faught E, Ayala R, Montouris GG, Leppik IE. Randomized controlled trial of zonisamide for the treatment of refractory partial-onset seizures. *Neurology* 2001; **57**: 1774–1779.

Glauser TA, Pellock JM. Zonisamide in pediatric epilepsy: review of the Japanese literature. *Journal of Child Neurology* 2002; **17**: 87–96.

Kim HL, Aldridge J, Rho JM. Clinical experience with zonisamide monotherapy and adjunctive therapy in children with epilepsy at a tertiary care referral center. *Journal of Child Neurology* 2005; **20**: 212–219.

Kyllerman M, Ben-Menachem E. Zonisamide for progressive myoclonus epilepsy: long-term observations in seven patients. *Epilepsy Research* 1998; **29**: 109–114.

Leppik IE. Practical prescribing and long-term efficacy and safety of zonisamide. *Epilepsy Research* 2006; **68S**; S17–S24.

Low PA, James S, Peschel T, Leong R, Rothstein A. Zonisamide and associated oligohydrosis and hyperthermia. *Epilepsy Research* 2004; **62**: 27–34.

Mimaki T. Clinical pharmacology and therapeutic drug monitoring of zonisamide. *Therapeutic Drug Monitoring* 1998; **29**: 593–597.

Patsalos PN. *Antiepileptic drug interactions: a clinical guide*, 3rd edition. Springer, London, UK; 2016.

Patsalos PN, Zugman M, Lake C, James A, Ratnaraj N, Sander JW. Serum protein binding of 25 antiepileptic drugs in a routine clinical setting: a comparison of free non-protein-bound concentrations. *Epilepsia* 2017; **58**: 1234–1243.

St. Louis EK, Gidal BE, Henry TR, Kaydanova Y, Krumholz A, McCabe PH, Montouris GD, Rosenfeld WE, Smith BJ, Stern JM, Waterhouse EJ, Schulz RM, Garnett WR, Bramley T. Conversions between monotherapies in epilepsy: expert consensus. *Epilepsy and Behavior* 2007; **11**: 222–234.

Suzuki Y, Imai K, Toribe Y, Ueda H, Yanagihara K, Shimono K, Okinaga T, Ono J, Nagai T, Matsuoka T, Tagawa T, Abe J, Morita Y, Fujikawa Y, Arai H, Mano T, Okada S. Long-term response to zonisamide in patients with West syndrome. *Neurology* 2002; **58**: 1556–1559.

Suzuki Y, Nagai T, Ono J, Imai K, Otani K, Tagawa T, Abe J, Shiomi M, Okada S. Zonisamide monotherapy in newly diagnosed infantile spasms. *Epilepsia* 1997; **38**: 1035–1038.

Wallander KM, Ohman I, Dahlin M. Zonisamide: pharmacokinetics, efficacy and adverse events in children with epilepsy. *Neuropediatrics* 2014; **45**: 362–369.

Weston J, Bromley R, Jackson CF, Adab N, Clayton-Smith L, Greenhalgh J, Hounsome J, McKay AJ, Tudor Smith C, Marson AG. Monotherapy treatment of epilepsy in pregnancy: congenital malformation outcomes in the child. *Cochrane Database Systematic Review* 2016; **11**: CD010224.

Z

SUGGESTED READING

ABBREVIATIONS

ACTH	adrenocorticotropic hormone
AED	antiepileptic drug
AMPA	α-amino-3-hydroxy-5-methyl-4-isoxazole propionic acid
AUC	area under the concentration versus time curve
bid	twice daily
BMI	body mass index
BUN	blood urea nitrogen
CBC	complete blood count
CCNU	1-(2-chlorethyl)-3-cyclohexyl-1-nitrosourea
Cmax	maximum plasma concentration
CNS	central nervous system
CO_2	carbon dioxide
CrCl	creatinine clearance
CYP	cytochrome P450
DEXA	dual energy X-ray absorptiometry
EAAC-1	excitatory amino-acid carrier-1
ECG	electrocardiogram
EEG	electroencephalogram
FDA	Food and Drug Administration
FDA PI	Food and Drug Administration Product Information
GABA	gamma-aminobutyric acid
GAT-1	GABA transporter-1
HCl	hydrogen chloride
HDL	high-density lipoprotein
HLA	human leukocyte antigen
im	intramuscular
iv	intravenous
LDL	low-density lipoprotein
MAOIs	monoamine oxidase inhibitors
NMDA	N-methyl-D-aspartate
PE	phenytoin equivalent
PEMA	phenyl-ethyl-malonamide
REM	rapid eye movement
SIADH	syndrome of inappropriate antidiuretic hormone secretion
tid	three times a day
Tmax	time to maximum concentration
UDP	uridine diphosphate
UGT	uridine glucuronyl transferase
UK SPC	United Kingdom Summary of Product Characteristics

INTERACTION TABLE

Interactions between antiepileptic drugs (AEDs): expected changes in plasma

PRE-EXISTING AED

AED added	BRV	CBZ	CLB	CZP	ESL-a	ESM	FBM	GBP	LCM	LTG
BRV	—	CBZ↓ CBZ-E⇑	↔	↔	NA	NA	NA	NA	↔	↔
CBZ	BRV↓	AI DMCLB⇑	CLB⇓	CZP⇓	ESL↓	ESM⇓	FBM⇓	↔	↔	LTG⇓
CLB	NA	CBZ↑ CBZ-E↑	—	NA	↔	NA	NA	NA	NA	↔
CZP	NA	↔	NA	—	NA	NA	↔	NA	NA	↔
ESL-a	NA	↔	↔	NA	—	NA	NA	↔	NA	LTG↓
ESM	NA	↔	NA	NA	NA	—	NA	NA	NA	↔
FBM	NA	CBZ↓ CBZ-E↑	CLB⇑ DMCLB⇑	CZP↑	?	?	—	NA	NA	LTG↑
GBP	NA	↔	NA	NA	↔	NA	FBM↑	—	NA	↔
LCM	NA	↔	NA	↔	NA	NA	NA	↔	—	↔
LTG	↔	↔	↔	CZP↓	↔	↔	↔	NA	↔	—
LEV	↔	↔	↔	↔	↔	↔	NA	↔	↔	↔
OXC	↔	CBZ↓	?	?	NCCP	?	?	NA	↔	LTG↓
PMP	NA	CBZ↓	CLB↓	↔	?	?	?	NA	NA	LTG↓
PB	BRV↓	CBZ⇓	CLB⇑ DMCLB⇑	CZP⇓	?	ESM⇓	↔	↔	LCM↓	LTG⇓
PHT	BRV↓	CBZ⇓	CLB⇓ DMCLB⇑	CZP⇓	ESL↓	ESM⇓	FBM⇓	↔	LCM↓	LTG⇓
PGB	NA	↔	NA	NA	NA	NA	NA	↔	NA	↔
PRM	?	CBZ⇓	?	CZP⇓	?	ESM⇓	?	NA	?	LTG⇓
RFN	NA	CBZ↓	↔	NA	NA	NA	NA	NA	NA	LTG↓
STP	?	CBZ⇑ DMCLB ⇑	CLB⇑	?	?	ESM↑	?	NA	NA	?
TGB	NA	↔	NA	NA	NA	NA	NA	NA	NA	↔
TPM	↔	↔	?	?	ESL↓	NA	?	NA	↔	↔
VPA	↔	CBZ-E⇑	↔	?	↔	ESM↑↓	FBM↑	↔	↔	LTG⇑
VGB	NA	CBZ↑↓	NA	NA	NA	NA	↔	NA	NA	↔
ZNS	NA	CBZ-E↑	?	?	NA	?	?	NA	NA	↔

BRV = brivaracetam; CBZ = carbamazepine; CBZ-E = carbamazepine-10,11-epoxide (active metabolite of CLB); ESL = eslicarbazepine (active metabolite of ESL-a); ESL-a = eslicarbazepine (active metabolite of OXC); LCM = lacosamide; LEV = levetiracetam; LTG = lamotrigine; PRM = primidone; RFN = rufinamide; STP = stiripentol; TGB = tiagabine; TPM = topiramate;

AI = autoinduction; NA = none anticipated; NCCP = not commonly co-prescribed; ↔ = no change; ⇓ = a usually clinically significant decrease in plasma level; ↑ = a usually minor (or inconsistent) increase in ★ = free (pharmacologically active) level may increase; ★★ = the effect on the active metabolite H-OXC concentrations (levels) when an AED is added to a pre-existing AED regimen

LEV	OXC	PMP	PB	PHT	PGB	PRM	RFN	STP	TGB	TPM	VPA	VGB	ZNS
↔	↔	NA	↔	PHT↑	↔	NA	NA	NA	NA	↔	↔	NA	↔
LEV↓	H-OXC↓	PMP⇓	↔	PHT↑↓	↔	PRM↓ PB↑	RFN↓	STP⇓	TGB⇓	TPM⇓	VPA⇓	↔	ZNS⇓
↔	↔	↔	↔	PHT↑	NA	PRM↑	↔	STP↑	?	NA	VPA↑	NA	NA
↔	NA	↔	↔	PHT↑↓	NA	↔	NA	NA	?	NA	↔	NA	↔
↔	NCCP	?	↔	PHT↑	NA	NA	NA	NA	NA	TPM↓	VPA↓	NA	?
↔	NA	?	↔	↔	NA	PRM↑	NA	NA	NA	NA	VPA↓	NA	NA
↔	↔	?	PB⇑	PHT⇑	NA	?	?	?	?	?	VPA⇑	VGB↓	NA
↔	NA	NA	↔	↔	PGB↓	NA	↔	NA	NA	↔	↔	NA	NA
↔	H-OXC↓	?	NA	↔	NA	NA	NA	NA	NA	↔	↔	NA	↔
LEV↓	↔	↔	↔	↔	↔	↔	↔	NA	NA	↔	VPA↓	NA	↔
—	NA	↔	↔	↔	↔	↔	NA	NA	NA	↔	↔	↔	NA
LEV↓	—	PMP⇓	PB↑	PHT↑	NA	?	RFN↓	?	?	TPM↓	↔	NA	NA
↔	OXC↑**	—	↔	↔	NA	?	?	?	?	↔	VPA↓	NA	↔
LEV↓	H-OXC↓	↔	AI	PHT↑↓	↔	NCCP	RFN↓	STP⇓	TGB⇓	TPM⇓	VPA⇓	↔	ZNS⇓
LEV↓	H-OXC↓	PMP⇓	PB↑	AI	PGB↓	PRM↓ PB↑	RFN↓	STP⇓	TGB⇓	TPM⇓	VPA⇓	↔	ZNS⇓
↔	NA	NA	↔	↔	—	NA	NA	NA	TGB↓	↔	↔	NA	NA
↔	?	?	NCCP↔	NA	—	RFN↓	STP⇓	TGB⇓	TPM⇓	VPA⇓	↔	ZNS⇓	
NA	NA	?	PB↑	PHT↑	NA	NA	—	NA	NA	↔	↔	NA	NA
NA	?	?	PB⇑	PHT⇑	NA	PRM⇑	?	—	?	?	VPA⇑	NA	?
↔	NA	NA	NA	↔	↔	NA	NA	NA	—	NA	VPA↓	NA	NA
↔	↔	PMP⇓	↔	PHT↑	↔	↔	↔	NA	?	—	VPA↓	NA	NA
↔	↔	↔	PB⇑	PHT↓*	NA	PB⇑	RFN↑	↔	↔	TPM↓	—	↔	↔
↔	NA	NA	↔	PHT↓	NA	↔	RFN↓	NA	NA	NA	↔	—	NA
NA	?	↔	↔	↔	NA	↔	?	?	NA	NA	↔	NA	—

metabolite of CBZ); CLB = clobazam; CZP= clonazepam; DMCLB = N-desmethylclobazam (active
acetate; ESM = ethosuximide; FBM = felbamate; GBP = gabapentin; H-OXC = 10-hydroxycarbazepine
OXC = oxcarbazepine; PB = phenobarbital; PGB = pregabalin; PHT = phenytoin; PMP = perampanel;
VGB = vigabatrin; VPA = valproic acid; ZNS = zonisamide.

↓ = a usually minor (or inconsistent) decrease in plasma level;

plasma level; ⇑ = a usually clinically significant increase in plasma level.

is not known; ? = unknown, an interaction could occur.

INDEX